Colorectal Surgery

Clinical Care and Management

Colorectal Surgery

Clinical Care and Management

EDITED BY

Bruce George

Oxford University Hospitals NHS Foundation Trust, Oxford, UK

Richard Guy

Oxford University Hospitals NHS Foundation Trust, Oxford, UK

Oliver Jones

Oxford University Hospitals NHS Foundation Trust, Oxford, UK

Jon Vogel

University of Colorado, Colorado, USA

WILEY Blackwell

This edition first published 2016 © 2016 by John Wiley & Sons Ltd

Registered office: John Wiley & Sons Ltd, The Atrium, Southern Gate, Chichester, West Sussex, PO19 8SQ, UK

Editorial offices: 9600 Garsington Road, Oxford, OX4 2DQ, UK
The Atrium, Southern Gate, Chichester, West Sussex, PO19 8SQ, UK
111 River Street, Hoboken, NJ 07030-5774, USA

For details of our global editorial offices, for customer services and for information about how to apply for permission to reuse the copyright material in this book please see our website at www.wiley.com/wiley-blackwell.

The right of the authors to be identified as the authors of this work have been asserted in accordance with the UK Copyright, Designs and Patents Act 1988.

Library of Congress Cataloging-in-Publication Data

Names: George, Bruce, 1960- , editor. | Guy, Richard, 1964- , editor. |
    Jones, Oliver, 1971- , editor. | Vogel, Jon, 1970- , editor.
Title: Colorectal surgery : clinical care and management / edited by Bruce
    George, Richard Guy, Oliver Jones, Jon Vogel.
Other titles: Colorectal surgery (George)
Description: Chichester, West Sussex, UK ; Hoboken, NJ : John Wiley & Sons
    Inc., 2016. | Includes bibliographical references and index.
Identifiers: LCCN 2015039644 | ISBN 9781118674789 (cloth)
Subjects: | MESH: Colonic Diseases–surgery. | Colon–surgery. | Colorectal
    Surgery–methods. | Rectal Diseases–surgery. | Rectum–surgery.
Classification: LCC RD543.C57 | NLM WI 650 | DDC 617.5/547–dc23 LC record available at
http://lccn.loc.gov/2015039644

A catalogue record for this book is available from the British Library.

Wiley also publishes its books in a variety of electronic formats. Some content that appears in print may not be available in electronic books.

Cover image: © Eraxion/Getty

Set in 9.5/13pt, MeridienLTStd by SPi Global, Chennai, India.
Printed and bound in Malaysia by Vivar Printing Sdn Bhd

1   2016

Contents

Section B: Inflammatory bowel disease, 73

Bruce George

Section C: Pelvic floor disorders, 141

Oliver Jones

List of contributors

Mohamed Abdelrahman
Research Fellow, Oxford University Hospitals NHS Foundation Trust, Oxford, UK

Shazad Ashraf
Consultant Colorectal Surgeon, University Hospital, Birmingham, UK

Sujata Biswas
Gastroenterology Registrar, Translational Gastroenterology Unit, Oxford University Hospitals NHS Foundation Trust, Oxford, UK

Emma Bracey
Surgical Fellow, Oxford University Hospitals NHS Foundation Trust, Oxford, UK

Nicolas Buchs
Colorectal Surgeon, University Hospitals of Geneva, Geneva, Switzerland

Marcus Chow
Medical Officer, Tan Tock Seng Hospital, Singapore

Christopher Cunningham
Consultant Colorectal Surgeon, Oxford University Hospitals NHS Foundation Trust, Oxford, UK

James East
Consultant Gastroenterologist, Oxford University Hospitals NHS Foundation Trust, Oxford, UK

Charles Evans
Consultant Colorectal Surgeon, University Hospitals of Coventry and Warwickshire, Coventry, UK

Myles Fleming
Colorectal Surgical Fellow, Auckland Hospital, Auckland, New Zealand

Luana Franceschilli
Colorectal Surgeon, University of Rome Tor Vergata, Rome, Italy

Bruce George
Consultant Colorectal Surgeon, Oxford University Hospitals NHS Foundation Trust, Oxford, UK

Kim Gorissen
Consultant Colorectal and Emergency Surgeon, Oxford University Hospitals NHS
Foundation Trust, Oxford, UK

Martijn Gosselink
Colorectal Surgeon, Erasmus Medical Centre, Rotterdam, The Netherlands

Richard Guy
Consultant Colorectal Surgeon, Oxford University Hospitals NHS Foundation Trust,
Oxford, UK

Roel Hompes
Consultant Colorectal Surgeon, Oxford University Hospitals NHS Foundation Trust,
Oxford, UK

Gareth Horgan
Consultant Gastroenterologist, Naas General Hospital, Dublin, Ireland

Oliver Jones
Consultant Colorectal Surgeon, Oxford University Hospitals NHS Foundation Trust,
Oxford, UK

Heman Joshi
Specialist Surgical Registrar, St Helens and Knowsley NHS Trust, Merseyside, UK

Rebecca Kraus
Colorectal Surgeon, University Hospital, Basel, Switzerland

Simon Leedham
Consultant Gastroenterologist, Translational Gastroenterology Unit, Oxford University
Hospitals NHS Foundation Trust, Oxford, UK; Wellcome Trust Centre for Human
Genetics, Oxford University, Oxford, UK

Ian Lindsey
Consultant Colorectal Surgeon, Oxford University Hospitals NHS Foundation Trust,
Oxford, UK

Richard Lovegrove
Colorectal Fellow, Mount Sinai Hospital, University of Toronto, Toronto, Canada

Marc Marti-Gallostra
Colorectal Surgeon, University Hospital Vall d'Hebron, Barcelona, Spain

Ami Mishra
Consultant Colorectal Surgeon, West Suffolk Hospital, Bury St. Edmunds, Suffolk, UK

Neil Mortensen
Professor of Colorectal Surgery, Oxford University Hospitals NHS Foundation Trust,
Oxford, UK

Alistair Myers
Colorectal Surgeon, Hillingdon Hospital NHS Foundation Trust, London, UK

Par Myrelid
Colorectal Surgeon, University Hospital of Linkoping, Linkoping, Sweden

Jonathan Randall
Consultant Surgeon, University Hospitals, Bristol, UK

Frederic Ris
Consultant Colorectal Surgeon, University Hospitals of Geneva, Geneva, Switzerland

Astor Rodrigues
Consultant Paediatric Gastroenterologist, Oxford University Hospitals NHS Foundation Trust, Oxford, UK

Silvia Silvans
Colorectal Surgeon, Hospital del Mar, Barcelona, Spain

Richard Tilson
Colorectal Foundation Doctor, Oxford University Hospitals NHS Foundation Trust, Oxford, UK

Christian Toso
Visceral Surgeon and Associate Professor, University Hospitals of Geneva, Geneva, Switzerland

Koen van Dongen
Colorectal Surgeon, Maashospital Pantein, Beugen, The Netherlands

Jon Vogel
Colorectal Surgeon and Associate Professor of Surgery, University of Colorado, Colorado, US

Lai Mun Wang
Consultant Histopathologist, Department of Cellular Pathology, Oxford University Hospitals NHS Foundation Trust, Oxford, UK

Sara Q. Warraich
Colorectal Foundation Doctor, Oxford University Hospitals NHS Foundation Trust, Oxford, UK

Kate Williamson
Gastroenterologist, Oxford University Hospitals NHS Foundation Trust, Oxford, UK

Massarat Zutshi
Colorectal Surgeon, Cleveland Clinic, Cleveland, US

Foreword

Mastering the art and science of surgery is becoming increasingly difficult. The explosion of knowledge and technology is a threat to even a relatively new specialty like colorectal surgery. Our medical students have little exposure to the subject and need instant tutorials, our trainees struggle with the increasing complexity of operative surgery, and consultant staff are beginning to subspecialize. Everyone is finding it difficult to keep up. If you agree then this accessible, readable, and very enjoyable book will help.

Although not in quite the same league as the Case Records of the Massachusetts General Hospital, we have a weekly academic meeting in Oxford at which one of the residents or consultant staff presents a "case of the week." The diagnosis, management, and outcome of each are poked, prodded, and recorded so that we can address our ignorance, learn from our mistakes, and look at controversies from every point of view.

This book distils some of these cases into 52 clinical vignettes arranged into groups of colorectal cancer, inflammatory bowel disease, proctology, and emergency surgery. For each group, there is a background chapter, and then the cases are presented with a discussion point, a series of learning points, and an important paragraph, "Could we have done better?" A particularly nice touch is the Letter from America in which one of our former residents looks at how US guidelines and practice might have differed from ours.

The Editors have done a great job choosing and putting together a terrific range of cases, some of which I remember only too well. And on reflection, yes, we could have done better.

Neil Mortensen, Oxford

SECTION A
Colorectal cancer

Bruce George
Oxford University Hospitals NHS Foundation Trust, Oxford, UK

Incidence

Colorectal cancer (CRC) is the second most common cause of cancer-related mortality in the Western world. Approximately 6% of the population will develop CRC during their lifetime.

Pathogenesis

Colorectal cancer develops through a stepwise accumulation of genetic and epigenetic alterations. There are three major molecular mechanisms involved in colorectal carcinogenesis:
- chromosomal instability
- microsatellite instability
- CpG island methylation.

Chromosomal instability

In the late 1980s, Vogelstein *et al.* described a series of genetic alterations resulting in change from normal colonocytes through adenoma to carcinoma. Key genes in this process include adenomatous polyposis coli (APC), k-ras and p53, all of which code for proteins critically involved in regulation of cell turnover. APC is a tumor suppressor gene on chromosome 5q21 (long arm of chromosome 5). The APC protein controls degradation of beta-catenin which is involved in the control of epithelial cell turnover. Mutation of the APC gene results in accumulation of beta-catenin which, in turn, alters expression of several genes affecting cell proliferation, differentiation, and apoptosis. Germline mutation in the APC gene results in familial adenomatous polyposis (FAP).

Colorectal Surgery: Clinical Care and Management, First Edition.
Edited by Bruce George, Richard Guy, Oliver Jones, and Jon Vogel.
© 2016 John Wiley & Sons, Ltd. Published 2016 by John Wiley & Sons, Ltd.

Microsatellite instability

Microsatellites are short repeat nucleotide sequences found throughout the genome and are prone to errors during replication. Mutations in mismatch repair genes result in an increased risk of CRC. Tumors associated with defects in DNA mismatch repair are characterized by increased microsatellite instability. Germline mutations in mismatch repair genes result in hereditary nonpolyposis colorectal cancer (HNPCC).

CpG island methylation

More recently, epigenetic influences such as DNA methylation have been found to be involved in tumorigenesis. Normally, only about 3–4% of all cytosines in DNA are methylated and methylation only occurs at cytosines at the 5′ end of guanine (CpGs). Clusters of CpGs tend to occur in the promoter region of many genes. Increased methylation of CpGs at the promoter end of tumor suppressor genes may result in reduced activation of the genes, resulting in increased tumor risk. Environmental factors may exert their influence on carcinogenesis through epigenetic mechanisms.

Awareness of the molecular changes in individual tumors is likely to become increasingly important in individualizing treatment. Sporadic tumors, for example, with features of high microsatellite instability, tend to respond poorly to 5-fluorouracil (5FU) chemotherapy.

Risk factors for colorectal cancer

Increasing age, a family history of CRC and long-term ulcerative colitis (UC) or Crohn's colitis are major risk factors for the development of CRC. Rare situations in which the risk is slightly increased include acromegaly, renal transplantation, and a history of abdominal irradiation.

Family history

Twin studies suggest that about 20% of CRC have an inherited predisposition. The mechanism of inherited risk is well characterized in patients with FAP (about 1% of all CRC) and HNPCC (about 3–5% of all CRC), but not in the remainder of those with a positive family history.

Familial adenomatous polyposis is an autosomal dominant condition resulting from mutation in the APC gene. The disease is characterized by the development of multiple polyps, usually over 100, in adolescence and, unless treated, inevitable progression to colon cancer. Extracolonic features include gastroduodenal polyps – with a lifetime risk of duodenal cancer of 12% – and desmoid tumors. The precise site of the mutation in the APC gene correlates with the clinical phenotype, for example the risk of developing desmoid tumors.

Hereditary nonpolyposis colorectal cancer is an autosomal dominant condition caused by a germline mutation in DNA mismatch repair genes. Loss of mismatch repair genes results in replication errors, increased mutations, and an increased risk of malignancy. The hallmark of HNPCC is microsatellite instability. Individuals with HNPCC tend to develop tumors at a younger age than those with sporadic tumors and are also at increased risk of other tumors, especially endometrial, gastric, ovarian, and urinary tract.

It is impractical to genetically test all family members of patients with CRC for HNPCC, and various criteria have been developed to identify patients and families likely to have HNPCC, the most common being the Amsterdam Criteria (Box A.1).

Box A.1 Amsterdam criteria for the diagnosis of HNPCC.

Amsterdam I

- At least three relatives with CRC, one of which should be a first-degree relative of the other two
- At least two successive generations affected
- At least one CRC diagnosed before the age of 50 years
- FAP excluded
- Tumors verified histologically

Amsterdam II

- At least three relatives with an HNPCC-associated cancer, one of which should be a first-degree relative of the other two
- At least two successive generations affected
- At least one CRC diagnosed before age 50 years
- FAP excluded
- Tumors verified histologically

Diet and lifestyle

A high-fiber diet has been postulated for many years to be associated with a reduced risk of CRC, although results from several meta-analyses show conflicting results. The EPIC study suggests that a high-fiber diet is associated with a 40% risk reduction. On the other hand, red meat, smoking, alcohol, and obesity have been associated with an increased risk. Increased physical exercise has been shown to be independently associated with a reduced risk.

Long-term aspirin therapy has been shown in several studies with over 20-year follow-up to be associated with a reduced risk, although a recent consensus group felt that further research was needed before aspirin could be recommended as chemoprevention for high-risk groups [1].

Pathology

Most CRCs are thought to arise from adenomatous polyps. A variety of polyps is found in the colon and rectum, varying in their premalignant potential (Box A.2).

Box A.2 Types of polyp in the colon and rectum.

- Adenoma
- Serrated lesions
- Hamartomatous
- Inflammatory
- Pseudo-polyps

The site, size, number, and shape of polyps are important in assessing risk. The majority of polyps are sessile or pedunculated, although the Paris classification is useful, particularly when assessing small flat lesions (Figure A.1).

When viewed colonoscopically using adjuncts such as chromoendoscopy ("dye spray") and high-definition imaging, different "pit patterns" may be observed on the surface of polyps, which may help to identify the type of polyp (Figure A.2).

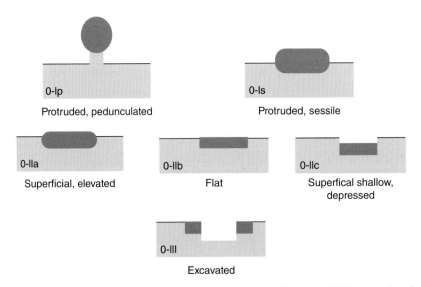

| 0-lp | 0-ls |
| Protruded, pedunculated | Protruded, sessile |

| 0-lla | 0-llb | 0-llc |
| Superficial, elevated | Flat | Superfical shallow, depressed |

| 0-lll |
| Excavated |

Figure A.1 Paris classification. *Source*: Participants in the Paris Workshop. 2003. Reproduced with permission of Elsevier.

Pit pattern type	Characteristics
I	roundish pils
II	stellaror papillary pits
III S	smallroundish or tubular pits (smaller than type I pits)
III L	large roundish or tubular pits (larger than type I pits)
IV	branch-like or gyrus-like pits
V	non-structured pits

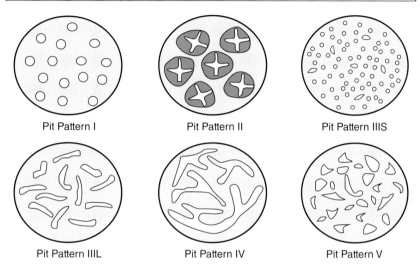

Pit Pattern I   Pit Pattern II   Pit Pattern IIIS

Pit Pattern IIIL   Pit Pattern IV   Pit Pattern V

Figure A.2 Polyp pit patterns. *Source*: Williams [2]. Reproduced with permission of Wiley.

Broadly speaking, pit patterns 1 and 2 tend to be associated with normal or nonneoplastic lesions, types 3 and 4 with adenomas, and type 5 with invasive malignancy.

Adenomatous polyps show cellular dysplasia and are potentially premalignant. Architecturally, they may be classified as tubular, tubulovillous or villous. Thus, larger villous lesions with high-grade dysplasia have a higher risk of malignant transformation.

Serrated lesions are being increasingly recognized, particularly since the advent of screening programs, although their natural history remains unclear. There are three types of serrated lesions.

- *Hyperplastic polyp.* These tend to be small sessile lesions mainly in the rectum and have no malignant potential.
- *Sessile serrated adenoma (SSA).* These tend to occur in the right colon, may be large in size but can be difficult to identify colonoscopically. They are associated with a risk of synchronous advanced neoplasms.
- *Traditional serrated adenoma (TSA).* These are more likely to be situated in the left colon and are easier to identify colonoscopically.

It is thought that SSAs and TSAs may progress to invasive malignancy by a distinct molecular pathway, involving BRAF mutation and epigenetic silencing of mismatch repair genes. The importance of thorough colonoscopic clearance and surveillance is being realized. Multiple hyperplastic polyposis syndromes are being increasingly recognized and have a 50% lifetime risk of CRC (see **Case 2**).

Appearance and distribution

Macroscopically, CRC may be polypoid, ulcerated or annular. The distribution of tumors is approximately as follows: 40% rectum or rectosigmoid junction, 25% sigmoid, 25% cecum or ascending colon, and the remainder (10%) in the transverse or descending colon.

Pathological features

Microscopically, tumors are adenocarcinomas with varying degrees of differentiation. Histological features associated with a poor prognosis include mucinous, signet ring, and neuroendocrine differentiation. Immunohistochemically, colorectal carcinomas tend to be CK20 positive and CK7 negative.

Colorectal cancer staging

The most common pathological staging systems in use are the Dukes and TNM (Tumor, Node, Metastases) systems (Table A.1). Dukes' original stages are as follows.
- A – tumor confined to the bowel wall without lymph node involvement
- B – tumor beyond the wall with no lymph node involvement
- C – any tumor with lymph node involvement

Later modifications included C1 (apical node not involved), C2 (apical node involved), and Dukes' D to indicate distant metastases.

The prognosis following CRC resection is largely dependent upon the pretreatment radiological staging [3, 4]. This can only be determined for TNM stages, in various permutations and combinations (Table A.2), as Dukes' staging relies on the histopathological examination of a resected specimen.

Clinical presentation

Colorectal malignancy may be detected in asymptomatic individuals, either through screening or incidentally during investigation of other problems. More commonly, tumors present due to symptoms related to the primary tumor or due to metastatic spread.

Symptoms of colorectal cancer

The classic symptoms of colorectal malignancy depend on the site of the tumor. Rectal tumors tend to present with overt rectal bleeding, passage of mucus or

Table A.1 TNM classification system for colorectal cancer.

T stage	N stage	M stage
T1 Tumor confined to the submucosa	**N0** No lymph nodes contain tumor cells	**M0** No metastases seen in distant organs
T2 Tumor has grown into (but not through) the muscularis propria	**N1** Tumor cells seen in up to 3 regional lymph nodes*	**M1** Metastases seen in distant organs
T3 Tumor has grown into (but not through) the serosa	**N2** Tumor cells seen in 4 or more regional lymph nodes**	
T4 Tumor has penetrated the serosa and peritoneal surface **T4a** Extension into adjacent structures or organs **T4b** Bowel perforation		

*A tumor nodule in the pericolic or perirectal adipose tissue without evidence of residual lymph node is regarded as a lymph node metastasis if it is >3 mm in diameter. If it is <3 mm in diameter, it is regarded as discontinuous tumor extension.

**If there are tumor cells in nonregional lymph nodes (i.e. in a region of the bowel with a different pattern of lymphatic drainage to that of the tumor), that is regarded as distant metastasis (pM1).

Source: American Joint Committee on Cancer [5].

Table A.2 Five-year survival rate based on TMN staging of colon and rectal cancers.

TMN	Colon 5-year survival rate	Rectal 5-year survival rate
T1, T2 N0	97.1%	94.4%
T3 N0	87.5%	78.7%
T4 N0	71.5%	61.4%
T1, T2 N1	87.1%	85.1%
T1, T2 N2	75.0%	63.9%
T3 N1	68.7%	63.3%
T3 N2	47.3%	43.7%
T4 N1	50.5%	47.1%
T4 N2	27.1%	29.5%

tenesmus. Sigmoid and descending colon lesions tend to present with darker blood mixed with stool or an alteration in bowel pattern. Cancers in the right colon are more likely to be "silent" and to present with anemia, weight loss or anorexia.

In clinical practice, many patients present with symptoms which may fit for CRC but could also be attributed to a variety of benign disorders. Identification of significant ("red flag") symptoms (Box A.3) has been attempted in order to expedite appropriate investigations, and to exclude those who probably do not warrant urgent referral. In the UK, these have been used to facilitate rapid assessment, although the efficacy is questioned and there may still be a tendency for overreferral.

Box A.3 "Red flag" symptoms suggesting CRC.

- Rectal bleeding for more than 6 weeks without anal symptoms
- Change of bowel habit to looser, more frequent stools for more than 6 weeks in a person over 60 years of age
- Change of bowel habit to looser/frequent stools for >6 weeks and rectal bleeding in a person over 40 years
- Right iliac fossa mass
- Rectal mass
- Unexplained iron deficiency anemia (<11 g/dL in men, <10 g/dL in nonmenstruating women)

The majority of patients presenting with significant symptoms require luminal investigation, either by colonoscopy or CT colonography ("virtual colonoscopy"). A recent UK multicenter trial compared colonoscopy to CT colonography in patients referred with bowel symptoms [6]. Detection rates for cancers and large polyps were similar (11%), although significantly more patients required additional investigation after CT colonography than after colonoscopy.

Emergency presentation

About 25% of patients with CRC present as an emergency, most commonly with colonic obstruction. Tumor perforation, major bleeding or anemia may also prompt emergency admission.

Symptoms due to metastatic disease

Approximately 25% of patients with CRC have metastatic disease at the time of presentation, often with nonspecific symptoms such as weight loss, anorexia, lethargy or anemia. Less commonly, patients present with focal symptoms due to metastases in the liver (such as capsular pain), lung or brain.

Incidental detection following other investigations

Potentially important colorectal lesions may be detected on radiological imaging during investigations for unrelated pathology. Focal colonic uptake on PET scans, for example, is quite often an indicator of significant pathology. In a recent study [7], CRC was diagnosed in 12 of 28 patients undergoing colonoscopy for PET scan abnormalities.

Screening (see Cases 1, 2 and 8)

Colorectal cancer may be "the most screenable but least screened" of the major cancers. Screening methods include stool tests for occult blood, flexible sigmoidoscopy, colonoscopy or CT colonography.

Guaiac fecal occult blood testing (FOBT) is the most widely used screening method. Blood in the stool is detected by peroxidase activity of the heme part of the hemoglobin molecule, which is not specific to human blood. A positive test usually triggers further assessment by colonoscopy, and this forms the basis of the UK's NHS Bowel Cancer Screening Programme (BCSP) for individuals aged 60–75 years. A Cochrane review of major screening trials worldwide concluded that screening by FOBT decreases mortality from colorectal cancer by about 16%, although there may not be a difference in all-cause mortality between screened and unscreened groups [8].

Newer occult blood tests which are specific to human hemoglobin, such as detection of globin, may yield better results than guaiac-based FOBT.

Colonoscopy as a primary screening modality is attractive in being both diagnostic and potentially therapeutic and is generally considered to be the gold standard investigation for colorectal neoplasia. Whilst not perfect, with a measurable "miss rate" for adenomas, and the requirement for oral bowel preparation carrying some risk, application to large populations has been proven in the NHS BCSP, and endoscopist expertise continues to improve.

Flexible sigmoidoscopy (FS) as a screening tool has been subject to a major UK-based trial [9], involving 55–64 year olds. Polyps detected at flexible sigmoidoscopy were removed and high-risk patients underwent colonoscopy. At median follow-up of 11 years, screening was associated with a 31% reduction in mortality from colorectal cancer and a 23% reduction in CRC incidence. FS has now been incorporated into the NHS BCSP for those aged 55 years and over. The American College of Gastroenterology recommends screening by colonoscopy from the age of 50 years at 10-yearly intervals [10].

Radiological imaging of the colon by CT colonography (virtual colonoscopy) may be used as a screening investigation, and is incorporated into the NHS BCSP for less fit patients and for those in whom colonoscopy was incomplete. There are few procedural risks but exposure to ionizing radiation is of slight concern (see **Case 14**). A head-to-head comparison of colonoscopy and CT colonography [11] showed broadly similar detection rates, with CT colonography slightly outperforming colonoscopy for larger lesions.

Investigation of colorectal cancer

Ideally, all patients with CRC should be assessed by full colonoscopy with biopsy of the primary tumor. Synchronous tumors may be detected in around 4% of cases. Convincing CT colonography may negate the requirement for colonoscopic biopsy, particularly for proximal colonic tumors. All rectal cancers should have histological confirmation.

Staging should be undertaken with CT scanning of the abdomen and chest in order to exclude metastatic disease. Rectal tumors usually require MRI for local staging, allowing assessment of T stage, N stage, vascular invasion, and the mesorectal margin. Endoanal ultrasound may be useful for assessing the T stage of small or early tumors. Liver MRI or PET-CT may be indicated for further clarification of disease stage.

Measurement of serum carcinoembryonic antigen (CEA) at the time of diagnosis is controversial and not universal, but may be useful for assessing response to treatment and during follow-up, particularly in the presence of liver metastases [12].

Decision making: the multidisciplinary team (MDT)

There is some evidence that outcomes may be improved by formal discussion in multidisciplinary meetings at which surgeons, radiologists, oncologists, and pathologists, amongst others, review individual cases. Burton *et al.* [13] showed that this process was associated with a lower R1 resection rate and Morris *et al.* [14] demonstrated better surgical and oncological outcomes.

Colonic cancer

Most patients without metastatic disease proceed to surgical resection. A small proportion of locally advanced colonic tumors may benefit from preoperative neoadjuvant chemotherapy, although good evidence and indications are lacking.

Malignant colonic obstruction (see Cases 4 and 10)

Surgical options for the management of malignant colonic obstruction have traditionally included defunctioning stoma, Hartmann's procedure or resection with on-table colonic lavage and primary anastomosis. Self-expanding metallic stents, usually inserted under endoscopic and radiological guidance, may rapidly relieve obstruction. In the elderly, unfit patient or those with advanced or metastatic disease, stenting is an attractive palliative option but stenting as a "bridge to surgery" with curative intent is more controversial. The aim is to relieve obstruction, allow correction of physiological abnormalities and then proceed to semi-elective surgery, potentially after bowel preparation. Such surgery is more likely to be undertaken laparoscopically and to be restorative. A recent metaanalysis of randomized trials describes technical and clinical success rates for stenting of 71% and 69%, respectively [15]. Potential complications include stent migration, blockage, and, more seriously, perforation, a clinical perforation rate of 7% and a silent perforation rate of 14% being reported in the metaanalysis. Stenting may cause tumor fracturing [16] and perhaps hematological and lymphatic dissemination.

Effects on local or distant recurrence have not been fully evaluated, although a Dutch study did not identify a major increased risk of recurrence [17], despite a high perforation rate. A study from Oxford, however, did identify a higher rate of local recurrence in patients treated by stenting before surgery compared to resection alone [18].

The randomized CReST trial (www.crest.bham.ac.uk) is evaluating short- and long-term outcomes from stenting as a bridge to surgery and may shed more light on these important questions.

Rectal cancer

The challenge of rectal cancer management in the absence of advanced metastatic disease is to achieve curative treatment with minimal morbidity. Total mesorectal excision, popularized by Heald [19], and preoperative radiotherapy [20, 21] have been associated with dramatic improvements in oncological outcome. Furthermore, improvements in preoperative imaging have permitted a more tailored approach to patient management.

Anterior resection remains the default treatment for rectal cancer. The MDT must identify:
- patients with early tumors amenable to local resection
- patients with tumors at risk of local recurrence who may require preoperative radiotherapy or chemoradiotherapy
- cases of complete clinical response after chemoradiotherapy
- patients who require abdominoperineal excision of the rectum (APER) or are "on the cusp" of ultra-low anterior resection or APER
- patients with potentially curative synchronous liver and rectal tumors
- patients with locally advanced or recurrent disease (see case 11).

Local excision

Local excision may be reasonably considered for early rectal tumors. Whilst the avoidance of major abdominal and pelvic surgery may be attractive and less morbid, the reduced radicality of the resection, and the lack of lymph node retrieval, may have consequences which must be discussed with the patient.

The risk of lymph node involvement in T1 tumors may be difficult to estimate but depends on tumor size, extent of penetration into the submucosa, and degree of differentiation.

Invasive tumor within a pedunculated polyp is assessed by the Haggitt system [22] (Figure A.3) (see **Case 1**). Invasion in a sessile polyp is assessed by the Kikuchi *et al.* [23] system (Figure A.4). This simply describes invasion into the upper third (sm1), the middle third (sm2) or the lower third (sm3) of the submucosa.

Disruption of a locally excised specimen or piecemeal removal of a sessile polyp by endoscopic mucosal resection (EMR) may prevent accurate Kikuchi

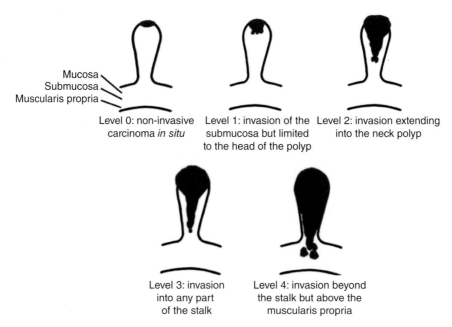

Mucosa
Submucosa
Muscularis propria

Level 0: non-invasive carcinoma *in situ*

Level 1: invasion of the submucosa but limited to the head of the polyp

Level 2: invasion extending into the neck polyp

Level 3: invasion into any part of the stalk

Level 4: invasion beyond the stalk but above the muscularis propria

Figure A.3 Haggitt system for cancer invasion in a pedunculated polyp. *Source*: Haggitt *et al.* [22]. Reproduced with permission of Elsevier.

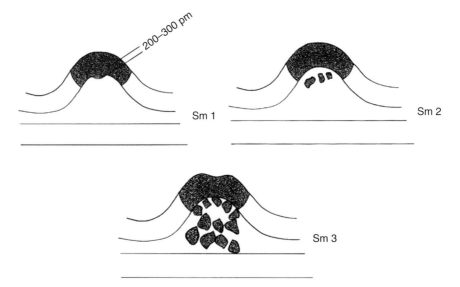

200–300 pm

Sm 1

Sm 2

Sm 3

Figure A.4 The Kikuchi classification for sessile malignant polyps. *Source*: Kikuchi *et al.* [23]. Reproduced with permission of Springer publications.

assessment. An alternative approach focuses on the depth and width of invasion beyond the muscularis mucosa.

Current opinion is that tumors suitable for local excision with curative intent should:

- be less than 3 cm diameter
- not be poorly differentiated
- have early T1 invasion only (sm1 or 2)
- have no evidence of nodal involvement on MRI.

Tumors which do not meet these criteria have a greater risk of tumor in lymph nodes and should generally be treated by conventional resection. A recent trial comparing local excision by transanal endoscopic microsurgery (TEM) with laparoscopic anterior resection for T1/T2 rectal tumors showed less morbidity following TEM. There were two local recurrences after TEM (2/28, 7%) compared to none after anterior resection, although this difference was not statistically significant [24].

Local excision may be employed as a compromise for patients who are medically unfit for major resection.

Preoperative radiotherapy (see Cases 5–7)

Preoperative radiotherapy (RT) may be delivered in short or long courses. Short-course RT is typically 5×5 Gy over 5 days followed by surgery the next week. Long-course RT is usually 45–50 Gy given over about 5 weeks with 5FU given during weeks 1 and 5. Surgery is undertaken about 6–8 weeks after completion of chemoradiotherapy. There is increasing evidence that a longer interval to surgery, perhaps out to 12 weeks, may be associated with more tumor shrinkage [25].

Several large trials have shown a significant reduction in local recurrence following surgery after short-course RT compared to surgery alone [20, 21, 26–28]. Only one of these trials – the Swedish rectal cancer trial – showed an improvement in overall survival.

Long-course chemoradiotherapy (CRT) has the advantage over short-course RT (with early surgery) of achieving tumor shrinkage ("downstaging"). This may permit surgical resection with negative margins – which might not have been achieved without CRT – with a significantly reduced risk of local recurrence. Downstaging by CRT may also increase the chance of sphincter-preserving surgery.

Complete clinical response

Around 10–15% of patients will achieve a complete pathological response to long-course CRT, with the result that no viable tumor cells are found in the surgical resection specimen. Such patients have a better prognosis [29]. The idea of avoiding major resectional surgery in patients with a complete clinical response has been popularized by Habr-Gama *et al.* from Brazil [30] although other groups have not been able to obtain such good results [31]. It is recommended that a "watch and wait" approach after an apparently complete clinical response should only be considered within a rigorous follow-up regime or, ideally, a clinical trial (see **Case 5**).

Need for APER

Patients with very low rectal tumors are at the highest risk of positive margins, and either a poor functional outcome following restorative surgery or the need for a permanent stoma. The vast majority of such patients will receive preoperative chemoradiotherapy.

A decision regarding feasibility of sphincter preservation versus APER requires detailed clinical assessment, review of MR scans, and discussion with the patient. If a decision is made to undertake an APER, the plane of dissection, position of threatened margins, and the method of perineal reconstruction should be planned in advance.

Metastatic disease

In patients with metastatic disease, the dominant treatment is usually chemotherapy. Surgery may only be indicated to alleviate symptoms from the primary tumor not controllable by conservative means. For patients with potentially curative synchronous liver and colonic tumors, 60–70% undergo resection of the primary as initial treatment. This may be associated with significant postoperative morbidity preventing subsequent chemotherapy or liver surgery. Furthermore, R1/R2 rates are higher when the surgeon is aware of metastatic disease [32]. Over the last decade, there has been a move towards a "liver first" approach [33] or, in selected cases, simultaneous liver resections if both are relatively straightforward (see **Case 9**). A similar approach has been adopted for metastatic rectal disease [34]. Clearly, the liver first approach is not appropriate if the primary tumor is causing obstructive symptoms due to the risk of complete obstruction occurring during chemotherapy or liver surgery.

Surgical treatment

Colonic resections

Oral bowel preparation is not required for cancers proximal to the splenic flexure, but many surgeons still prefer to prepare the bowel prior to surgery for left-sided tumors. Venous thromboembolism (VTE) prophylaxis (usually with compression hosiery and subcutaneous fractionated heparin injections) should be administered, and prophylactic antibiotics given just prior to surgery.

The majority of colonic resections can be undertaken laparoscopically, although obstructing, perforated or locally advanced tumors may be better undertaken by open techniques. For right-sided and transverse colonic tumors, resection is by right or extended right hemicolectomy. Distal transverse and descending colonic tumors may be resected by left hemicolectomy or extended right/subtotal colectomy. Subtotal colectomy may also be indicated for synchronous right and left-sided tumors, for obstructing cancers, and should be considered in patients with HNPCC. Sigmoid tumors are usually treated by high anterior resection with anastomosis of descending colon to upper rectum. Whatever resection is chosen, *en bloc* lymph node removal by high ligation of the relevant vessels should be ensured and a "harvest" of at least 12 lymph nodes is recommended for adequate nodal staging.

Rectal resections

Bowel preparation is more universally accepted for rectal resections, and antibiotic and VTE prophlaxis should be given.

Rectal cancer surgery may present considerable surgical challenges. The principles of surgery for patients with potentially curative disease include:
- high-quality surgical excision with clear margins
- safe restoration of gastrointestinal continuity where appropriate
- preservation of bladder and sexual function.

The main rectal operations undertaken are:
- local peranal excision
- anterior resection
- Hartmann's procedure
- abdominoperineal excision (APER).

Local excision of early rectal cancer is most commonly undertaken by TEM. Posterior approaches to the rectum, e.g. transsphincteric (York–Mason) or transsacral (Kraske), are now very rarely undertaken for cancer, although these approaches remain useful in excision of presacral and retrorectal tumors and tail-gut cysts.

Anterior resection is the standard surgical procedure for most rectal tumors. The procedure may be undertaken by open techniques or a variety of minimally invasive methods, including totally laparoscopic, laparoscopically assisted, robotic or hybrid combinations.

For most anterior resections, the splenic flexure should be fully mobilized in order to achieve maximal length for a tension-free anastomosis. Rectal mobilization should be in the mesorectal plane with visualization and preservation of ureters and presacral hypogastric sympathetic nerves. Parasympathetic nervi erigentes may be seen anterolateraly at the level of the prostate but may be more difficult to see in an obese man with a narrow pelvis.

Dissection in the mesorectal plane is attractive as it is relatively bloodless and allows preservation of the mesorectal fascia. Oncologically, a total mesorectal excision (TME) is considered optimal treatment as viable tumor cells may be found within the mesorectum as far as 4 cm below the lower border of the tumor [35].

The level of distal rectal transaction depends on the precise site of the tumor. Patients with upper and mid rectal tumors should undergo TME with rectal transection at, or just above, the pelvic floor and it is important to ensure a clear margin of rectal wall below the tumor.

Tumors of the distal sigmoid and rectosigmoid can reasonably be resected with a 5 cm distal clearance.

For low rectal tumors, a 2 cm distal margin is considered standard [36], although a 1 cm margin is considered reasonable for very low tumors to permit sphincter preservation. Ueno demonstrated distal intramural spread beyond 1 cm in just 2.3% of cases, most of which were poorly differentiated [37]. Furthermore, a recent metaanalysis showed no difference in local recurrence or survival in patients with a distal margin less than 1 cm compared to more than 1 cm [38].

Tumors in the lower rectum may be treated by ultralow anterior resection with coloanal anastomosis or by APER, and deciding between these options may be very difficult. Factors involved in the decision making include certainty of distal tumor clearance, bowel function with an ultra-low join, especially after radiotherapy, and the need for a permanent colostomy. It may be appropriate to seek a second surgical opinion on the appropriate operation. Recently, transanal ("bottom-up") TME has become popular in a few centers, allowing a safe distal clearance under direct vision and a low coloanal anastomosis.

Abdominoperineal excision (APER) is indicated for tumors that are considered too low to resect with restoration of continuity with clear margins and reasonable bowel function. APER may be a difficult operation and, historically, resection margin involvement, tumor perforation, and long-term survival are all worse after APER compared to anterior resection [39]. Over recent years, however, the concept of extralevator excision (ELAPE), with avoidance of "waisting" of the specimen at the level of the pelvic floor, has gained popularity either in the conventional Lloyd-Davies position or, most elegantly, in the prone position. For ELAPE, compared with standard APER, lower margin positivity and low local recurrence rates have been reported [40].

Hartmann's procedure is occasionally indicated in frail elderly patients who would be technically appropriate for an anterior resection but who are not considered suitable for restoration of continuity, either in terms of their perceived inability to withstand the morbidity of an anastomotic leak, or to tolerate the likely poor function of a low anastomosis.

Postoperative management

Following elective colorectal surgery, most patients should be part of an enhanced recovery after surgery (ERAS) program. The process should start preoperatively with patient education, stoma teaching if necessary, and carbohydrate drink loading. Operative factors to facilitate ERAS include minimally invasive techniques, local or regional analgesia, and avoidance of drains and nasogastric tubes. Early mobilization, early return to diet, and avoidance of excess intravenous fluids and opiate analgesia are some of the important postoperative ERAS measures.

Follow-up after resection

Pathological findings should be discussed at an MDT meeting in order to decide on the need for adjuvant therapy and to plan appropriate follow-up [41].

Several studies have compared intensive versus less intensive follow-up regimes. Although most have shown no major differences, a Cochrane meta-analysis suggested a reduction in all-cause mortality with intensive follow-up. Generally, regular clinical follow-up and CEA measurements with CT at 1, 2, 3, and 5 years, and colonoscopy at 1 year and subsequently 3–5 yearly are recommended for Dukes' B and C (stage 2/3) disease up to 5 years. Early tumors (Dukes' A) probably just need colonoscopic follow-up. There are no specific guidelines beyond 5 years.

Other tumors

Tumors of the appendix

Tumors of the appendix are rare but biologically diverse, and are traditionally subdivided into those of epithelial and nonepithelial origin. Nonepithelial tumors are extremely rare and include GISTs, sarcomas, and lymphomas. Epithelial tumors may be usefully considered in three groups – adenomas, carcinomas and carcinoids – although distinction between the groups is not absolute.

Appendiceal tumors are most commonly identified incidentally following appendicectomy. Some are detected on radiological scanning or at surgery for unrelated reasons and a small number of patients present with abdominal distension due to the "jelly belly" of pseudomyxoma peritonei.

Adenomas

Appendiceal adenomas are most commonly identified incidentally following appendicectomy, but increasing numbers of adenomas and serrated polyps are seen in association with the appendix orifice on accurate colonoscopy. Endoscopic removal of these polyps may be challenging and hazardous, and laparoscopic cecectomy may sometimes be necessary.

Adenomas may undergo cystic degeneration with mucous filling of cysts leading to the clinical entity of mucocele. Rupture of mucoceles due to a cystadenoma is thought to be a potential cause of pseudomyxoma peritonei (PMP). Appendiceal mucoceles may be due to:

- mucosal hyperplasia (no risk of PMP)
- a fecolith with obstruction and accumulation of mucus (no risk of PMP)
- mucinous cystadenoma
- mucinous cystadenocarcinoma.

Care should always be taken to avoid rupture during removal of a mucocele of the appendix due to the risk of PMP if the mucocele turns out to be due to an underlying mucinous cystadenoma. Following appendicetomy for a mucinous neoplasm, recommended follow-up would be by abdominal CT or MR at 1 year if there was intraoperative spillage of mucin or if high-grade dysplasia was seen pathologically.

Carcinomas

Adenocarcinoma of the appendix is similar clinicopathologically to colonic adenocarcinoma and should be managed along the same lines. Well-differentiated mucinous adenocarcinoma is associated with mucin production and may progress to PMP. Poorly differentiated mucinous tumors have a poor prognosis.

Carcinoid tumors

Most classic carcinoid (neuroendocrine) tumors are small, located at the tip of the appendix, and are found incidentally in an appendicectomy specimen. Indeed, the vast majority are adequately treated by appendicectomy. Risk factors for carcinoid tumors with the potential to behave in a malignant fashion are:

- size over 2 cm
- invasion into the mesoappendix
- a positive resection margin
- vascular invasion.

If any of these adverse features are present, management should be discussed at a dedicated neuroendocrine tumor MDT. Right hemicolectomy, mainly for adequate lymph node removal and assessment, may be recommended.

Carcinoid tumors with a more aggressive biology include mucinous carcinoid (also called goblet cell carcinoid) and mixed carcinoid-adenocarcinoma. Such tumors tend to be managed along the lines of a standard adenocarcinoma.

Anal tumors

Tumors of the anal canal are defined according to their precise location. Tumors involving the anorectal junction are considered rectal tumors if the epicenter of the tumor is at least 2 cm above the dentate line, and anal cancers if the tumor is within 2 cm of the dentate line. Anal canal tumors are defined as such down to the anal verge. Anal margin tumors are defined as cancers within 5 cm of the anal margin.

The majority of anal tumors are squamous cell carcinomas. Anal margin (perianal) squamous cell carcinomas are keratinizing whilst the anal canal tumors from the distal end of the anal canal are nonkeratinizing. Tumors arising in the

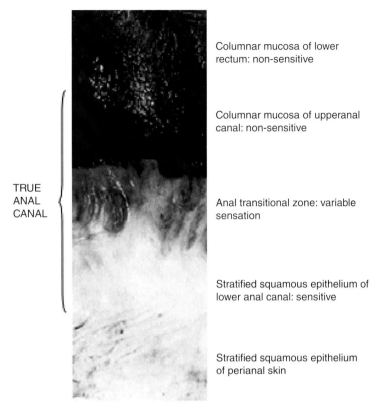

Columnar mucosa of lower
rectum: non-sensitive

Columnar mucosa of upperanal
canal: non-sensitive

TRUE
ANAL
CANAL

Anal transitional zone: variable
sensation

Stratified squamous epithelium of
lower anal canal: sensitive

Stratified squamous epithelium
of perianal skin

Figure A.5 Histological representation of the anal canal including the anal transition zone. *Source*: George [42]. Reproduced with permission of Elsevier.

transitional zone are defined as transitional tumors (also known previously as cloacogenic or basaloid tumors) (Figure A.5). Adenocarcinomas may arise from the upper columnar-lined part of the anal canal or from adjacent anal glands. The lymphatic drainage of the anal canal above the dentate line is to the perirectal, internal iliac or inferior mesenteric nodes, whilst below the dentate line the drainage is to the superficial inguinal lymph nodes.

Anal tumors are rare although the incidence appears to be rising. A higher incidence of anal squamous cell carcinoma (ASCC) is associated with human papillomavirus infection (HPV), genital warts, high numbers of sexual partners, anoreceptive intercourse, cigarette smoking, female gender, and infection with human immunodeficiency virus (HIV).

Clinical presentation

Anal intraepithelial neoplasia (AIN)
A high index of suspicion is needed for the diagnosis of AIN because patients may simply present with perianal irritation. Any unusual anal lesions should be

biopsied. Low-grade AIN may appear similar to anal condylomata but AIN III lesions are frequently flat and plaque-like.

Bowen's disease

This is defined as squamous dysplasia at the anal margin and is distinct from AIN because it represents dysplasia in the perianal skin rather than the anal canal. Clinical presentation is with white or red areas in the perianal skin which may be contiguous with anal canal dysplasia.

Anal canal and anal margin cancer

The most common symptoms of anal cancer are bleeding (45%), pain, and the sensation of a rectal mass (30%). Other symptoms include pruritus ani and anal discharge and, if the anal sphincters are involved with tumor, fecal soiling, tenesmus, and incontinence. Patients can present with enlarged inguinal lymph nodes but without anal symptoms, and around 20% of patients present without any tumor-related symptoms at all.

Rarely, an incidental anal squamous cell carcinoma (SCC) or AIN may be found unexpectedly in a skin tag or hemorrhoidectomy specimen.

Management

AIN

The aim of management of AIN is to prevent the development of invasive cancer. The long-term risks of progression of AIN I/II and AIN III are different and are therefore managed with different strategies. The risk of progression to invasive cancer in AIN I/II is low in immunocompetent patients, whilst AIN III in an immunocompromised patient with HIV has a high risk of progression. Patients with HIV should be managed with a different strategy from immunocompetent patients.

AIN I or II

Observation is the mainstay of management of low-grade dysplasia (AIN I and AIN II), mainly because of the high recurrence rates seen after attempts to eradicate the dysplasia. High recurrence rates probably occur because of the persistence of HPV infection outside the margins of the dysplasia.

AIN III

All patients with AIN III should be considered for HIV testing. The modalities of treatment for AIN III that have been studied include surgery with local excision, immunomodulation therapy, ablation and photodynamic therapy, but surgery remains the main method of treatment along with observation.

HIV-positive patients with AIN

These patients have a significantly high risk for developing invasive anal cancer and should be monitored with regular long-term follow-up with a recommended review every 4–6 months and biopsy of any suspicious lesions.

Anal margin (perianal) cancers (see Case 12)

Anal margin squamous cell carcinomas are histologically perianal skin cancers, which usually have a more favorable outcome than anal canal tumors. Data on optimal management of these tumors are lacking, but the current treatment recommendation is for local excision for T1 tumors (<2 cm diameter) provided that adequate margins (>5 mm) can be achieved without compromising sphincter function. For patients with T2 or higher T stages, or lymph node involvement, chemoradiotherapy is recommended.

Anal canal cancer

Assessment of anal canal tumors should be undertaken in an appropriate MDT. Abdominal examination must include palpation of inguinal nodes and digital rectal examination. Examination under anesthetic is helpful to allow adequate biopsies to be taken.

All patients with invasive anal cancer should be staged with a CT scan of the chest, abdomen, and pelvis to assess distant metastatic spread. Patients should also have a pelvic MRI scan to allow accurate assessment of anal anatomy and aid the detection of pelvic and inguinal lymph node involvement. PET-CT or fine needle aspiration cytology may be required to complement assessment of enlarged inguinal nodes.

Treatment

Chemoradiotherapy

The current standard treatment for anal canal cancers is concurrent radiotherapy and chemotherapy with mitomycin C (MMC) and 5-fluorouracil (5FU). Distant metastatic disease is uncommon in anal cancer (<10% of patients) but there is no effective treatment for distant metastases at present.

Surgery

Options for surgery in the management of anal cancer are now limited to initial assessment and biopsy, colostomy formation and, uncommonly, salvage APER.

Defunctioning colostomy formation may be required before chemoradiotherapy, particularly in cases of fecal incontinence or contiguous vaginal involvement with the potential for fistulation. The rate of pretreatment colostomy is between 5% and 8% and the majority of these rarely go on to have a reversal of the stoma.

Post chemoradiotherapy, a colostomy may be required to manage late toxicity related to chemoradiotherapy, such as anal stenosis, fistulation or incontinence.

Abdominoperineal excision of the rectum is reserved for local recurrence of tumors or persistence of tumor following chemoradiotherapy. During the first 3 years after chemoradiotherapy, approximately 20–25% of patients will have local disease relapse [26]. Salvage surgery results in a 5-year survival rate of 40–60% in those suitable for surgery.

Prognosis and survival

Survival at 5 years following anal canal cancer treatment varies from 70% for stage 1 to 20% for stage 4. Inguinal node involvement, fixation of tumor to the pelvic side-wall, and positive margins are associated with a poor prognosis.

Follow-up

The aim of follow-up after chemoradiotherapy is to detect disease recurrence that is amenable to further potentially curative treatment, in the form of aggressive salvage surgery. Most recurrences following chemoradiotherapy occur within the first 3 years of treatment, which means that follow-up should be more intense during this time-period. Typical follow-up protocols include 3-monthly clinical examination and 6-monthly pelvic MR and abdomen/chest CT for the first 3 years post treatment. The frequency and intensity of follow-up can be reduced after 3 years.

References

1 Cuzick J, Otto F, Baron JA, *et al*. Aspirin and non-steroidal anti-inflammatory drugs for cancer prevention: an international consensus statement. *Lancet Oncol* 2009; **10**(5):501–7.

2 Williams JG, Pullan RD, Hill J, *et al*. Management of the malignant colorectal polyp: ACPGBI position statement. *HYPERLINK "http://www.ncbi.nlm.nih.gov/pubmed/23848492" Colorectal Dis* 2013; **15**(2):1–38. doi:10.1111/codi.12262.

3 Gunderson LL, Jessup JM, Sargent DJ, Greene FL, Stewart A. Revised tumor and node categorization for rectal cancer based on surveillance, epidemiology, and end results and rectal pooled analysis outcomes. *J Clin Oncol* 2010; **28**(2):256–63.

4 Gunderson LL, Jessup JM, Sargent DJ, Greene FL, Stewart AK. Revised TN categorization for colon cancer based on national survival outcomes data. *J Clin Oncol* 2010; **28**(2):264–71.

5 American Joint Committee on Cancer 2009. *Colon and Rectum Cancer Staging*, 7th edn. Chicago: AJCC.

6 Atkin W, Dadswell E, Wooldrage K, *et al*. Computed tomographic colonography versus colonoscopy for investigation of patients with symptoms suggestive of colorectal cancer (SIGGAR): a multicentre randomised trial. *Lancet* 2013; **381**(9873):1194–202.

7 Treglia G, Calcagni ML, Rufini V, *et al*. Clinical significance of incidental focal colorectal (18)F-fluorodeoxyglucose uptake: our experience and a review of the literature. *Colorectal Dis* 2012; **14**(2):174–80.

8 Hewitson P, Glasziou P, Watson E, Towler B, Irwig L. Cochrane systematic review of colorectal cancer screening using the fecal occult blood test (hemoccult): an update. *Am J Gastroenterol* 2008; **103**(6):1541–9.

9 Atkin WS, Edwards R, Kralj-Hans I, *et al*. Once-only flexible sigmoidoscopy screening in prevention of colorectal cancer: a multicentre randomised controlled trial. *Lancet* 2010; **375**(9726):1624–33.

10 Rex DK, Johnson DA, Anderson JC, Schoenfeld PS, Burke CA, Inadomi JM. American College of Gastroenterology guidelines for colorectal cancer screening 2009 [corrected]. *Am J Gastroenterol* 2009; **104**(3):739–50.

11 Pickhardt PJ, Choi JR, Hwang I, *et al*. Computed tomographic virtual colonoscopy to screen for colorectal neoplasia in asymptomatic adults. *N Engl J Med* 2003; **349**(23):2191–200.

12 Locker GY, Hamilton S, Harris J, *et al*. ASCO 2006 update of recommendations for the use of tumor markers in gastrointestinal cancer. *J Clin Oncol* 2006; **24**(33):5313–27.

13 Burton S, Brown G, Daniels IR, Norman AR, Mason B, Cunningham D. MRI directed multidisciplinary team preoperative treatment strategy: the way to eliminate positive circumferential margins? *Br J Cancer* 2006; **94**(3):351–7.

14 Morris E, Haward RA, Gilthorpe MS, Craigs C, Forman D. The impact of the Calman-Hine report on the processes and outcomes of care for Yorkshire's colorectal cancer patients. *Br J Cancer* 2006; **95**(8):979–85.

15 Tan CJ, Dasari BV, Gardiner K. Systematic review and meta-analysis of randomized clinical trials of self-expanding metallic stents as a bridge to surgery versus emergency surgery for malignant left-sided large bowel obstruction. *Br J Surg* 2012; **99**(4):469–76.

16 Gorissen KJ, Tuynman JB, Fryer E, *et al*. Local recurrence after stenting for obstructing left-sided colonic cancer. *Br J Surg* 2013; **100**:1805–9.

17 Sloothaak DA, van den Berg MW, Dijkgraaf MG, *et al*. Oncological outcome of malignant colonic obstruction in the Dutch Stent-In 2 trial. *Br J Surg* 2014; **101**(13):1751–7.

18 Gorissen KJ, Tuynman JB, Fryer E, *et al*. Local recurrence after stenting for obstructing left-sided colonic cancer. *Br J Surg* 2013; **100**(13):1805–9.

19 MacFarlane JK, Ryall RD, Heald RJ. Mesorectal excision for rectal cancer. *Lancet* 1993; **341**(8843):457–60.

20 Kapiteijn E, Marijnen CA, Nagtegaal ID, *et al*. Preoperative radiotherapy combined with total mesorectal excision for resectable rectal cancer. *N Engl J Med* 2001; **345**(9):638–46.

21 Martling A, Holm T, Johansson H, Rutqvist LE, Cedermark B. The Stockholm II trial on preoperative radiotherapy in rectal carcinoma: long-term follow-up of a population-based study. *Cancer* 2001; **92**(4):896–902.

22 Haggitt RC, Glotzbach RE, Soffer EE, Wruble LD. Prognostic factors in colorectal carcinomas arising in adenomas: implications for lesions removed by endoscopic polypectomy. *Gastroenterology* 1985; **89**(2):328–36.

23 Kikuchi R, Takano M, Takagi K, *et al*. Management of early invasive colorectal cancer. Risk of recurrence and clinical guidelines. *Dis Colon Rectum* 1995; **38**(12):1286–95.

24 Chen YY, Liu ZH, Zhu K, Shi PD, Yin L. Transanal endoscopic microsurgery versus laparoscopic lower anterior resection for the treatment of T1-2 rectal cancers. *Hepato-gastroenterology* 2013; **60**(124):727–32.

25 Petrelli F, Sgroi G, Sarti E, Barni S. Increasing the interval between neoadjuvant chemoradiotherapy and surgery in rectal cancer: a meta-analysis of published studies. *Ann Surg* 2013; Nov 20 (epub ahead of print).

26 Cedermark B, Johansson H, Rutqvist LE, Wilking N. The Stockholm I trial of preoperative short term radiotherapy in operable rectal carcinoma. A prospective randomized trial. Stockholm Colorectal Cancer Study Group. *Cancer* 1995; **75**(9):2269–75.

27 Swedish Rectal Cancer Trial. Improved survival with preoperative radiotherapy in resectable rectal cancer. *N Engl J Med* 1997; **336**(14):980–7.

28 Sebag-Montefiore D, Stephens RJ, Steele R, *et al.* Preoperative radiotherapy versus selective postoperative chemoradiotherapy in patients with rectal cancer (MRC CR07 and NCIC-CTG C016): a multicentre, randomised trial. *Lancet* 2009; **373**(9666):811–20.

29 Martin ST, Heneghan HM, Winter DC. Systematic review and meta-analysis of outcomes following pathological complete response to neoadjuvant chemoradiotherapy for rectal cancer. *Br J Surg* 2012; **99**(7):918–28.

30 Habr-Gama A, Perez RO, Proscurshim I, *et al.* Patterns of failure and survival for nonoperative treatment of stage c0 distal rectal cancer following neoadjuvant chemoradiation therapy. *J Gastrointest Surg* 2006; **10**(10):1319–28; discussion 28–9.

31 Glynne-Jones R, Hughes R. Critical appraisal of the 'wait and see' approach in rectal cancer for clinical complete responders after chemoradiation. *Br J Surg* 2012; **99**(7):897–909.

32 Hamady ZZ, Malik HZ, Alwan N, *et al.* Surgeon's awareness of the synchronous liver metastases during colorectal cancer resection may affect outcome. *Eur J Surg Oncol* 2008; **34**(2):180–4.

33 Mentha G, Roth AD, Terraz S, *et al.* 'Liver first' approach in the treatment of colorectal cancer with synchronous liver metastases. *Digest Surg* 2008; **25**(6):430–5.

34 Buchs NC, Ris F, Majno PE, *et al.* Rectal outcomes after a liver-first treatment of patients with stage IV rectal cancer. *Ann Surg Oncol* 2015; **22**(3):931–7.

35 Scott N, Jackson P, al-Jaberi T, Dixon MF, Quirke P, Finan PJ. Total mesorectal excision and local recurrence: a study of tumour spread in the mesorectum distal to rectal cancer. *Br J Surg* 1995; **82**(8):1031–3.

36 Monson JR, Weiser MR, Buie WD, *et al.* Practice parameters for the management of rectal cancer (revised). *Dis Colon Rectum* 2013; **56**(5):535–50.

37 Ueno H, Mochizuki H, Hashiguchi Y, *et al.* Preoperative parameters expanding the indication of sphincter preserving surgery in patients with advanced low rectal cancer. *Ann Surg* 2004; **239**(1):34–42.

38 Bujko K, Rutkowski A, Chang GJ, Michalski W, Chmielik E, Kusnierz J. Is the 1-cm rule of distal bowel resection margin in rectal cancer based on clinical evidence? A systematic review. *Ind J Surg Oncol* 2012; **3**(2):139–46.

39 den Dulk M, Putter H, Collette L, *et al.* The abdominoperineal resection itself is associated with an adverse outcome: the European experience based on a pooled analysis of five European randomised clinical trials on rectal cancer. *Eur J Cancer* 2009; **45**(7):1175–83.

40 Holm T, Ljung A, Haggmark T, Jurell G, Lagergren J. Extended abdominoperineal resection with gluteus maximus flap reconstruction of the pelvic floor for rectal cancer. *Br J Surg* 2007; **94**(2):232–8.

41 Cunningham D, Atkin W, Lenz H-J, *et al.* Colorectal cancer. *Lancet* 2010; **375**(9719):1030–47.

42 George B. Anal and perianal disorders. *Medicine* 2015; **43**:314–319.

CASE 1

A screen-detected colonic conundrum

Ami Mishra

West Suffolk Hospital, Bury St. Edmunds, Suffolk, UK

A 68-year-old man received a kit through the post for the bowel cancer screening program. He decided to enrol and performed the test, sending it off the same day. His results came back and he was invited for colonoscopy (see Section A, page 9). He was completely asymptomatic with no change in bowel habit or rectal bleeding. He had no family history of bowel cancer and apart from treated hypertension was otherwise well.

At colonoscopy, two small hyperplastic polyps were found in the rectum and a 3 cm pedunculated polyp in the distal sigmoid. The pedunculated polyp was removed by the endoscopist using a snare and diathermy. The polypectomy site was tattooed. No other lesion was found up to the cecum.

The polyp was examined by a histopathologist and found to contain an adenocarcinoma within a tubulovillous adenoma (Figure 1.1). The pathology report was as follows.

- Macroscopic description: a 28 mm pedunculated polyp.
- Microscopic description: this is a 13 mm mucinous adenocarcinoma arising within a tubulovillous adenoma with background low- and high-grade dysplasia.
- Haggitt level 3 (invasion into stalk of polyp). The maximum thickness of invasive tumor from the muscularis mucosae is 6 mm.
- Lymphovascular invasion is not seen.
- The stalk resection margin is tumor free and is 1 mm from the tumor.
- Complete resection: yes.
- TNM: pT1, L0, V0, R0

In the first instance, a staging CT scan of the chest, abdomen, and pelvis was organized. This showed no residual abnormality in the colon and no evidence of abnormal lymph nodes or distant metastasis.

Colorectal Surgery: Clinical Care and Management, First Edition.
Edited by Bruce George, Richard Guy, Oliver Jones, and Jon Vogel.
© 2016 John Wiley & Sons, Ltd. Published 2016 by John Wiley & Sons, Ltd.

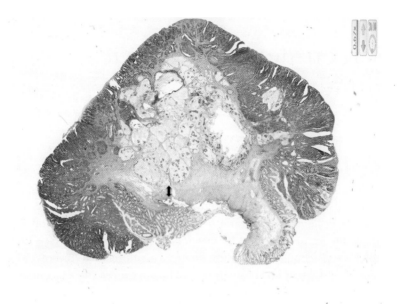

Figure 1.1 Polypectomy specimen with invasive mucinous adenocarcinoma extending into stalk (Haggitt level 3).

DECISION POINT

Does he need any further treatment? What would you do?

This is a borderline decision. The patient has an early invasive tumor arising within a polyp. Although completely excised, there is a risk of tumor in lymph nodes, which may result in tumor recurrence. This must be balanced against the risks of surgical resection. T1 tumors are subclassified using the Haggitt or Kikuchi systems depending on whether the lesion is pedunculated or sessile (see pages 11–12).

Usually a Haggitt level 3 polyp which has been completely excised would not need any additional treatment. However, the MDT was influenced by the mucinous appearance and extension of 6 mm beyond the muscularis mucosae. Our estimate of lymph node positivity risk was 20–25%. The recommendation was that the patient should undergo a laparoscopic high anterior resection.

Following the MDT meeting, the situation was discussed in detail with the patient. The patient was against major surgical resection, despite understanding the risk of residual malignant nodes. He was concerned about the risks of surgery, in particular anastomotic leakage and the small risk of needing a temporary stoma which we quoted as about a 10% risk. He opted for close colonoscopic and radiological follow-up.

Colonoscopy and CT scanning 12 months post polypectomy were normal. He remains well 18 months after the polypectomy.

LEARNING POINTS

- The NHS Bowel Cancer Screening Program (www.cancerscreening.nhs.uk) has now been rolled out across the United Kingdom although the strategy is slightly different across the different countries. In England, the fecal occult blood (FOB) test is offered every 2 years to everyone aged 60–74. The participant is sent a kit with three flaps that each contains two windows onto which the stool specimen is placed. The kit is then sent back. The result is normal (0 positive spots), unclear (1–4 positive) or abnormal (5 or 6 positive spots). Unclear tests require retesting whilst participants with an abnormal result are offered colonoscopy.
- Following local excision of rectal or colonic tumors, further surgery is required if the lesion is T2 or at the margin of resection (R1). There is some debate as to whether 1 mm or 2 mm is required to be a clear margin.
- For T1 lesions, further surgery to remove lymph nodes should be considered if:
  - Kikuchi sm3 (23% risk nodal involvement)
  - Haggitt 4
  - depth over 2000 microns (2 mm)
  - poorly differentiated
  - lymphovascular invasion
  - tumor budding.

Could we have done better?

It remains unclear if the correct decision was made, as the patient has been followed up for just 18 months. The decision made by MDTs tends to be oncologically "correct" without addressing patient wishes, except when more extreme patient views are brought to the MDT discussion. A better MDT recommendation might have been "borderline favoring surgical resection, pending discussion with patient and assessment of fitness."

LETTER FROM AMERICA

The National Cooperative Cancer Network (NCCN; www.nccn.org) supports the use of polypectomy alone for malignant pedunculated polyps with a negative resection margin, moderate or well-differentiated neoplastic cells, and the absence of lymphovascular invasion. While studies have shown the value of submucosal invasion depth measurement, this variable is not part of the decision-making process advocated by the NCCN.

Jon Vogel and Massarat Zutshi

CASE 2

Serrated Pathways

Sujata Biswas[1], Lai Mun Wang[2] & Simon Leedham[1,3]

[1] Translational Gastroenterology Unit, Oxford University Hospitals NHS Foundation Trust, Oxford, UK
[2] Department of Cellular Pathology, Oxford University Hospitals NHS Foundation Trust, Oxford, UK
[3] Wellcome Trust Centre for Human Genetics, Oxford University, Oxford, UK

A 67-year-old lady attended for colonoscopy as part of the UK Bowel Cancer Screening Program due to positive guaiac fecal occult blood testing. She had no past medical problems, took no medications, and was a nonsmoker. There was no relevant family history.

Colonoscopy revealed six right-sided flat serrated lesions, two of which were greater than 10 mm (Figure 2.1) and which were removed by endoscopic mucosal resection. Histology confirmed two large sessile serrated adenomas (SSAs) and further small hyperplastic polyps.

The WHO has defined three criteria for the diagnosis of serrated polyposis syndrome (SPS):

- the presence of more than five hyperplastic polyps proximal to the sigmoid colon of which two are greater than 10 mm in diameter
- >20 hyperplastic polyps throughout the colon
- any hyperplastic polyps proximal to the sigmoid colon in a patient with a first-degree relative with SPS.

Thus, a diagnosis of serrated polyposis syndrome was made.

DECISION POINT

How often should the patient undergo surveillance colonoscopy and what genetic counseling should she seek?

There is no formal UK guidance for surveillance but the American consensus guidelines suggest surveillance colonoscopy annually. They also suggest biennial endoscopic surveillance of the retained colorectal segment following resection due to rapid recurrence of polyps and neoplasia. All polyps greater than 5 mm should be resected.

American guidelines suggest screening colonoscopy be performed in first-degree relatives aged 40 years or over, or beginning at an age 10 years younger than the age at diagnosis of the youngest affected relative.

Colorectal Surgery: Clinical Care and Management, First Edition.
Edited by Bruce George, Richard Guy, Oliver Jones, and Jon Vogel.
© 2016 John Wiley & Sons, Ltd. Published 2016 by John Wiley & Sons, Ltd.

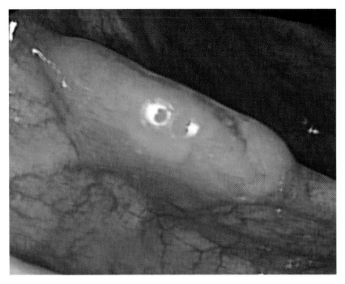

Figure 2.1 Endoscopic image of serrated polyp.

Next colonoscopy after 2 years showed multiple flat polyps in the right colon and four polyps greater than 5 mm were removed. Again histology confirmed sessile serrated adenomas without dysplastic features.

She returned for colonoscopy 1 year later and there was an unusual villous lesion at the ileocecal valve (Figure 2.2). This was biopsied and showed a serrated polyp with high-grade dysplasia. There was also the histological suspicion of desmoplastic stroma. BRAF V600E mutation was detected. Immunohistochemistry showed loss of MutL homolog 1 (MLH1) and postmeiotic segregation increased 2 (PMS2) expression consistent with an unstable lesion. CT staging scan showed no abnormalities and after discussion at the multidisciplinary meeting, surgical resection was recommended.

DECISION POINT

What operation would you do?

There is no clear evidence to help decide between right hemicolectomy and subtotal/total colectomy for SPS. Factors to be considered include the accuracy of polyp assessment at future colonoscopy, family history, age, and burden of surgery in the individual patient. It was felt that a right hemicolectomy was reasonable in this lady.

This patient underwent laparoscopic right hemicolectomy. Pathology confirmed serrated adenocarcinoma, T1N0R0, with lymphatic space invasion. There were three sessile serrated polyps within the specimen, one with high-grade dysplasia 6 cm from the tumor.

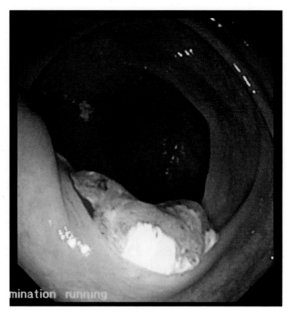

Figure 2.2 Endoscopic image of ileocecal lesion at colonoscopy.

DECISION POINT

What is the prognosis of serrated pathway tumors?

Prognosis may be dependent on the molecular profile of the lesion. MSI tumors tend to have a good prognosis because they are often found at an early stage and contain numerous tumor-infiltrating lymphocytes. However, lesions that do not progress via MLH1 (MSI-negative tumors) give rise to tumors which are aggressive and difficult to treat.

Targeted EGF-receptor therapy such as cetuximab is generally not effective in serrated cancers because the majority have activating BRAF or KRAS mutations downstream of the EGFR pathway that cetuximab targets. There is no literature on adjuvant therapy specific to serrated cancer and no distinction is made from treatment of conventional colorectal cancer.

This patient did not undergo adjuvant therapy.

LEARNING POINTS

- The serrated pathway is emerging as a distinct and important carcinogenesis pathway and is thought to be responsible for up to 30% of colorectal cancer.
- Multiple flat lesions at colonoscopy should alert the endoscopist to consider the diagnosis of serrated polyposis syndrome.
- SPS is associated with a significant cancer risk and American guidelines recommend patients be surveyed with colonoscopy on an annual basis.
- All polyps greater than 5 mm should be resected.
- Any dysplastic lesion should undergo surgical resection given the high risk of malignant change.
- A careful multidisciplinary decision needs to be made with regard to surgery and adjuvant therapy.

Could we have done better?

There are no major criticisms in the management of this case. Ideally, the decision between right hemicolectomy and total colectomy might have been made on the basis of the molecular profile of the individual tumor, but evidence for this in clinical practice is awaited.

LETTER FROM AMERICA

Guidelines for surveillance after colorectal polypectomy are summarized by Lieberman [1]. Annual colonoscopy is recommended for patients with serrated polyposis syndrome.

Jon Vogel and Massarat Zutshi

Reference

1 Lieberman DA. American Gastroenterological Association. Colon polyp surveillance: clinical decision tool. *Gastroenterology* 2014; **146**(1):305–306.

CASE 3

Large tubulovillous adenoma of the rectum treated by TEM

Richard Tilson[1], Shazad Ashraf[2] & Christopher Cunningham[1]

[1] Oxford University Hospitals NHS Foundation Trust, Oxford, UK
[2] University Hospital, Birmingham, UK

A 67-year-old gentleman was referred by his GP complaining of a 3-month history of a change in bowel habit. He had initially noticed increased looseness of his stool together with passage of mucus and blood. The patient was otherwise well with no systemic symptoms or weight loss. His past medical history included hypertension and a previous TIA. He was a smoker of 10 cigarettes per day. There was no significant family history of colorectal cancer.

On digital rectal examination, there was an easily palpable soft mass in the low rectum. Rigid sigmoidoscopy in clinic confirmed a large friable soft lesion occupying most of the lumen of the lower rectum. It was not possible to pass the rigid scope past the lesion.

A colonoscopy was performed which revealed an extensive near circumferential rectal polyp starting at 3–4 cm above the anorectal junction and extending up to 12–15 cm. The macroscopic appearance was thought to be benign although the bulk of the lesion made assessment difficult and precluded endoscopic removal. Endoscopic biopsies characterized this lesion as a tubulovillous adenoma with evidence of focal high-grade dysplasia (5%).

Endorectal ultrasound revealed an enormous villous lesion in the mid rectum arising from the right lateral wall but filling the entire mid and upper rectum. No definite invasion was demonstrated but the lesion was incompletely visualized due to length. MRI evaluation demonstrated no invasive component (Figure 3.1). Staging CT showed no evidence of regional lymph node spread or distant metastases.

DECISION POINT

How should this lesion be managed?

The options considered were either local excision via a per-anal approach or an anterior resection. Although clearly an extensive lesion, it was thought to be non-invasive and that local excision by Transanal endoscopic microsurgery (TEM) would be preferable to a major resection.

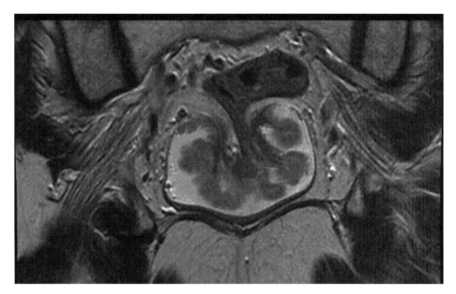

Figure 3.1 MRI image demonstrating "intussuscepting lesion."

At TEM, a large, polypoid tumor was found to extend circumferentially from the distal rectum up to the rectosigmoid junction, with the bulk of disease on the right wall. The lesion was removed primarily by circumferential submucosal dissection although there were some areas of full-thickness dissection, including one area just above the peritoneal reflection anteriorly. The resultant defect was repaired with no residual defect or excessive tension. At the time of the operation, there was no obvious breach of the peritoneum.

The patient was given postoperative intravenous antibiotics. One day after surgery, the patient was well with a soft abdomen and only slightly raised inflammatory markers. His rectal catheter was removed. On day two, however, his abdomen was found to be tender and his inflammatory markers rose significantly (CRP>156, WCC 18).

An urgent CT (Figure 3.2) with rectal contrast revealed no extraluminal leak of contrast but there was evidence of free gas within the peritoneal cavity and mesorectum.

DECISION POINT

What would you do now?

The options were to treat conservatively with IV antibiotics or to intervene surgically, probably by laparoscopy, wash-out, and defunctioning stoma. He was reexamined and found to be systemically well with tenderness localized to the left iliac fossa. It is quite common to get a fever after extensive TEM procedures, although the free gas and high white count were a concern. A decision was made to treat conservatively but to monitor closely.

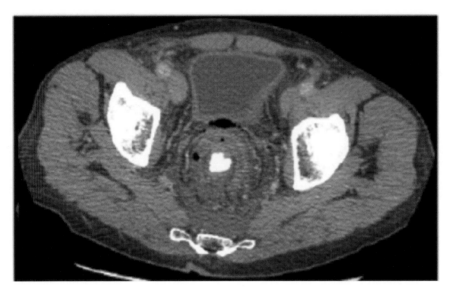

Figure 3.2 CT demonstrating free air between rectum and bladder.

He was treated with IV broad-spectrum antibiotics. Over the subsequent days, the patient's pain settled considerably with normalization of his inflammatory markers. The patient was discharged on the seventh postoperative day.

The pathology report showed an extensive sessile tubulovillous adenoma with focal high-grade dysplasia (5%). The patient was well at 3-month follow-up appointment with no further complications. His preoperative symptoms had resolved completely.

LEARNING POINTS

- Transanal endoscopic microsurgery (TEM) is appropriate for benign rectal lesions and carefully selected early tumors (see page 13).
- Endoluminal rectal ultrasound is useful to assess smaller lesions, but MR is probably better at identifying invasion in large lesions.
- Minimally invasive techniques such as TEM are not risk free but their complication profile is more favorable than radical surgery for rectal lesions.
- "TEM fever" is common following resection of large rectal lesions by TEM and usually settles with conservative management provided there are no clinical features of generalized peritonitis or severe systemic sepsis.

Could we have done better?

Extensive rectal lesions extending above the peritoneal reflection are obviously at risk of breaching the peritoneal cavity when resected by TEM. Assessment by laparoscopy following TEM may help to identify breeches of the peritoneal cavity which might benefit from repair, drain or defunctioning.

Another point to consider is the theoretical risk of upstaging of malignant lesions on peritoneal breach when doing full-thickness excisions in the upper/anterior rectum. In a study by Chen *et al.* [1], comparing TEM with laparoscopic anterior resection (LAR) for T1/T2 rectal cancer, local recurrence was noted in two patients undergoing TEM versus none in the LAR group, although this was not statistically significant. The same study demonstrated more rapid postoperative recovery and a better morbidity profile in the TEM group.

Reference

1 Chen YY, Liu ZH, Zhu K, Shi PD, Yin L. Transanal endoscopic microsurgery versus laparoscopic low anterior resection for the treatment of T1-2 rectal cancers. *Hepatogastroenterology* 2013; **60**(124):727–732.

CASE 4

To stent or not to stent?

Jonathan Randall
University Hospitals, Bristol, UK

A 79-year-old man presented to Accident and Emergency with a 2-day history of vomiting. He described crampy lower abdominal pain since the morning and on further questioning he had not opened his bowels properly for more than 5 days. He had had no previous abdominal surgery or investigations. He suffered chronic obstructive airways disease as a lifelong smoker, which was managed in the community with inhalers. On examination, his abdomen was distended and tympanic, although soft on palpation. Rectal examination revealed a collapsed empty rectum. The abdominal radiograph showed distended large bowel loops and more central small bowel loops. A CT scan of the chest, abdomen, and pelvis was performed the next morning and showed an obstructing distal sigmoid cancer but no evidence of metastatic disease (Figure 4.1). The cecum was distended to 9 cm.

He was reexamined and confirmed to have a distended but soft and nontender abdomen. He was rehydrated with IV fluids and correction of a low potassium.

DECISION POINT

How would you treat this man?

This patient has mechanical large bowel obstruction, with CT evidence of a stenosing sigmoid tumor. The appearances were not those of pseudoobstruction. The treatment options considered were stenting as bridge to surgery in a few weeks time or straight to surgery (see pages 10–11). He was considered suitable for the CREST trial of stenting versus surgery (www .birmingham.ac.uk/research/activity/mds/trials/bctu/trials/coloproctology/crest).

He was given the relevant patient information, but after lengthy discussions he elected to undergo a colonic stenting procedure rather than participate in the trial. He was swayed by the high mortality and stoma risk of emergency surgery in the elderly.

He underwent colonic stent insertion using a combination of fluoroscopic and colonoscopic guidance. A guidewire was passed through the obstructing tumor. The stent was then placed over the guidewire and released to slowly open the lumen. In this case, it was noted that the obstruction was near complete and

---

Colorectal Surgery: Clinical Care and Management, First Edition.
Edited by Bruce George, Richard Guy, Oliver Jones, and Jon Vogel.
© 2016 John Wiley & Sons, Ltd. Published 2016 by John Wiley & Sons, Ltd.

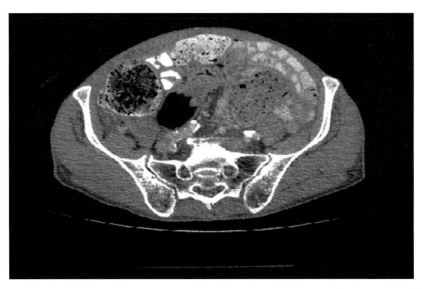

Figure 4.1 A distal sigmoid tumor visible on CT with distended large bowel loops upstream full of feculent matter.

guidewire negotiation was difficult although eventually the stent was successfully deployed.

During and immediately after the procedure the patient passed small quantities of flatus and liquid stool. However, despite laxatives in the days after the procedure, he remained distended and complained of continuing lower abdominal pain. A plain abdominal X-ray showed persisting fecal loading above the stent (Figure 4.2). A contrast enema was performed that demonstrated a patent stent although only a small lumen could be demonstrated. In the hours after the enema, he complained of increasing abdominal pain, mostly on the right side. Examination showed evidence of generalized tenderness with guarding in the lower abdomen. In view of the technically difficult stent insertion, the nonresolution of obstruction and the significant abdominal tenderness, it was decided to undertake a laparotomy.

A laparotomy was performed and a colonic perforation at the site of stenting was found with fecal contamination. A thorough wash-out and Hartmann's procedure was performed.

The patient had a prolonged stay in hospital. Repeat CT scans identified small collections that were unsuitable for drainage and required prolonged courses of antibiotics. He was eventually discharged home with a package of care. The histology showed moderately differentiated adenocarcinoma, pT4N1 (1/25 lymph nodes), R0, Dukes C1. Given his preexisting co-morbidities alongside a long and complicated hospital stay, postoperative chemotherapy was not appropriate. He continues to be followed up and his last CT showed no evidence of recurrence.

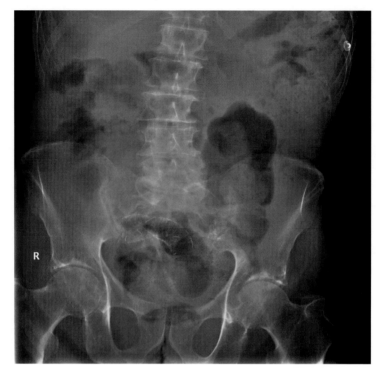

Figure 4.2 Abdominal X-ray 2 days after stent insertion. The stent is just visible over the sacrum but there are still some dilated large bowel loops containing fecal residue.

Could we have done better?

This patient had a stormy postoperative course following a Hartmann's procedure after stent failure and perforation. Although the stenting procedure was technically difficult, it appeared to be successful at the time. This case highlights the risks associated with stent insertion as well as the predictably high morbidity of an emergency Hartmann's procedure in the elderly. The precise place of colonic stenting remains debatable, especially in younger patients with potentially curative disease (see section A, pages 10–11). It is disappointing that we were not able to enrol this patient in the appropriate trial.

LEARNING POINTS

- Patients presenting with large bowel obstruction need rehydration and correction of electrolyte disturbances.
- Stenting can be considered in the palliative setting or as a "bridge to surgery."
- Colonic stenting is successful in about 70% of cases.
- Perforation rates following stenting are about 7% (overt) to 14% (silent).
- Long-term oncological risks of stenting require longer term evaluation.

LETTER FROM AMERICA

ASCRS clinical practice guidelines for colon cancer (2012): Obstructing left-sided colon cancers may be approached in a variety of ways. These include (1) endoscopic stent and subsequent nonemergent resection, (2) resection with anastomosis, (3) resection with anastomosis and proximal bowel diversion, and (4) Hartmann's procedure. The choice of surgery depends on the condition of the patient and the operative findings. Hartmann's procedure is recommended for the most dire situations and resection and primary anastomosis for patients at the other end of the clinical spectrum. Successful initial endoscopic stenting may improve the chances for subsequent successful completion of a minimally invasive resection without ostomy.

Jon Vogel and Massarat Zutshi

CASE 5

Advanced rectal cancer: Brazil or Japan?

Oliver Jones

Oxford University Hospitals NHS Foundation Trust, Oxford, UK

A 69-year-old, sexually active man presented with tenesmus and rectal bleeding. On rigid sigmoidoscopy, he had an obvious rectal cancer 6 cm from the anal verge. He had a colonoscopy and biopsies which confirmed adenocarcinoma and that there was no other synchronous proximal lesion.

A CT scan showed no metastatic disease. An MRI scan showed a bulky mid-rectal cancer which was staged as T3N2. There was an obturator node which was suspicious for tumor involvement measuring 12 mm which was moderately FDG avid on PET scanning. There were further mildly FDG avid nodes in the mesorectum threatening the mesorectum (Figure 5.1).

The patient was discussed in the MDT meeting and a decision made to offer long course chemoradiotherapy. The patient underwent treatment with chemoradiotherapy for 6 months.

On end-of-treatment CT scanning, there was no evidence of residual disease. He underwent a flexible sigmoidoscopy and there was no residual luminal cancer visible, just a scar. Biopsies from the scar showed no residual tumor (Figure 5.2). He underwent repeat PET scanning which showed a reduction in size of the obturator node and loss of uptake. There was otherwise no uptake within the pelvis, confirming an apparent complete response.

DECISION POINT

Should this patient undergo resectional surgery and if so, should he be offered a low anterior resection or an abdominoperineal resection? Also, what should be done about the obturator node which would be outside the normal TME plane of resection?

The options considered at the MDT were:

• no intervention with close surveillance

• standard resection with low anterior resection or APR

• standard resection plus lateral node dissection to remove the obturator node.

Colorectal Surgery: Clinical Care and Management, First Edition.
Edited by Bruce George, Richard Guy, Oliver Jones, and Jon Vogel.
© 2016 John Wiley & Sons, Ltd. Published 2016 by John Wiley & Sons, Ltd.

(continued)

It was felt that a conventional TME resection was the more appropriate recommendation. An extended resection to include the lateral pelvic nodes was not thought to be beneficial and would probably increase the morbidity, especially relating to bladder and sexual function. Although popular in Japan for low rectal tumors, an extended lateral dissection is rarely undertaken in the West. The general view is that although lateral pelvic nodes are a poor prognostic feature, radical dissection does not offer an improved oncological benefit. This view was further supported by the apparently good clinical and radiological response.

The option of no surgery but close surveillance was considered reasonable, although still unorthodox in the UK. Impressive results have been reported from a Brazilian group. It was felt reasonable to offer this to the patient provided he appreciated that it was not standard care and that close surveillance was imperative.

The options were discussed in detail with the patient. He was not at all keen on a permanent stoma and very concerned about potential sexual dysfunction. He felt that anterior resection would potentially leave him unable to continue to work. He decided on the option of no surgery and close surveillance.

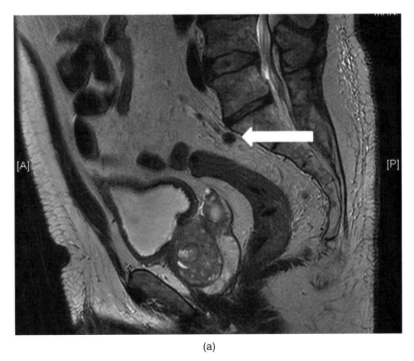

(a)

Figure 5.1 (a) MRI (sagittal) of pelvis, showing tumor 6 cm from the anal verge and probable involved lymph node just inferior to aortic bifurcation (*white arrow*).

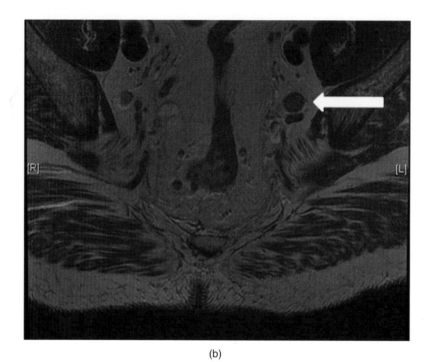

(b)

Figure 5.1 (b) MRI of pelvis, showing left obturator lymph node (*white arrow*).

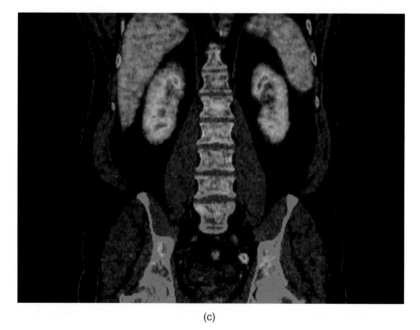

(c)

Figure 5.1 (c) PET scan showing moderately active rectal cancer and enhanced uptake in left obturator node.

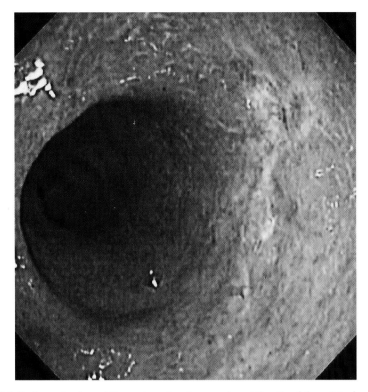

Figure 5.2 Endoscopic view of the rectum showing scarring at the site of the original cancer, with no evidence of residual tumor.

DECISION POINT

What frequency of endoscopic surveillance, CT, and MRI surveillance would be appropriate?

There is no consensus on how patients with a complete clinical response should be followed up. The ongoing "Deferral of surgery" trial (www.royalmarsden.nhs.uk/research/clinical-trials/pages/deferral-of-surgery.aspx) has 3-monthly MRI and sigmoidoscopy, with yearly CT, which is what we opted to do.

Two years on from the completion of downstaging chemoradiotherapy, the patient remains well and disease free.

LEARNING POINTS

- Involved lymph nodes in the pelvic side-wall are a poor prognostic feature and probably an important cause of local recurrence after conventional treatment. Although popular in Japan, an extended lateral lymph node dissection has not been demonstrated to confer a better oncological outcome and probably increases surgical morbidity.

- About 10–15% of patients will achieve a complete pathological response to long course chemoradiotherapy, such that no viable tumor cells are found in the surgical resection specimen. Such patients have a better prognosis.
- The option of avoiding major resectional surgery in patients with a complete clinical and radiological response has been popularized by Habr-Gama *et al.* from Brazil. If this approach is adopted then a rigorous follow-up protocol must be followed aiming to identify recurrent tumor while it is curable. The risk is that at the point of relapse, the disease is found to be locally advanced or metastatic and therefore incurable. We are awaiting ongoing trials investigating whether this strategy will have the same cure rate as immediate surgery. In the meantime, provided the patient is aware of these risks and a robust follow-up protocol is used, most clinicians would agree this is a reasonable option.

LETTER FROM AMERICA

The management of this patient would not be supported by ASCRS clinical practice guidelines for rectal cancer (2013): "Patients with an apparent complete clinical response to neoadjuvant therapy should be offered a definitive resection." Neither the NCCN nor the ASCRS currently recommends observation alone for complete responders to neoadjuvant therapy.

Jon Vogel and Massarat Zutshi

CASE 6

Marginal decisions

Oliver Jones

Oxford University Hospitals NHS Foundation Trust, Oxford, UK

A 41-year-old, sexually active man presented with rectal bleeding and a change in bowel habit. He underwent a colonoscopy and a rectal cancer was diagnosed with a lower border 10 cm from the anal verge. Biopsies confirmed adenocarcinoma. He underwent a staging CT scan of the chest, abdomen, and pelvis, which suggested that there was no metastatic disease, and an MRI of the pelvis.

The MRI scan suggested that this was a T2 tumor with the circumferential margin not threatened by the tumor itself. There was, however, a lymph node measuring 13 × 8 mm touching the mesorectal fascia (Figure 6.1). The case was discussed at the multidisciplinary meeting where the consensus was that the node was probably not involved.

DECISION POINT

Should this patient have neoadjuvant treatment or go straight to surgery?

This was felt to be a difficult decision. Our standard approach is to recommend long course chemotherapy when the surgical margin of excision is threatened. In this case, the main tumor was not threatening the margin. The lymph node in question was close to the margin but thought to probably not be involved. It was therefore decided to recommend "straight to surgery."

The options were discussed with the patient and the recommendations of the MDT made known to him. The decision was made to proceed straight to surgery.

The splenic flexure was fully mobilized and the IMA and IMV taken high via a single port laparoscopic approach. A Pfannenstiel incision was then made to complete the pelvic dissection. A total mesorectal excision was undertaken and a decision made to defunction with a loop ileostomy.

The postoperative histology confirmed that this was a T3N1 tumor with a single node involved, corresponding to the node seen on MRI. This was within 0.5 mm of the circumferential margin and so was classified as an R1 resection.

The patient was discussed in the MDT and treated with 6 months of postoperative chemotherapy (oxaliplatin and capecitabine). He completed the course

Colorectal Surgery: Clinical Care and Management, First Edition.
Edited by Bruce George, Richard Guy, Oliver Jones, and Jon Vogel.
© 2016 John Wiley & Sons, Ltd. Published 2016 by John Wiley & Sons, Ltd.

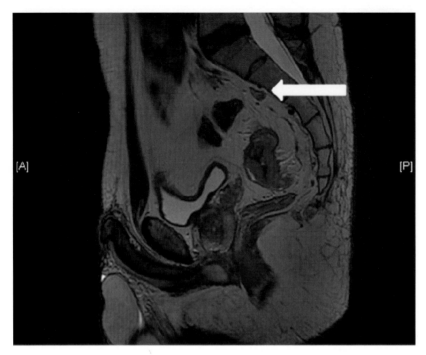

Figure 6.1 Sagittal MRI scan showing lymph node at the circumferential resection margin.

of treatment except for the final cycle of oxaliplatin which was not given due to severe peripheral neuropathy. End-of-treatment scans showed no evidence of local or distant recurrence. He underwent a contrast enema which confirmed no evidence of anastomotic leak and underwent an uneventful reversal of ileostomy.

Nine months after surgery, the patient remains well and is disease free. He has good bowel function with minimal urgency. He has normal bladder function and some slight reduction in erectile function. There is no evidence of disease recurrence.

Could we have done better?

In hindsight, this man should have received preoperative long course chemoradiotherapy (LCRT). The place of LCRT for mesorectal lymph nodes at the predicted surgical margin is controversial and not generally considered an absolute indication for LCRT. A selective approach to LCRT must balance the risks of an R1 margin with the risks of excessive use of radiotherapy. It is possible that PET-CT may have helped with assessment of the positive lymph node in this case. The sensitivity of PET-CT for lymph node assessment is only about 30% and therefore would probably not have altered management.

LEARNING POINTS

- R1 resection in rectal cancer patients is a bad prognostic factor. R1 resections are associated with an increased local relapse, distant metastasis, and as such a decreased overall survival. The aim is to identify those who are likely to have an R1 prior to surgery, as LCRT is significantly more effective in reducing local relapse when given prior to surgery rather than in the adjuvant setting.

LETTER FROM AMERICA

The ASCRS rectal cancer clinical practice guidelines note that the role of CT-PET in the staging of rectal cancer "remains to be determined." In cases in which the IMA nodes are clinically negative, division of the superior rectal artery at its origin from the IMA is advocated (rather than division of the IMA at its origin). This approach will afford the same oncological value and may decrease risk of sympathetic nerve injury. A "site-specific" TME, with a 5 cm distal mesorectal margin, is advocated for high rectal cancer such as the one presented in this case. In the USA, a defunctioning ostomy is typically reserved for cases that involve preoperative radiotherapy and/or a coloanal anastomosis.

Jon Vogel and Massarat Zutshi

CASE 7

Locally advanced rectal cancer invading prostate

Richard Guy[1], Roel Hompes[1] & Rebecca Kraus[2]

[1] Oxford University Hospitals NHS Foundation Trust, Oxford, UK
[2] University Hospital, Basel, Switzerland

A 67-year-old man, with no significant past medical history, presented with a short history of uncomfortable flatulence and rectal bleeding. Colonoscopy revealed a malignant-looking mass 4 cm from the anal verge, confirmed as invasive adenocarcinoma on biopsies. A pelvic MRI scan demonstrated extramural extension of tumor and possible invasion into an enlarged prostate plus a 7 mm diameter mesorectal node (Figure 7.1). There was no evidence of distant metastases on CT and radiological staging was T3N1M0.

The case was discussed at the colorectal MDT and long course chemoradiotherapy (CRT) recommended. The patient was entered into the ARISTOTLE Trial (investigating the addition of irinotecan to standard capecitabine chemoradiotherapy). He was randomized to the experimental arm and planned for 45 Gy in 25 fractions concurrently with capecitabine 650 mg/m^2 bd on days of radiotherapy treatment and irinotecan 60 mg/m^2 weekly from day 2. During the fourth week of his CRT, his neutrophil count fell to 0.7 and all chemotherapy was discontinued. He was admitted with fever and malaise and required IV antibiotics on a neutropenic sepsis protocol. He also suffered with nausea, diarrhea, mucositis, and fatigue.

On imaging 6 weeks following completion of chemoradiotherapy (CRT), the patient seemed to have responded relatively poorly to treatment, with an MRI tumor regression grade of 5. The anterior margin remained threatened, with appearances in keeping with infiltration into the posterior prostate.

At MDT, a recommendation was made to wait longer in order to see if further regression occurred and to seek opinion on surgical options. A further scan almost 3 months later showed that the tumor had reduced in signal and volume compared with the initial MRI scan but had increased in volume since the 6-week interim scan. Treated tumor was seen to extend beyond the wall and had broad contact with the prostate between 10 and 1 o'clock. There was low signal, presumed fibrosis, extending along the anterior rectal wall and posterior aspect of the prostate to the level of the anorectal junction.

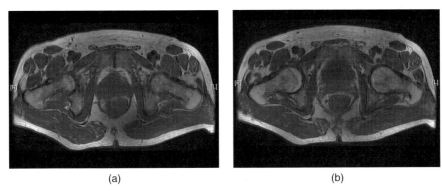

(a)   (b)

Figure 7.1 Pelvic MRI scan at presentation. Axial slices through the tumor show prostatic encroachment (a) and an enlarged pathological mesorectal lymph node (b).

DECISION POINT

What would you do now?

The overall assessment was that the tumor had not responded dramatically to downsizing chemoradiotherapy, was close to the prostate, but there was no evidence of distant disease. The surgical questions were as follows.

- What should the planned plane of dissection be anteriorly? Options considered were a standard mesorectal excision, to "shave the prostate" or to radically resect the prostate *en bloc*

- Could a sphincter-saving reconstruction be undertaken?

It was considered oncologically safest to recommend a pelvic clearance with APR and *en bloc* cystoprostatectomy. Reconstruction with a coloanal anastomosis was considered unwise after radiotherapy and a pelvic clearance. Similarly, although theoretically feasible, bladder preservation and continent urethral reconstruction was considered too high risk.

The patient proceeded to abdominoperineal resection with *en bloc* cystoprosta-tectomy. As all the pathology was in the anterior rectum, the perineal plane of dissection chosen posteriorly was the intersphincteric plane, in order to reduce the ultimate size of the perineal defect, with wider excision anterolaterally.

A double-barreled "wet" sigmoid colostomy was fashioned in the left iliac fossa, with the ureters separately anastomosed to the blind efferent limb of the stoma (Figure 7.2). The pelvis and perineal defects were reconstructed with a right vertical rectus abdominis myocutaneous (VRAM) flap.

Histopathological examination of the resected specimen showed residual microscopic foci of moderately differentiated adenocarcinoma within a 10 mm tumor scar. There was invasion beyond the muscularis propria into subserosa and a broad area of fibrous extension involving the prostatic capsule on the left side but no tumor invasion into the prostatic capsule itself. The histological measurement from tumor to nonperitonealized circumferential margin was 4 mm. There was extramural venous but no lymphatic invasion and 10 lymph nodes examined were negative for tumor (ypT3 N0 L0 V1 R0, Dukes' B). Tumor

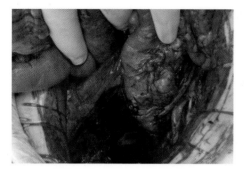 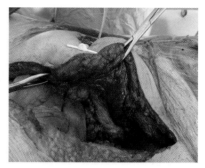

Figure 7.2 Operative view of ureterosigmoid anastomosis (*left*) and loop "wet" colostomy (*right*).

regression grade was 2. There was an incidental $10 \times 6 \times 5$ mm focus of prostatic adenocarcinoma of Gleason pattern $3 + 3$ in the right lateral peripheral zone with perineural infiltration but no extraprostatic extension.

Could we have done better?

The main debate postoperatively was whether or not *en bloc* resection of the bladder and prostate had been really necessary. The final pathology showed no rectal tumor involving the prostate but did show evidence of fibrosis consistent with the presence of tumor prior to chemoradiotherapy. Accurate radiological assessment of the extent of tumor after downsizing chemoradiotherapy is extremely difficult. Even when reviewed in hindsight with knowledge of the final pathology, no clear plane could be seen between rectal tumor and prostate. It would certainly have been a risk oncologically to just remove the rectum. Trying to surgically "shave" the prostate under these circumstances is usually futile and risks recurrence.

LEARNING POINTS

- There is some evidence that a longer interval to surgery is associated with more tumor shrinkage [1].
- Doubt about prostatic invasion by rectal cancer should usually be assumed to mean that there is invasion, especially following chemoradiotherapy.
- Attempting to find a plane between prostate and rectal cancer under these circumstances is unsuccessful and prostatic "shaving" is to be avoided.
- Double-barreled wet colostomy avoids the need for a second stoma and leaves a rectus abdominis muscle available for a VRAM flap.

LETTER FROM AMERICA

In cases such as these, preoperation long course chemoradiotherapy is used. Repeat staging would often be performed although not specifically endorsed by the National Cooperative Cancer Network. Eight to 10 weeks after completion of neoadjuvant therapy, an exenteration that includes the bladder and prostate would be performed as the authors described. Typically, an ileal conduit with urostomy would be favored over implantation of the ureters into the colostomy.

Jon Vogel and Massarat Zutshi

Reference

1 Petrelli F, Sgroi G, Sarti E, Barni S. Increasing the interval between neoadjuvant chemoradiotherapy and surgery in rectal cancer: a meta-analysis of published studies. *Ann Surg* 2015; Dec 9 (epub ahead of print).

CASE 8

Low rectal cancer and synchronous polyps

Richard Guy
Oxford University Hospitals NHS Foundation Trust, Oxford, UK

A 66-year-old woman underwent a BCSP colonoscopy following positive FOBT. Past medical history included appendicectomy, cesarean section, and hysterectomy, and she was fit and well. Digital rectal examination revealed a 4 cm diameter rectal cancer with a lower limit 3 cm above the anorectal junction on the left posterior wall. At colonoscopy, the cancer was confirmed and a 20 mm plaque-like polyp (Paris classification 0-IIa; see page 4) was seen just below it (Figure 8.1), as well as an 8 mm polyp anteriorly in the rectum and a 15 mm pedunculated polyp in the distal sigmoid. In the ascending colon, there was a 40 mm lateral spreading nongranular-type lesion. This was not removable endoscopically but considered entirely benign by an expert colonoscopist – and a tattoo was placed distally (anal side).

Biopsies of the presumed rectal cancer confirmed invasion. CT imaging showed no evidence of metastatic disease. MRI of the rectum showed a 4 cm diameter tumor in the low rectum on the left posterolateral wall with early extramural invasion and enlarged nodes with a benign appearance. The cancer was staged as T3N0 with no threatened margins.

DECISION POINT

How would you proceed?

Would you remove all the rectal polyps – what about the one below the cancer? Could this be incorporated within your resection?

Are you satisfied with the opinion on the right-sided polyp or would you like definitive histology?

It was considered that this was an operable rectal cancer with no need for preoperative radiotherapy/chemoradiotherapy. The main surgical challenge was the distal benign-looking sessile polyp which extended close to the anorectal junction. If a standard low anterior resection was to be undertaken with 1–2 cm distal clearance, the staple line might sit right on or through the polyp. A more distal resection incorporating this polyp would probably necessitate a transanal TME and peranal coloanal anastomosis (or even APR) with potential associated morbidity and, for a benign polyp, this was felt to be overtreatment. The difficult polyp in the right colon

---

Colorectal Surgery: Clinical Care and Management, First Edition.
Edited by Bruce George, Richard Guy, Oliver Jones, and Jon Vogel.
© 2016 John Wiley & Sons, Ltd. Published 2016 by John Wiley & Sons, Ltd.

(*continued*)

was at the limits of endoscopic resection but was accepted as being benign. Low anterior resection and right hemicolectomy, with two anastomoses, was also considered but felt to be excessive. The option of preliminary colonoscopic removal of the benign polyp followed by anterior resection was considered. There would be a theoretical risk of cancer cells implanting into the polypectomy site, although this was considered to be very low. The consensus was to resect the distal polyp by endoscopic submucosal resection (EMR) initially, with low anterior resection a few weeks later, and colotomy at the same time for removal of the right-sided polyp.

The patient underwent colonoscopic EMR of the two rectal polyps (Figure 8.2). Both were reported histologically to be tubular adenomas with low-grade dysplasia.

Three weeks later, the patient underwent surgery. The splenic flexure was first approached laparoscopically medial to lateral but access onto the IMV and a submesenteric dissection proved particularly difficult. Omental detachment from the transverse colon was commenced but it was wrapped around the flexure and distal transverse colon with obliteration of the lesser sac, necessitating conversion to laparotomy. The left colon was fully mobilized and high ligation of the IMA performed. The rectum was mobilized in the mesorectal plane and then staple-transected at the anorectal junction as a "close shave" following luminal wash-out, to obtain a good TME specimen.

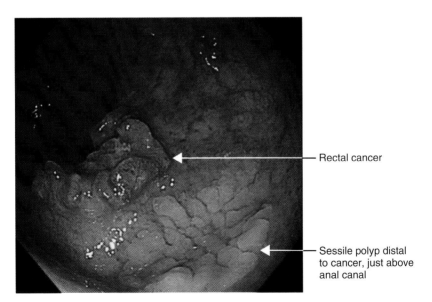

— Rectal cancer

— Sessile polyp distal to cancer, just above anal canal

Figure 8.1 Endoscopic image of the rectal cancer (*arrow*) with adjacent polyp and plaque-like lesion below (*arrow*).

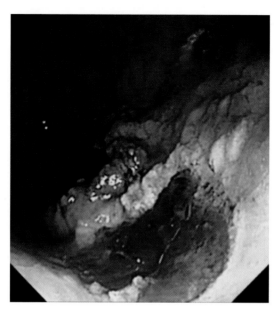

Figure 8.2 Appearance following EMR of both polyps – note how close to the lower end of the cancer the EMR margin appears.

The transverse colon and right colon were mobilized and on-table colonoscopy precisely identified the right-sided polyp. A longitudinal colotomy was made distal to it and, following a submucosal lifting injection with a saline-adrenaline solution, the polyp was removed as a single specimen, and the colotomy repaired transversely. A low stapled colorectal anastomosis was undertaken and defunctioned with a loop ileostomy. The patient made an uneventful recovery.

Histopathological examination of the rectal cancer showed a Dukes' B T3 N0 (0/43 nodes) V1 R0 cancer. The right-sided polyp was a benign tubulovillous adenoma. The patient did not receive adjuvant chemotherapy and, after a satisfactory water-soluble contrast enema examination, the ileostomy was closed without complication.

Could we have done better?

Transanal TME, including the cancer and distal polyp in the resection specimen, with either a stapled or hand-sewn coloanal anastomosis to the dentate line, might have been feasible and would have avoided the need to carry out, and potential risks of, polypectomy prior to cancer resection, but this might have been offset by inferior function.

LEARNING POINTS

- Significant colorectal polyps should probably be removed prior to cancer resection if there is any suspicion that they will not be included in the resection specimen.
- The risk of tumor seeding into a polypectomy site distal to a cancer is very low and rarely reported.

LETTER FROM AMERICA

In the USA, preoperative long course chemoradiotherapy remains the standard of care for rectal adenocarcinoma in the mid or low rectum with a clinical stage of 2 (T3 or T4) or 3 (any T, N+). If possible, preoperative endoscopic removal of the right colon lesion would be the preferred route rather than operative colotomy. In some centers, an alternative approach to the right colon polyp would be laparoscopic-assisted colonoscopic polypectomy. Ultimately, TME with sutured coloanal anastomosis and defunctioning loop ileostomy would be the favored approach to deal with all of the described rectal pathology.

Jon Vogel and Massarat Zutshi

CASE 9

Liver or rectum first?

Nicolas Buchs, Frederic Ris & Christian Toso
University Hospitals of Geneva, Geneva, Switzerland

A 52-year-old man, with no significant past medical or family history, presented with a short history of rectal bleeding. Digital rectal examination revealed a hard mass 6 cm from the anal verge. Colonoscopy confirmed a mainly posterior tumor, involving three quadrants, 9 cm in length but not causing obstruction. The rest of the colonoscopy was normal. Biopsies of the tumor confirmed adenocarcinoma. A CT scan showed two liver lesions in segments VII and VII compatible with liver metastases, and FDG avid on PET (Figure 9.1). Rectal MRI staged the mid-rectal tumor as T3N2, showing a large presacral node threatening the mesorectal margin (Figure 9.2).

DECISION POINT

How would you now proceed? Would you advise treatment for the rectum or liver disease in the first instance?

This is often a conundrum which provokes much discussion and can be difficult to resolve. Although clearly stage 4 disease (T3N2M1), both the liver and rectal disease were considered resectable and so aggressive treatment with potentially curative intent was considered appropriate. The main discussion was about the "order of play." Targeting either of the sites without dealing with the other site risked losing control of the disease. The three options considered were:

- standard approach (rectum first, then chemotherapy, and then liver resection)

- reverse strategy (liver-oriented chemotherapy first, then liver resection, and finally rectal resection)

- simultaneous strategy (combined rectal and liver resections during the same procedure, and chemotherapy).

It was felt that the risk of synchronous resection was too high, mainly on account of potential blood loss and mesenteric hypoperfusion associated with liver surgery. Combined liver and bowel resection was thought to be appropriate only if both are straightforward (e.g. right-sided colonic tumor and nonextended liver resection). After MDT discussion, the consensus was to proceed with the "reverse" strategy.

The patient received four cycles of FOLFOX chemotherapy (oxaliplatin, 5FU, and folinic acid), which were well tolerated. Following completion of

Colorectal Surgery: Clinical Care and Management, First Edition.
Edited by Bruce George, Richard Guy, Oliver Jones, and Jon Vogel.
© 2016 John Wiley & Sons, Ltd. Published 2016 by John Wiley & Sons, Ltd.

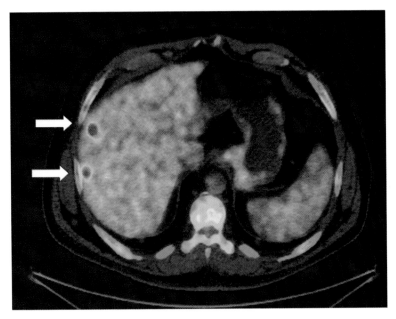

Figure 9.1 PET-CT scan showing two liver metastases (*arrowed*).

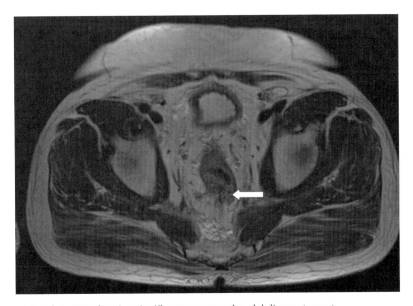

Figure 9.2 Pelvic MRI showing significant mesorectal nodal disease (*arrow*).

chemotherapy, radiological evaluation showed a good response of the primary tumor and liver metastases, with no new disease. He proceeded to a minimally invasive liver resection, without complications. Ten weeks after the liver surgery, he received long course chemoradiotherapy to the pelvis (42 Gy over 6 weeks). MR imaging 6 weeks after chemotherapy showed a decrease in size of both the primary tumor and presacral marginal node. Some 12 weeks after completion of chemoradiotherapy, he underwent laparoscopic-assisted low anterior resection and loop ileostomy, an *en bloc* extended cuff of presacral fascia being taken at the level of the threatening node. The final histology report showed a ypT3N0 cancer with negative margins (R0).

Three weeks later, he re-presented with general malaise and an offensive anal discharge. Flexible sigmoidoscopy showed ischemia of the last 2–3 cm of colon just above the anastomosis, with a line of demarcation between pink and pale pink mucosa. A CT scan showed evidence of an anastomotic leak and pre-sacral collection. This required a difficult relaparotomy and disconnection of the coloanal anastomosis with formation of an end colostomy. Despite this complication, he made a satisfactory recovery and was able to commence chemotherapy 8 weeks later.

Could we have done better?

The oncological outcome was good but the surgical outcome was unfortunate and, ultimately, he is unlikely to have coloanal continuity restored. The best he can hope for is closure of ileostomy to bring the colon back into circuit. It is possible that if the anterior resection had been performed first, in the traditional way, this complication may have prevented liver resection with inevitable disease progression.

LEARNING POINTS

- A reverse or "liver first" approach can be considered in patients with potentially (R0) resectable rectal and liver cancers, with or without initial downstaging chemotherapy.
- This case highlights the potential morbidity associated with rectal cancer surgery and supports the liver-first approach to resectable liver disease.

CASE 10

Beware bad livers!

Kate Williamson

Oxford University Hospitals NHS Foundation Trust, Oxford, UK

A 65-year-old woman presented to clinic with bright red rectal bleeding, and a 2-month history of change in bowel habit, tending to constipation, and abdominal discomfort. She had some associated generalized abdominal discomfort. Past medical history included alcoholic cirrhosis, diagnosed 2 years previously. A transjugular intrahepatic portosystemic shunt (TIPS) had been inserted 1 year previously for medically refractory ascites, and a recent ultrasound had shown it to be patent with good Doppler flow. On clinical examination, she was obese (BMI 34 kg/m^2) with spider nevi and palmar erythema, but not jaundice. The abdomen was soft and nontender, and digital rectal examination unremarkable.

Flexible sigmoidoscopy and CT colonography revealed an obstructing descending colonic tumor, biopsies of which confirmed adenocarcinoma (Figure 10.1).

A staging CT scan showed no evidence of metastatic disease. Liver function tests showed: bilirubin 33 μmol/L, albumin 40 g/L, prothromin time 15.9 seconds, hemoglobin 15.5 g/dL, and platelets 110×10^9/L. A week later she presented as an emergency with abdominal pain, distension, and absolute constipation. A colonic stent was successfully inserted.

DECISION POINT

Would you now offer resection? Should she be managed conservatively?

It was accepted that this lady's co-morbidity, in particular cirrhosis, increased the risks of surgery. However, she was relatively young with no evidence of metastatic disease and her CT abdomen had not shown evidence of portal hypertension (no ascites, decompressed collaterals). In view of this, the MDT recommended proceeding to surgery.

Open left hemicolectomy was undertaken. She had a stormy postoperative course, requiring intensive care for 5 days. Complications included hypotension requiring inotropes, wound infection and dehiscence requiring topical negative pressure therapy and decompensation of the underlying cirrhosis, with hepatic encephalopathy and ascites. Serum bilirubin rose to 43 μmol/L, prothrombin

Colorectal Surgery: Clinical Care and Management, First Edition.
Edited by Bruce George, Richard Guy, Oliver Jones, and Jon Vogel.
© 2016 John Wiley & Sons, Ltd. Published 2016 by John Wiley & Sons, Ltd.

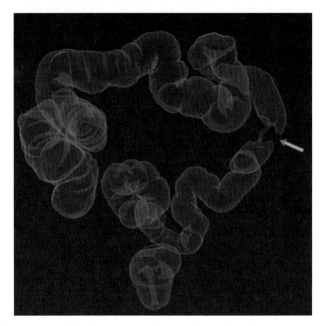

Figure 10.1 Reconstructed CT colonography showing desending colon cancer.

time to 25 seconds, and albumin dropped to 24 g/L. She was discharged on day 37 and made a slow recovery. The resection specimen showed a moderately differentiated adenocarcinoma with serosal invasion (pT3), with lymphatic and vascular invasion, and nodal involvement (N1, Dukes' C).

DECISION POINT

Would you recommend adjuvant chemotherapy?

It was felt that the patient was too frail, with advanced liver disease, to undergo standard platinum-based chemotherapy for her Dukes' C cancer, and she was not offered chemotherapy.

Liver synthetic function gradually returned to baseline, although she was unable to walk more than 20 meters. She was still alive 12 months postoperatively.

Could we have done better?

It is not clear whether surgical resection has improved her survival or quality of life compared with simply leaving her with a colonic stent, and one wonders whether operation was appropriate given her co-morbidities. She was given perioperative antibiotic prophylaxis but no additional antibiotics and she was not given lactulose. Although lacking a strong evidence base, patients with cirrhosis undergoing gastrointestinal surgery should probably receive an extended course of prophylactic antibiotics and lactulose to reduce the risk of infections and encephalopathy, respectively.

LEARNING POINTS

- At least 30% of cirrhotic patients have a significant postoperative complication, the main ones being ascites, encephalopathy, renal failure, bleeding, and infection.
- Operative mortality in patients with cirrhosis may be predicted using the Child–Turcotte–Pugh Score (CTP) (Table 10.1) or the Model for End Stage Liver Disease (MELD). The MELD score is based on age, ASA grade, bilirubin, creatinine, INR, and etiology of cirrhosis and may be readily calculated online. If one combines the various studies looking at CTP score as a predictor of mortality, the general surgical mortality rates are as follows.
  - CTP A: 10%
  - CTP B: 30%
  - CTP C: 76–82%

Table 10.1 Child–Turcotte–Pugh Score.

	1 point	2 points	3 points
Bilirubin (mol/L)	<34	34–50	>50
Albumin (g/L)	>35	28–35	<28
INR	<1.7	1.7–2.3	>2.3
Ascites	Absent	Mild/ on diuretics	Moderate–severe
Hepatic encephalopathy	Absent	Grade I–II/ on laxatives	Grade III–IV

CTP A = 5–6 points; B = 7–9 points; C = 10–15 points.
INR, international normalized ratio.
Source: Papatheodoridis [1]. Reproduced with permission of Wiley.

Reference

1 Cholongitas E, Papatheodoridis GV, Vangeli M, Terreni N, Patch D, Burroughs AK. Systematic review: The model for end-stage liver disease–should it replace Child-Pugh's classification for assessing prognosis in cirrhosis? *Aliment Pharmacol Ther* 2005; **22**(11–12):1079–89. Article first published online: 2 Nov 2005. doi: 10.1111/j.1365-2036.2005.02691.x

CASE 11

Anastomotic recurrence?

Bruce George

Oxford University Hospitals NHS Foundation Trust, Oxford, UK

A 72-year-old man presented with fresh rectal bleeding. Past medical history included a myocardial infarct 12 years previously and controlled hypertension. Colonoscopy demonstrated a 1.5 cm polypoid sigmoid tumor not amenable to colonoscopic removal, and biopsies showed invasive adenocarcinoma. Staging investigations showed no evidence of distant disease, although the primary tumor could not convincingly be seen radiologically.

He proceeded to laparoscopic high anterior resection and, other than a superficial wound infection at the umbilicus, he made a good postoperative recovery. Histopathology demonstrated an early polyp cancer (T1, [sm3], N0[0/8 nodes], R0).

A routine follow-up CT scan 1 year later showed some thickening at the anastomosis, possibly due to postoperative changes, but possibly indicating tumor recurrence. A subsequent MR scan showed an extramural mass adjacent to the anastomosis. Colonoscopy showed a 4 mm inflammatory polyp at the anastomosis, but no evidence of luminal recurrence, and biopsies of this showed chronic inflammatory cells only. A PET scan showed increased uptake in this region with an SUV of 12.1 (Figure 11.1).

DECISION POINT

What would you do now? Are you convinced that this is recurrent disease?

The MR and PET-CT scans are suggestive of local recurrence adjacent to the anastomosis, but this was considered unusual following resection of an early (T1N0) tumor 15 months earlier. The colonoscopic appearances did not really support recurrence. The case was discussed in detail at the MDT meeting and the options considered were:

- continued surveillance with repeat scans in 3 months

- further investigations to look for local recurrence

- treat aggressively as presumed local recurrence.

Radiologically guided percutaneous biopsy of the perianastomotic mass was considered hazardous and not likely to yield a representative sample. Surveillance only risked "missing the boat" as this was considered to be a potentially curative localized recurrence. It was decided to recommend a further resection. The next question was whether to proceed directly to surgery or to "downsize" with chemoradiotherapy, despite lack of histological evidence. As the radiology was convincing, the oncologists agreed to proceed with chemoradiotherapy.

Colorectal Surgery: Clinical Care and Management, First Edition.
Edited by Bruce George, Richard Guy, Oliver Jones, and Jon Vogel.
© 2016 John Wiley & Sons, Ltd. Published 2016 by John Wiley & Sons, Ltd.

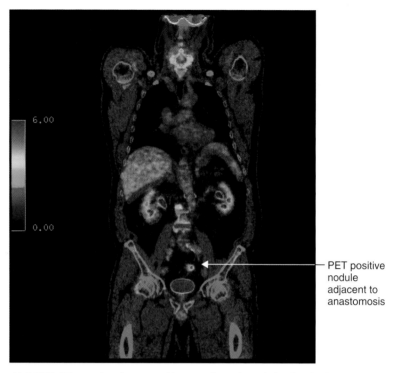

Figure 11.1 PET-CT scan showing area of increased uptake in left side of pelvis, adjacent to previous anastomosis.

The patient received chemoradiotherapy over 5 weeks, after which a repeat MRI scan showed shrinkage of the perianastomotic mass, although abnormal soft tissue still touched the predicted mesorectal excision margin. It was decided to hold off surgery until 12 weeks after radiotherapy in the hope of obtaining the maximum downsizing effect.

At operation, there was considerable fibrosis around the previous anastomosis, but no evidence of distant disease. A "re-do" anterior resection was carried out with an anastomosis 5 cm beyond the area of perianastomotic fibrosis, covered by a loop ileostomy.

Pathological examination showed no evidence of malignancy in the resected specimen and no additional therapy was recommended by the MDT.

The patient's recovery was complicated by an anastomotic leak and a prevertebral collection, too small for radiological drainage. Blood cultures grew *E. coli* sensitive to co-amoxiclav and gentamicin, and with antibiotics his general condition improved, although he continued to complain of severe low back pain. He was readmitted with persistent pain and fever and imaging showed gas in the L5–S1 disk/epidural space, requiring 6 weeks of intravenous antibiotics. Subsequent review over 12 months revealed persistent vertebral inflammatory changes but no evidence of recurrent disease and contrast enema examination plus flexible sigmoidoscopy have shown a healthy anastomosis.

Could we have done better?

Local recurrence after a high anterior resection for a T1 tumor would have been unusual and it is still uncertain whether this was the case, or whether the chemoradiotherapy "sterilized" it. Only eight lymph nodes were retrieved in the original specimen and it is, therefore, possible that this did represent nodal persistence or recurrence. Perhaps a more radical resection, despite the knowledge that this was an early tumor, would have been preferable. As far as the presumed recurrence is concerned, it seems unlikely that any more proof could have been obtained. The severity of the anastomotic leak was probably not appreciated and the patient's complaints of persistent back and hip pain probably should have prompted more aggressive treatment.

LEARNING POINTS

- The diagnosis of recurrent tumor after surgery for colorectal carcinoma may be difficult – it is not always feasible to obtain histological proof of recurrence and treatment may have to proceed without histological proof.
- Spinal infections associated with anastomotic leak are rare but require prolonged courses of parenteral antibiotics.

LETTER FROM AMERICA

The ASCRS clinical practice guidelines for colon cancer note that multimodality therapy for colon cancer local recurrence offers the greatest chance for cure. The American Cancer Society includes guidance suggesting that colon cancer resections that include less than 12 lymph nodes should be treated as if they were the next stage higher. In this case, raising the stage by one level would be unlikely to have changed initial management as adjuvant chemotherapy is seldomly indicated for stage 2 colon cancer. In some centers, endoscopic ultrasound-guided biopsy of the suspected local recurrence may have been done to confirm local recurrence prior to embarking on additional cancer therapy.

Jon Vogel and Massarat Zutshi

CASE 12

Challenging warts

Emma Bracey & Bruce George

Oxford University Hospitals NHS Foundation Trust, Oxford, UK

A 42-year-old heterosexual male presented with a 4-week history of anal pain, discharge, and a lump near the anus. Three years previously, he had undergone banding of hemorrhoids and excision of some anal warts. His past medical history included psoriasis and sarcoidosis. On examination, he was obese (BMI 41.2 kg/m^2). Perianal inspection revealed three lesions close to the anal margin (Figure 12.1). Digital rectal examination, proctoscopy, and rigid sigmoidoscopy were normal.

DECISION POINT

What would you do next? Would you remove all the lesions?

It was felt that a precise diagnosis of these lesions was important. The clinical decision centered around whether excision or incision/punch biopsy would be most appropriate. It was decided to excise all three lesions with a close margin.

The lesions were excised under general anesthesia and postoperative healing was slow, with some wound breakdown. On histological examination, the polypoid lesion (A) showed a focus of invasive squamous cell carcinoma (SCC) on a background of condyloma acuminata. The ulcerated lesion (B) showed a moderately differentiated SCC on a background of anal intraepithelial neoplasia 3 (AIN 3). Lateral excision margins were clear but, in specimen B, AIN extended to the deep margin. The other lesion (C) was a fibroepithelial polyp. Immunohistochemistry for human papilloma virus (HPV) was negative for specimen B. Occasional nuclei showed weak positivity for HPV in specimen A.

DECISION POINT

What would you do now? Is further surgery indicated?

Several members of the MDT considered that, as the lesions were at the anal margin, they should be treated by wide surgical excision, with avoidance of chemoradiotherapy if possible. Others (mainly the surgeons) felt that wide excision in a large male with a funnel-shaped anal area and wounds which had proved slow to heal would be challenging, with a high chance of wound breakdown and sepsis. Furthermore, the proven multifocal nature of the disease suggested the need for a more generalized therapy. It was therefore agreed that external beam radiotherapy would be appropriate.

Colorectal Surgery: Clinical Care and Management, First Edition.
Edited by Bruce George, Richard Guy, Oliver Jones, and Jon Vogel.
© 2016 John Wiley & Sons, Ltd. Published 2016 by John Wiley & Sons, Ltd.

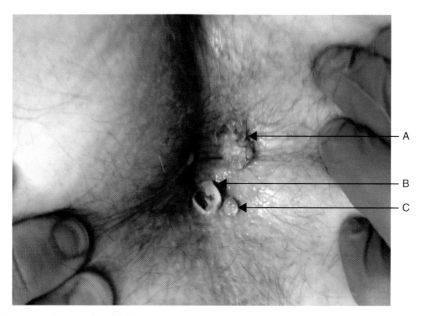

Figure 12.1 Three perianal lesions.

The patient underwent long course radiotherapy but shortly after completion, he suffered severe perianal skin excoriation and fecal leakage, which eventually resolved. At follow-up 10 months later, he remains well with no clinical or radiological evidence of recurrent disease.

Could we have done better?

In hindsight, the ulcerated lesion (B) should probably have been biopsied only (using a punch biopsy), rather than excised. This would have allowed a diagnosis to be made and then wide excision to be undertaken as primary treatment, perhaps avoiding the need for radical radiotherapy.

LEARNING POINTS

- Anal margin squamous cell carcinomas have a more favorable outcome than anal canal tumors. The current treatment recommendation is for local excision for T1 tumors (<2 cm diameter) provided that adequate margins (>5 mm) can be achieved without compromising sphincter function. For patients with T2 or higher T stages, or lymph node involvement, chemoradiotherapy is recommended.
- The management of anal tumors should be coordinated by an appropriate MDT with involvement of plastic surgeons and specialists in genitourinary medicine as required.

LETTER FROM AMERICA

The NCCN guidelines for perianal (anal margin) squamous cell carcinoma advise biopsy to confirm invasive cancer and local excision for T1N0, well-differentiated tumors. If "adequate margins" are achieved, observation is recommended. If the margins of excision are inadequate, reexcision is recommended or chemoradiotherapy may be considered. First-line chemoradiotherapy is also recommended for T2 or larger tumors, tumors that are not well differentiated, and those with lymph node involvement.

Jon Vogel and Massarat Zutshi

CASE 13

An unusual right iliac fossa mass

Bruce George

Oxford University Hospitals NHS Foundation Trust, Oxford, UK

A 58-year-old woman presented with pain and a mass in the right iliac fossa. Ultrasound and CT imaging showed a 19 cm mass with compression of the right ureter and liver metastases (Figure 13.1). The initial impression was that this was probably an ovarian tumor and she was referred to the gynecological oncology team. Ca-125 was modestly raised at 160, but CEA was normal.

DECISION POINT

How would you establish the diagnosis? Should a biopsy be performed?

It was felt that the overall picture was not typical of ovarian malignancy: the Ca-125 was not as high as would be expected in the presence of metastatic ovarian malignancy and there was neither omental disease nor ascites. The possibility of sarcoma was considered. The radiological appearances, however, were not diagnostic of a particular type of sarcoma, e.g. liposarcoma, which would have obviated the need for biopsy. It was therefore felt that a histological diagnosis was important and the right iliac fossa mass was easily accessible to percutaneous biopsy. Despite the risk of tumor seeding along the biopsy track, this was felt to be justified. Liver biopsy and laparoscopic biopsies were also considered but were felt to carry a slightly higher risk.

Percutaneous biopsy of the mass was undertaken. This showed features of a spindle cell neoplasm. Immunohistochemical staining was positive for cKIT, indicating a diagnosis of gastrointestinal stromal tumor (GIST). Following discussion at the local sarcoma MDT, treatment with imatinib, a tyrosine kinase inhibitor, was initiated.

The patient tolerated the imatinib well with no significant side-effects. A PET-CT scan 6 months following commencement of treatment showed a significant improvement with no increased FDG uptake in either the liver or primary mass, and she continued on imatinib. Four months later, repeat PET-CT showed a small area of avid FDG uptake within the primary tumor (Figure 13.2).

Colorectal Surgery: Clinical Care and Management, First Edition.
Edited by Bruce George, Richard Guy, Oliver Jones, and Jon Vogel.
© 2016 John Wiley & Sons, Ltd. Published 2016 by John Wiley & Sons, Ltd.

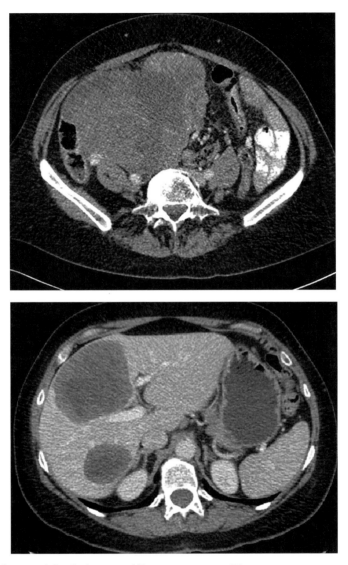

Figure 13.1 Large abdominal mass and liver metastases on CT scan.

DECISION POINT

Would you simply continue with medical therapy or is surgical resection now indicated?

Would you resect the pelvic mass and the liver disease?

It was thought that the PET-positive focus was probably due to "selection" of a clone of imatinib-resistant cells. In recent years, understanding of the tumor biology of GISTs has improved enormously. The most common oncogenic mutation responsible for tumor proliferation is in exon 11, which is associated with an excellent response to imatinib. Mutations

(continued)

at other sites or cKit-negative tumors are associated with a less favorable response to imatinib. Indeed, it is becoming apparent that different areas within tumors may have different mutational characteristics. Therapeutic options considered at this stage were second-line tyrosine kinase inhibitors (e.g. sunatinib) or surgical resection. Despite some reluctance to embark on a major pelvic resection in a patient with liver metastases, it was felt that this was justified and potentially curative.

At operation, there was no evidence of liver disease. The pelvic tumor was attached to the sigmoid colon and densely adherent to the right pelvic side-wall at the level of the distal ureter. Radical resection was undertaken, with *en bloc* resection of the tumor mass, adjacent sigmoid colon, lower 3 cm of ureter and right ovary and fallopian tube. The right ureter was reimplanted into the bladder and a colorectal anastomosis made. Postoperative recovery was uneventful and a cystogram on day 10 showed no evidence of urinary leakage. Histology confirmed features of a GIST. The patient remains well 9 months postoperatively with no evidence of tumor recurrence.

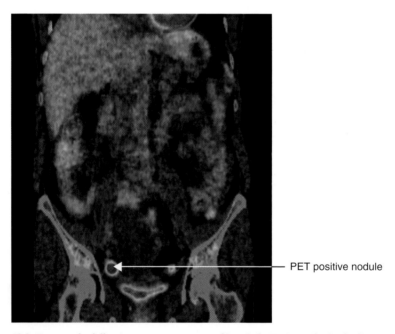

PET positive nodule

Figure 13.2 Ten months following commencement of imatinib, FDG uptake in the liver was absent, with only a small area of avidity in the pelvis.

Could we have done better?

A laparoscopic biopsy of the abdominal mass might have been oncologically preferable to a percutaneous biopsy in view of the potential for tumor seeding along the needle track. Following a percutaneous biopsy, ideally the track should be excised or incorporated within the surgical incision. The pathology report showed no evidence of tumor involving the ureter and, in theory, ureteric excision could have been avoided, but in practice it is usually better to err on the side of caution and resect.

LEARNING POINTS

- GISTs should be considered in the differential diagnosis of any unusual abdominal mass.
- Dramatic responses to tyrosine kinase inhibitors may be seen with these tumors.
- Percutaneous biopsy of an abdominal mass risks tumor seeding, potentially converting a curable into a noncurable situation.

SECTION B
Inflammatory bowel disease

Bruce George
Oxford University Hospitals NHS Foundation Trust, Oxford, UK

Introduction

The term "inflammatory bowel disease" refers to Crohn's disease and ulcerative colitis (UC). Whilst these conditions share many common features, they also have many differences in diagnosis, disease course, and medical treatment. However, it is probably true that it is in surgery that the differences between the conditions are most marked.

Crohn's disease

Epidemiology
The prevalence of Crohn's disease is about 2–5 per 1000 of the population in northern Europe and Scandinavia and appears to be increasing. The prevalence is lower in southern Europe and rare in Africa, the Far East, and South America.

Pathogenesis
The pathogenesis involves a complex interaction between genetic susceptibility, environmental factors, infective agents, and the immune system. This is reviewed in more detail elsewhere [1].

Macroscopic pathology
Inflammatory changes of Crohn's may affect any part of the gastrointestinal tract, but are most commonly seen in the ileocecal region, small bowel, and large bowel. Areas of inflammation separated by normal bowel are characteristic, giving rise to skip lesions. Viewed from the luminal aspect, the macroscopic features include ulceration and strictures. Ulceration ranges from small aphthous ulcers, through longitudinal serpiginous discontinuous ulcers to deep fissuring

Colorectal Surgery: Clinical Care and Management, First Edition.
Edited by Bruce George, Richard Guy, Oliver Jones, and Jon Vogel.
© 2016 John Wiley & Sons, Ltd. Published 2016 by John Wiley & Sons, Ltd.

ulceration. Edematous islands of mucosa surrounded by intercommunicating fissures lead to the characteristic cobblestone appearance seen at endoscopy. Viewed from the serosal side, either by the surgeon or in the pathology laboratory, macroscopic features include bowel wall thickening, fat wrapping, and enlarged mesenteric lymph nodes.

Microscopic pathology

The hallmark microscopic features are focal ulceration, transmural inflammation in the form of lymphoid aggregates, and granulomas. Granulomas are seen in less than 50% of cases.

Complications

Stricturing disease may progress to intestinal obstruction. Fistulating disease may result in abscess formation adjacent to the bowel or fistulation into another structure such as bladder, vagina, skin or another segment of bowel.

Extraintestinal manifestations of Crohn's (see Clinical features) occur in about one-third of patients. Long-standing disease is also associated with an increased risk of malignancy, including colorectal adenocarcinoma (see **Case 17**), small bowel adenocarcinoma, lymphoma, and anal neoplasia (see **Case 20**).

Clinical features

The clinical features of Crohn's disease depend on the age of presentation, the site of disease, the severity/behavior of the intestinal disease, and the presence or absence of extraintestinal manifestations. Presentation may vary from the classic triad of abdominal pain, weight loss, and diarrhea to bizarre presentations such as cerebral abscesses or skin rashes. Nonspecific symptoms such as malaise, fever, and anorexia are common.

A variety of classifications of Crohn's disease exist [2], the most widely used today being the Montreal classification.

Extraintestinal manifestations occur in about one-third of patients (Table B.1). Most tend to mirror disease activity in the colon, apart from ankylosing spondylosis and primary sclerosing cholangitis which run independent courses.

Table B.1 Extraintestinal manifestations of Crohn's disease.

System	Manifestation
Musculoskeletal	Arthropathy Ankylosing spondylosis
Eye	Uveitis Episcleritis
Skin	Erythema nodosum Pyoderma gangrenosum
Hepatobiliary	Primary sclerosing cholangitis
Hematological	Increased risk of venous thromboembolism

Diagnosis

Diagnosis depends on the integration of clinical features with radiological imaging, endoscopic appearances, histopathology, and laboratory data.

Colonoscopy with ileal intubation is required in the vast majority of patients with Crohn's disease. Upper GI endoscopy is recommended in all children/adolescents with suspected IBD (see **Case 14**), but is not routinely employed in adult practice. Capsule endoscopy is being increasingly used in the assessment of small bowel disease.

Computed tomography or MR enterography or enteroclysis (-clysis implies that luminal contrast is given via an enteric tube) have replaced traditional barium studies in most centers. MR is preferable in young patients due to the lack of radiation exposure and is particularly useful in assessing perianal disease. Abdominal ultrasound is more operator dependent than CT/MR but is useful in younger patients when local expertise exists.

There is no single biomarker for Crohn's disease. C-reactive protein and the fecal granulocyte proteins lactoferrin and calprotectin may add supportive evidence for the diagnosis of IBD, but are more useful in monitoring disease activity.

Natural history

The annual incidence of hospital admission is 20%; 50% of patients require surgery within 10 years of diagnosis and 50% experience postoperative recurrence within 10 years [3]. Although difficult to predict accurately, certain factors such as young age of onset, early need for steroids, perianal disease, and repeated small bowel resections are associated with a more aggressive natural history. It is postulated and hoped that early mucosal healing with optimum medical therapy may improve the natural history.

Medical treatment of Crohn's disease

The management of Crohn's disease involves a mixture of general supportive care, medical therapy, nutritional therapy, endoscopy, and surgery. Involvement with local or national patient support groups may be helpful (www .crohnsandcolitis.org.uk). All patients should be supported to stop smoking. Nutritional deficiencies including anemia should be addressed.

Medical treatment typically utilizes a short-term agent (e.g. steroids) combined with a long-term maintenance drug such as a thiopurine or methotrexate. The major groups of drugs used to treat Crohn's disease are summarized in Table B.2, with choice of drug dependent on disease site, severity and a weighing up of the efficacy, likely side-effects, and complications.

Absolute contraindications to anti-TNF therapy may be remembered by the acronym STOIC.

S: Sepsis or infection, including pelvic or perianal
T: TB

O: Optic neuritis (or other demyelinating disorder)

 I: Infusion reaction (previous sensitivity to anti-TNF drug or murine products)

C: Cancer (past or present) or Cardiac failure (moderate or severe)

Surgical treatment

Surgery is indicated for complications of the disease, principally strictures and fistulae, and failure of medical therapy. Data suggest that over 80% of patients with Crohn's disease will eventually require surgery during their lifetime [4]. More recent data suggest that the need for major abdominal surgery is decreasing [5], perhaps due to improvements in medical therapy. Many doctors and patients fear surgery due to the perceived high risks, including anastomotic leakage, fistulae, pain, altered body image, and short bowel syndrome. The factors that make surgery for Crohn's disease dangerous are well established. Several studies have shown that sepsis, steroids, and malnutrition are independent risk factors for anastomotic leakage [6]. The challenge to physicians and surgeons is to accept

Table B.2 Drugs used to treat Crohn's disease.

Group	Common examples	Uses	Comments
Steroids	Prednisolone Budesonide Hydrocortisone	Induction of remission for moderate and severe disease. Not for long-term use	Useful to induce remission but should not be used long term
Thiopurines	Azathioprine 6-Mercaptopurine	Maintaining remission	Regular FBC monitoring required. Dose requirement and side-effect profile may be predicted by measurement of drug metabolism (TPMT activity)
Methotrexate	Methotrexate	Maintaining remission, usually if thiopurine resistant or intolerant	Regular LFT monitoring required
Antibiotics	Metronidazole Ciprofloxacin	Short-term infections. Possible role in reducing postoperative recurrence	
Biologics (anti-TNF)	Infliximab Adalimumab	Efficacy in acute treatment and maintenance established in major trials	

FBC, full blood count; LFT, liver function test; TNF, tumor necrosis factor; TPMT, thiopurine methyltransferase.

that most patients with Crohn's disease will require surgery at some stage and that a critical part of overall patient management is to undertake surgery when conditions are favorable, rather than when multiple risk factors exist.

Principles

Preoperative
- Reduce risk factors by improving nutrition, weaning steroids, and draining sepsis (see **Case 15**).
- Ensure up-to-date imaging/colonoscopy, especially to ensure no distal obstruction to proposed anastomoses.
- Ensure MDT discussion and appropriate involvement of dieticians and stomatherapists in preoperative preparation.

Operative
- Use laparoscopic techniques as much as reasonably possible.
- Preserve bowel length by minimal resections or use of stricturoplasty (see **Case 16**).
- Avoid anastomoses if more than one major risk factor present.

Postoperative
- Thorough evaluation of suspected postoperative leaks (see **Cases 46 and 48**).
- Caution to avoid reoperating on hostile abdomen.
- Consider drug treatment to reduce risk of recurrent Crohn's (see **Cases 14–16 and 18**).

Stricturing small bowel disease (see Case 16)
Isolated stricturing disease of the small bowel tends to be distal and usually amenable to a limited resection. Extensive stricturing disease presents a greater surgical challenge. An important principle is to preserve bowel length whenever possible, especially bearing in mind the likelihood of recurrent small bowel disease in the future. Minimal resection with just 2–3 cm of macroscopically normal bowel at each end is preferable to more extensive resections [7]. The concept of stricturoplasty (SP) to facilitate gut preservation was initially described by Lee and Papaioannou [8]. In the simplest technique, the bowel is opened longitudinally over the stricture and closed transversely, resulting in widening of the stricture segment. Obvious concerns are the risk of leakage due to suturing through diseased bowel and the risk that failure to remove the diseased segment would lead to earlier recurrence. A systematic review of stricturoplasty [9], assessing over 1000 patients worldwide undergoing over 3000 stricturoplasties, reported a low surgical complications rate (4% septic complications) and a surgical recurrence rate of 23%, which compares favorably to recurrence rates after resectional surgery. Longer strictures may be widened with the Finney technique.

There is slight concern about the risk of small bowel tumors developing at SP sites. A few cases have been reported although this seems to be so rare as to not represent a significant objection to SP. When undertaking SP, some mucosal ulceration is commonly seen on the mesenteric side of the small bowel. Our policy is not to biopsy routinely unless there are any unusual features.

Ileocecal disease (see Cases 14, 15, and 50)

The most common site of Crohn's disease is the terminal ileum. Historical data suggest that 80% of patients with distal ileal disease require surgery with 5 years of diagnosis and up to 91% with longer follow-up [10]. Standard indications for surgery are obstruction due to stricturing disease, fistulae or failure of medical therapy. There is an increasing vogue for earlier surgery when the general condition of the patient is good, rather than after prolonged medical therapy. Fibrotic stricturing disease is less likely to respond to medical therapy than inflammatory, phlegmonous disease. MRE and inflammatory markers may be helpful in deciding between medical and surgical treatment.

The standard operation for terminal ileal disease is a laparoscopic ileocecal resection. In a multicenter RCT by McLeod *et al.* [11], no difference was noted in complication rates or endoscopic recurrence between end-to-end and side-to-side anastomoses. In the general surgical literature, a recent Cochrane metaanalysis suggests that stapled anastomoses are associated with a lower leak rate than hand-sewn anastomoses (1.4% versus 6%, p<0.02) [12].

Postoperatively, the question of medical prophylaxis to reduce the risk of Crohn's recurrence should be addressed. All patients should be advised and supported to stop smoking. There is some evidence that 5-ASA drugs, thiopurines, and infliximab may reduce recurrent Crohn's rates. Common practice is to give thiopurines to patients considered to be at moderate risk and anti-TNF to patients at very high risk. Where uncertainty exists, it is common practice to undertake a colonoscopy at 6–12 months and base subsequent medical therapy on the peri-anastomotic appearances.

Crohn's colitis (see Cases 17 and 18)

Surgery for Crohn's colitis is usually indicated for persisting symptoms despite optimum medical therapy. Approximately 50% of patients with colitis require surgery within 10 years and 25% require a permanent stoma. The choice of surgery depends on the distribution of inflammation and the presence or absence of proctitis or anal disease. Long-standing Crohn's colitis is associated with an increased risk of malignancy of a similar order of magnitude as is seen in UC.

Segmental colectomy may be appropriate for an isolated segment of inflammation or stricture in the colon, but represents less than 10% of operations done for colonic Crohn's. A meta-analysis suggests no difference in operative complications or ultimate stoma rates for segmental versus complete colectomy but indicates a slightly earlier time to recurrence in the segmental resection group [13]. Strictures in the colon should be resected rather than widened by SP for diagnostic certainty and because of the much higher risk of malignancy in the colon compared to small bowel. Extensive colitis with rectal sparing and no significant anal pathology may be treated by colectomy and ileorectal anastomosis. Provided that sphincter function is preserved then reasonable functional results may be obtained. Although disease recurrence is quite high [14], several years of useful stoma-free function may be obtained.

Defunctioning ileostomy may be considered as treatment of Crohn's colitis (or severe anal disease; see later in this chapter). Inflammation in Crohn's disease (unlike UC) is dependent on some luminal antigenic stimulus for continued inflammation. Diverting the fecal stream with an ileostomy may be used to decrease colonic inflammation. About 20% of patients with Crohn's colitis achieve sufficient reduction in inflammation subsequently to have ileostomy reversal with reasonable function [15]. For the majority of patients, a defunctioning ileostomy is a helpful psychological stepping stone to proctocolectomy. Proctocolectomy with permanent ileostomy may still be needed. Proctectomy in the mesorectal or perimuscular plane depends on surgeon preference. Pelvic autonomic nerve injury is theoretically more likely in the mesorectal plane, although this plane is more familiar and less vascular. If there is minimal perianal disease then the perineal dissection should be in the intersphincteric plane. If there is extensive perianal disease then a wider excision is required, often with myocutaneous flap reconstruction.

Anal disease (see Cases 19 and 20)

About 30% of patients with Crohn's have significant anal pathology at some stage. The more distal the intestinal inflammation, the more likely there is to be anal disease. Anal pathology is extremely variable in severity and the natural history is difficult to predict. Tags and fissures represent mild disease, although fistulae, strictures, and ulceration may create severe disease.

Management depends on thorough disease assessment, including colonoscopy and small bowel imaging. Assessment of the anorectum relies on clinical examination, endoanal ultrasound, MRI, and EUA with biopsies. Key factors in planning treatment are:
- proctitis
- severity of disease, e.g. complex/simple fistula/sepsis
- patient symptoms and expectations.

Fissure

Fissures in Crohn's tend to be less symptomatic than non-Crohn's fistulae. If symptomatic, they should be treated along standard "sphincter-preserving" lines.

Tags

Perianal tags are common. It is generally best to avoid surgical excision. Steroid injection into the soft tissue of the tag and adjacent area may be helpful. If very symptomatic, surgical excision may be considered provided there is no proctitis and the patient has realistic expectations, including the risk of very slow wound healing.

Stricture

Anorectal strictures associated with adjacent inflammatory disease tend to cause more symptoms, respond less well to nonsurgical management, and have a higher risk of proctectomy. Preliminary management typically involves gentle stricture dilatation, drainage of any associated sepsis, and biopsy to check for associated malignancy. Subsequent management will depend on the response to initial treatment. Strictures associated with fistulating disease have a poor prognosis and should be managed along the lines of fistulating disease (see below).

Fistulae (see Cases 19 and 20)

Fistulae and abscess represent acute and chronic manifestations of the same disease process. Management of fistulating disease in Crohn's may be usefully considered in four potential phases [16].

1 First aid: drainage of perianal abscesses with seton placement if there is an obvious fistula.

2 Bridging treatment: typically this phase involves leaving seton drains in place, short course antibiotics, and optimization of medical therapy. Failure of this phase necessitates a search for sepsis with an MRI or EUA. Occasionally, a defunctioning stoma is necessary to bridge to a calm controlled situation.

3 Quality of life treatment: ranges from long-term seton to attempt at definitive cure. Medical therapy, especially anti-TNF, may give symptomatic relief though sustained fistula healing is less likely. Multiple or complex fistulae associated with deep ulceration or strictures are extremely unlikely to be healed surgically.

4 Planning for proctectomy: if attempts to heal anal fistulae are unrealistic, then long-term defunctioning or proctectomy may be needed.

Ulcerative colitis

Epidemiology

The prevalence of UC is about 1–2 per 1000 in the population of the Western world. Peak incidence is in young adults.

Pathogenesis

The pathogenesis of UC is not fully understood. As with Crohn's disease, there is evidence of an interaction between genetic and environmental factors [17].

Genetic factors

There is genetic overlap between UC and Crohn's disease. About 10–25% of patients with IBD will have a first-degree relative with either UC or Crohn's disease. In recent years, several genes have been identified which are associated with UC, including HLA DR2 and the MHC class II region of chromosome 6 (also known as IBD3).

Extrinsic factors

Intriguingly, smoking and a previous appendicectomy both appear to be marginally protective against the development of UC.

Macroscopic pathology

Ulcerative colitis is characterized by continuous inflammation extending from the dentate line proximally, though when viewed from the serosal side at surgery, it may look relatively normal.

Extensive loss of mucosa in UC may result from severe inflammation. The remaining inflamed mucosa looks prominent and gives rise to the appearance of inflammatory polyps or pseudopolyps. Adenomatous polyps may also occur as in the rest of the population or may occur in association with UC.

Microscopic pathology

Inflammation in UC is diffuse and limited to the mucosa. Characteristic features include crypt abscesses, crypt distortion, loss of goblet cells, and Paneth cell metaplasia.

Acute complications

Acute complications such as massive hemorrhage or perforation are extremely rare. Severe acute attacks of colitis may be complicated by toxic dilatation of the colon. This is defined as a colonic diameter over 6 cm or cecal diameter over 9 cm.

Chronic complications

Strictures rarely occur in UC, but are well described. In practice, strictures in UC should raise suspicion of malignancy or Crohn's disease.

Long-standing UC is associated with an increased risk of developing colorectal carcinoma. Pancolitis, disease for over 8 years, a family history of colorectal cancer, primary sclerosing cholangitis, and postinflammatory pseudopolyps are associated with an increased risk of malignancy. One study reported a 2.5% risk of malignancy at 20 years and 7.6% risk at 30 years [18].

Extraintestinal manifestations are similar to those seen in Crohn's disease (see Table B.1).

Clinical features

Diarrhea with or without blood is the major symptom of UC. Crampy abdominal pain, urgency, tenesmus, and incontinence may also be seen. With more extensive, severe inflammation, systemic symptoms occur, including fever, malaise, and tachycardia.

A number of scoring systems of severity exist but from a surgeon's perspective, it is important to recognize acute severe colitis (see **Case 21**); see Box B.1.

Box B.1 Truelove and Witt's criteria of acute severe colitis (ASC).

Bloody diarrhea of six or more stools per 24 hours and ONE of the following:
- fever over 37.8°C
- pulse rate over 90
- hemoglobin less than 10.5 g/dL
- ESR over 30 mm/h

Diagnosis

The diagnosis of UC is usually made on the basis of a characteristic history, exclusion of an infective cause by stool cultures, and characteristic findings at colonoscopy and biopsy. CRP and ESR are commonly raised. pANCA is often raised in UC but not of use for diagnostic purposes.

Stool cultures exclude common pathogens such as salmonella, shigella, *E.coli* 0157:H7, and campylobacter. In high-risk cases, *C. diff* should be considered and in patients with recent travel, amebiasis or giardiasis considered. In at-risk patients with limited proctitis, sexually transmitted disease including gonorrhea and HSV should be considered. The main noninfective differential diagnoses include radiation proctitis/ colitis, ischemia, and Crohn's.

Colonoscopic features of UC include loss of normal vascular pattern, bleeding, erosions, and ulcers. Travis *et al.* have produced a simple validated scoring system to improve recording of colonoscopic findings (Table B.3) [19].

Imaging is not usually required in mild and moderate forms of UC. Plain abdominal radiology is required in the assessment of patients with acute severe

Table B.3 Scoring system for endoscopic appearances in ulcerative colitis.

	Anchor points	Definition
Vascular pattern	Normal (0)	Normal
	Patchy obliteration (1)	Patchy obliteration
	Obliterated (2)	Complete obliteration
Bleeding	None (0)	No visible blood
	Mucosal (1)	Spots/streaks of coagulated blood on
	Luminal mild (2)	surface
	Luminal moderate or	Some free liquid blood in lumen
	severe (3)	Frank blood in the lumen or visible oozing
Erosions and ulcers	None (0)	No visible erosions or ulcers
	Erosions (1)	Tiny (<5 mm) defects in mucosa
	Superficial ulcer (2)	Larger (>5 mm) superficial ulcers
	Deep ulcer (3)	Deeper excavated defects

colitis to look for features of toxic colitis or markers of disease severity. In situations where there is diagnostic uncertainty, cross-sectional imaging by CT may be required.

Medical treatment of acute UC

Mild and moderate attacks are generally treated with 5-ASA drugs, usually topically delivered with oral supplementation if necessary. Oral steroids are indicated if the disease is refractory to oral/topical 5-ASAs. Maintenance is with oral/topical 5-ASA drugs, although thiopurines may also be needed to maintain remission. Infliximab is occasionally required for steroid refractory/dependence despite thiopurines or when thiopurines are not tolerated.

Acute severe colitis (ASC) (see **Case 21**) is an emergency requiring hospital admission and specialist gastroenterology treatment with early surgeon involvement. Prior to widespread steroid use, ASC had a mortality of over 25%. The landmark trial by Truelove and Witts showed that high dose steroids compared to placebo reduced mortality from 24% to 7% [20]. The UK IBD audit showed that the mortality from this condition is still about 1%.

Current treatment relies on high-dose IV and rectal steroids. If after 3 days there is no major improvement, then second-line rescue therapy with either infliximab or ciclosporin may be added. If there is no substantial improvement by 5–7 days then urgent colectomy with ileostomy is indicated. On day 3 of treatment of ASC with high-dose steroids, if stool frequency >8/day or stool frequency 3–8/day + CRP >45, the chance of requiring a colectomy is 85% [21].

Surgical treatment of acute UC

Surgery is required in about 20–30% of patients with UC [22]. Acute indications for surgery include massive bleeding and perforation which are very rare. Fulminant colitis and toxic dilatation are almost absolute indications for surgery. If the patient's general condition is reasonable, it is reasonable to start medical therapy with high-dose steroids and monitor closely over 12–24 hours. If there is a clear improvement over this short period then emergency surgery may be averted.

Failure of ASC to settle with optimum medical therapy is a much more common indication for urgent surgery (see **Cases 21 and 24**). There is increasing evidence that prolonged medical therapy with delayed surgery is associated with a poor outcome.

Chronic indications for surgery are failure of medical therapy and dysplasia (see **Case 22**). Patients with UC have an increased risk of developing colorectal cancer. Surveillance colonoscopy is recommended after 8–10 years of extensive colitis, ideally using dye spray to enhance assessment (see **Case 22**).

Urgent colectomy (see Case 21)

In the acute situation the standard operation is colectomy, with end ileostomy and preservation of rectum. Laparoscopic colectomy reduces morbidity compared to open surgery. There is some debate about how to deal with the retained rectal stump: exteriorization as a mucus fistula, stapled closure at the pelvic brim or subcutaneous stapled closure. A longer stump potentially gives rise to symptoms whilst a shorter one risks staple line breakdown with intraabdominal sepsis. There are no trials comparing techniques and the decision probably needs to be tailored to the individual. In all cases, leaving a large rectal catheter for 3–5 days is advisable.

Elective surgery

In elective situations the surgical options are as follows.

- Colectomy and ileostomy (as in acute situation): this allows weaning off steroids whilst allowing subsequent pouch reconstruction. Elective procedure when the patient cannot be weaned off steroids and ultimately wishes to proceed to pouch reconstruction. Any diagnostic uncertainty between UC and Crohn's can also often be resolved.
- Proctocolectomy and permanent ileostomy: removes all disease but at the expense of a permanent stoma.
- Colectomy and ileorectal anastomosis (see **Case 23**): initially described in the 1950s [23]. The operation fell into disrepute due to the high cancer risk in the remaining rectum and the advent of IPAA. A recent Swedish study, however, suggests that IRA may be a reasonable option in carefully selected patients [24].
- Proctocolectomy and ileoanal pouch reconstruction (see **Cases 21 and 24**). This is explored in more detail below.
- Proctocolectomy and continent Kock pouch ileostomy (see **Case 25**): rarely performed today as it has a high risk of morbidity. It is occasionally indicated in motivated, counseled patients with a permanent ileostomy to achieve ileostomy continence.

Factors to consider when discussing potential pouch surgery

Is the pathology definitely UC?

Review of the pathology report and discussion at an IBD MDT meeting is recommended.

Are there any factors that increase the risk of pouch surgery (see Cases 21, 23, and 24)?

- Indeterminate colitis is associated with poorer outcome, pouch failure, and "late emergence of Crohn's disease." Most large units are happy to offer pouch surgery to patients with indeterminate colitis in the absence of additional risk factors.
- PSC increases the risk of pouchitis and poor pouch function.

- Poor anal sphincter function is likely to result in worse function. Objective assessment by anorectal physiology and endoanal ultrasound in some patients may be needed.
- Patients with major medical co-morbidity may be better served by proctectomy and permanent ileostomy.
- Steroids increase risk of septic complications after pouch surgery. Ideally, pouches should be formed after weaning off steroids.

Does the patient have realistic expectations of outcome?

Bowel function after pouch surgery will not be normal. Typical bowel frequency is 4–8×/day and once overnight. The failure rate is 10–20%, increasing with longer follow-up. A useful *aide-mémoire* is the 4-4-2 rule: 4 of every 10 patients do well with satisfactory bowel function; 4 of 10 do "ok" with manageable bowel habit, but typically need to take constipating drugs, modify diet or use pads; 2 of 10 do badly (one reverting to an ileostomy and one "muddling along" with very poor bowel function).

Have special issues such as fertility or erectile dysfunction been discussed?

A recent meta-analysis by Rajaratnam *et al.*, studying six papers, showed the relative risk of female infertility after pouch surgery to be 3.91 (95% confidence interval 2.06–7.44), although they concede that due to publication bias, this may be an overestimate [25].

Lindsey *et al.* showed that after proctectomy, 82.7% of men had normal erectile function [26]. Complete impotence occurred in 3.8% (all over 50 years of age) and partial impotence in 13.5%. No patients in their study reported ejaculatory difficulties.

Operative technique

Open or laparoscopic

Several studies have compared open with laparoscopic and laparoscopically assisted techniques of pouch construction. Most have demonstrated improved cosmesis and short-term outcomes with minimally invasive techniques but no differences in complications or function [27,28].

Obtaining adequate small bowel length

Complete mobilization of the small bowel mesentery up to the level of the duodenum and pancreas is usually sufficient to gain enough small bowel length for a pouch. Additional tricks include incising the peritoneum over the superior mesenteric vessels and placing the pouch in the pelvis with the mesentery posteriorly [29]. Beart's group have described a technique of dissection close to the bowel wall on the right side to permit preservation of the right and middle colic vessels [30]. This may increase mobilization by allowing division of the ileocolic vessels whilst preserving blood supply to the ileum. The need to do this must be anticipated prior to colectomy.

Plane of rectal dissection

There are no trials comparing dissection in the mesorectal plane with close rectal dissection. Close rectal dissection probably reduces the risk of nerve damage but is potentially a more bloody dissection.

Stapled or hand-sewn with mucosectomy

The most commonly undertaken technique of pouch–anal anastomosis is the stapled technique leaving 1–2 cm of diseased columnar mucosa. A long rectal cuff must be avoided. The more difficult operation of mucosectomy and hand-sewn anastomosis removes all the diseased mucosa, at least theoretically, though it may be associated with poorer function. A relative indication for mucosectomy is dysplasia or carcinoma in the rectum. The hand-sewn technique may be necessary if there are technical stapling problems intraoperatively and for re-do pouch surgery.

Pouch design

The original pouch design was a triple limb S pouch. However, this was associated with emptying problems due to a long or kinked efferent segment. Other subsequent pouch designs include the large volume W pouch, the H, and the J. Comparative studies have not shown major differences. The double limb J pouch is the most commonly undertaken, is simple to construct and seemingly minimizes emptying problems.

Defunctioning ileostomy

This probably reduces the major consequences of anastomotic dehiscence and pouch failure though this must be weighed against the complications of an ileostomy and subsequent closure. In our own institution, about 80% of pouches are defunctioned.

Pouch follow-up

Daytime leakage is 5% at 1 year post surgery, increasing to about 11% after 20 years. Corresponding figures for nocturnal leakage are 12% and 21%. Late complications, excluding pouchitis, occur in about 29% of patients and the ultimate failure rate requiring ileostomy formation is around 10%, but increases with long-term follow-up.

In the absence of overriding obstetric factors, more colorectal surgeons favor LSCS, although the objective evidence to support this is weak.

Systematic follow-up of patients after pouch surgery is often haphazard. A recent review of 1200 pouch patients from the Netherlands reported alarmingly high rates of dysplasia and carcinoma [31]; 25 (1.83%) patients developed dysplasia or carcinoma, mostly around the anal transition zone. Prior dysplasia or carcinoma were major risk factors. It is recommended that pouch patients who had dysplasia or carcinoma in the proctocolectomy specimen should have close surveillance with visualization and biopsy from the anal transition zone.

Management of poor pouch function (see Case 24)

Pouchitis is an idiopathic inflammation of an ileoanal pouch. It is more common after surgery for extensive UC, in nonsmokers, and in patients with PSC. The diagnosis depends on a combination of clinical features (increased bowel frequency with blood, urgency or fever), endoscopic features of inflammation and histological features of both acute and chronic inflammation. Several scoring systems are available (Table B.4).

About 30% of patients with a pouch for UC develop pouchitis at some stage. Of these, 60% develop recurrent pouchitis and about 5% develop chronic pouchitis. A Cochrane metaanalysis indicates that ciprofloxacin is superior to metronidazole in the treatment of acute pouchitis [32]. In chronic pouchitis, VSL-3 has been shown to be superior to placebo in maintaining remission achieved by antibiotics.

If true idiopathic pouchitis has been excluded in the problem pouch, then the assessment of poor pouch function can be usefully considered in three phases.

Table B.4 Pouchitis scoring system. A score of over 7 with at least one point from each domain is required for a strict definition of pouchitis.

Clinical features	Endoscopic features	Pathological features
Stool frequency:	Edema 1	Acute histological inflammation
Post-op usual 0	Granularity 1	Polymorphonuclear leukocyte
1–2/day > usual 1	Friability 1	infiltration:
3+/day > usual 2	Loss of vascular pattern 1	Mild 1
Rectal bleeding:	Mucous exudates 1	Moderate 2
None/rare 0	Ulceration 1	Severe 3
Daily 1		Ulceration per low power field:
Urgency or abdominal cramps:		<25% 1
None 0		25–50% 2
Occasional 1		>50% 3
Usual 2		
Fever >37.8°C		
Absent 0		
Present 1		

Phase 1

- Has pouch function always been poor or is it a recent deterioration?
- Are there features of Crohn's on the colectomy specimen?
- Were there features suggestive of pouch sepsis immediately after surgery?
- Are stool cultures normal?
- Are clinical examination, digital examination, and pouchoscopy all normal?

This approach may direct specific treatment, including dilatation of a pouch-anal stricture and treatment of pouchitis and cuffitis.

Phase 2

If there is no improvement, second-phase investigations are required. A simple *aide-mémoire* is to consider the pouch as a box. You should look in the box, outside the box, above the box, below the box, and check that the box can be emptied.

Box	Investigations	Possible causes
INSIDE	Pouchoscopy and biopsy Pouchogram	Chronic pouchitis Irritable pouch Small-volume pouch Infection, e.g. CMV, *C.diff*
OUTSIDE	MR or CT	Peri-pouch sepsis/fistula Unrelated pathology, e.g. fibroid
BELOW	Anorectal physiology and ultrasound Pouchogram EUA and biopsy	Pouch-anal stenosis Cuffitis Pouch-vaginal fistula Sphincter weakness Long rectal cuff
ABOVE	MRE Endoscopy	Adhesions Crohn's of small bowel Bacterial overgrowth NSAIDs Pre-pouch ileitis Celiac
EMPTYING	Dynamic evacuating "proctogram"	Anismus Prolapsed/intussusceptions

CMV, cytomegalovirus; CT, computed tomography; EUA, examination under anesthesia; MR, magnetic resonance; MRE, magnetic resonance enterography; NSAID, nonsteroidal antiinflammatory drug.

Phase 3

Revisional pouch surgery is occasionally appropriate though perhaps only in large-volume units. "Indefinite diversion" may be better than re-do surgery or pouch excision. In highly motivated individuals, a continent Kock ileostomy may be considered.

References

1 Baumgart DC, Sandborn WJ. Crohn's disease. *Lancet* 2012; **380**(9853):1590–605.

2 Vermeire S, van Assche G, Rutgeerts P. Classification of inflammatory bowel disease: the old and the new. *Curr Opin Gastroenterol* 2012; **28**(4):321–6.

3 Peyrin-Biroulet L, Loftus EV Jr, Colombel JF, Sandborn WJ. The natural history of adult Crohn's disease in population-based cohorts. *Am J Gastroenterol* 2010; **105**(2):289–97.

4 Mekhjian HS, Switz DM, Melnyk CS, Rankin GB, Brooks RK. Clinical features and natural history of Crohn's disease. *Gastroenterology* 1979; **77**(4 Pt 2):898–906.

5 Vester-Andersen MK, Prosberg MV, Jess T, *et al*. Disease course and surgery rates in inflammatory bowel disease: a population-based, 7-year follow-up study in the era of immunomodulating therapy. *Am J Gastroenterol* 2014; **109**(5):705–14.

6 Alves A, Panis Y, Bouhnik Y, Pocard M, Vicaut E, Valleur P. Risk factors for intra-abdominal septic complications after a first ileocecal resection for Crohn's disease: a multivariate analysis in 161 consecutive patients. *Dis Colon Rectum* 2007; **50**(3):331–6.

7 Fazio VW, Marchetti F, Church M, *et al*. Effect of resection margins on the recurrence of Crohn's disease in the small bowel. A randomized controlled trial. *Ann Surg* 1996; **224**(4):563–71; discussion 71–3.

8 Lee EC, Papaioannou N. Minimal surgery for chronic obstruction in patients with extensive or universal Crohn's disease. *Ann Roy Coll Surg England* 1982; **64**(4):229–33.

9 Tichansky D, Cagir B, Yoo E, Marcus SM, Fry RD. Strictureplasty for Crohn's disease: meta-analysis. *Dis Colon Rectum* 2000; **43**(7):911–19.

10 Farmer RG, Whelan G, Fazio VW. Long-term follow-up of patients with Crohn's disease. Relationship between the clinical pattern and prognosis. *Gastroenterology* 1985; **88**(6):1818–25.

11 McLeod RS, Wolff BG, Ross S, Parkes R, McKenzie M. Recurrence of Crohn's disease after ileocolic resection is not affected by anastomotic type: results of a multicenter, randomized, controlled trial. *Dis Colon Rectum* 2009; **52**(5):919–27.

12 Choy PY, Bissett IP, Docherty JG, Parry BR, Merrie A, Fitzgerald A. Stapled versus handsewn methods for ileocolic anastomoses. *Cochrane Database Syst Rev* 2011; **9**:CD004320.

13 Tekkis PP, Purkayastha S, Lanitis S, *et al*. A comparison of segmental vs subtotal/total colectomy for colonic Crohn's disease: a meta-analysis. *Colorectal Dis* 2006; **8**(2):82–90.

14 Williams JG, Wong WD, Rothenberger DA, Goldberg SM. Recurrence of Crohn's disease after resection. *Br J Surg* 1991; **78**(1):10–19.

15 Edwards CM, George BD, Jewell DP, Warren BF, Mortensen NJ, Kettlewell MG. Role of a defunctioning stoma in the management of large bowel Crohn's disease. *Br J Surg* 2000; **87**(8):1063–6.

16 Singh B, Mc CMNJ, Jewell DP, George B. Perianal Crohn's disease. *Br J Surg* 2004; **91**(7):801–14.

17 Abraham C, Cho JH. Inflammatory bowel disease. *N Engl J Med* 2009; **361**(21):2066–78.

18 Rutter MD, Saunders BP, Wilkinson KH, *et al*. Thirty-year analysis of a colonoscopic surveillance program for neoplasia in ulcerative colitis. *Gastroenterology* 2006; **130**(4):1030–8.

19 Travis SP, Schnell D, Krzeski P, *et al*. Reliability and initial validation of the ulcerative colitis endoscopic index of severity. *Gastroenterology* 2013; **145**(5):987–95.

20 Truelove SC, Witts LJ. Cortisone in ulcerative colitis; final report on a therapeutic trial. *BMJ* 1955;**2**(4947):1041–8.

21 Travis SP, Farrant JM, Ricketts C, *et al*. Predicting outcome in severe ulcerative colitis. *Gut* 1996; **38**(6):905–10.

22 Leijonmarck CE, Persson PG, Hellers G. Factors affecting colectomy rate in ulcerative colitis: an epidemiologic study. *Gut* 1990; **31**(3):329–33.

23 Aylett S. The surgery of diffuse ulcerative colitis; including a review of 100 cases of colitis treated by total colectomy and ileorectal anastomosis. *Postgrad Med J* 1959; **35**(400):67–74.

24 Andersson P, Norblad R, Soderholm JD, Myrelid P. Ileorectal anastomosis in comparison with ileal pouch anal anastomosis in reconstructive surgery for ulcerative colitis – a single institution experience. *J Crohn's Colitis* 2014; **8**(7):582–9.

25 Rajaratnam SG, Eglinton TW, Hider P, Fearnhead NS. Impact of ileal pouch-anal anastomosis on female fertility: meta-analysis and systematic review. *Int J Colorectal Dis* 2011; **26**(11):1365–74.

26 Lindsey I, George BD, Kettlewell MG, Mortensen NJ. Impotence after mesorectal and close rectal dissection for inflammatory bowel disease. *Dis Colon Rectum* 2001; **44**(6):831–5.

27 Hemandas AK, Jenkins JT. Laparoscopic pouch surgery in ulcerative colitis. *Ann Gastroenterol* 2012; **25**(4):309–16.

28 Schiessling S, Leowardi C, Kienle P, *et al.* Laparoscopic versus conventional ileoanal pouch procedure in patients undergoing elective restorative proctocolectomy (LapConPouch Trial) – a randomized controlled trial. *Langenbeck's Arch Surg* 2013; **398**(6):807–16.

29 Uraiqat AA, Byrne CM, Phillips RK. Gaining length in ileal-anal pouch reconstruction: a review. *Colorectal Dis* 2007; **9**(7):657–61.

30 Goes RN, Nguyen P, Huang D, Beart RW Jr. Lengthening of the mesentery using the marginal vascular arcade of the right colon as the blood supply to the ileal pouch. *Dis Colon Rectum* 1995; **38**(8):893–5.

31 Derikx LA, Kievit W, Drenth JP, *et al.* Prior colorectal neoplasia is associated with increased risk of ileoanal pouch neoplasia in patients with inflammatory bowel disease. *Gastroenterology* 2014; **146**(1):119–28.e1.

32 Holubar SD, Cima RR, Sandborn WJ, Pardi DS. Treatment and prevention of pouchitis after ileal pouch-anal anastomosis for chronic ulcerative colitis. *Cochrane Database Syst Rev* 2010; **6**:CD001176.

CASE 14

A problem teenager

Astor Rodrigues

Oxford University Hospitals NHS Foundation Trust, Oxford, UK

A 13 ¾-year-old boy was referred with a 3-month history of explosive nonbloody loose stools, crampy central abdominal pains prior to defecation, lethargy, and possibly weight loss. There was no past medical or family history. The initial impression was that of either a chronic gastrointestinal infection or inflammatory bowel disease.

Stool cultures were negative. Blood tests confirmed mild iron deficiency anemia, but normal inflammatory markers and celiac serology. Fecal calprotectin was markedly elevated.

He underwent an upper GI endoscopy and colonoscopy under GA. Gastroscopy revealed patchy erythema in the antrum and 4–5 discrete tiny aphthoid ulcers in the duodenum. Ileocolonoscopy showed moderate terminal ileal involvement with mucosal swelling, friability, and mucopus, but normal colonic appearances. Histology confirmed chronic gastritis, patchy acute duodenitis, and ileal inflammation with ulceration without granulomata identified.

Magnetic resonance enterography (MRE) showed nonstricturing, nonpenetrating terminal ileal thickening, and no other small bowel involvement.

DECISION POINT

How should he be treated?

The diagnosis of Crohn's disease was considered robust. Exclusive enteral nutrition (EEN) versus steroid treatment were discussed with his parents, both of whom were doctors. EEN avoids the side-effects of steroids and helps to maintain/improve nutrition, although may be difficult for the patient to tolerate. After discussion with the boy's parents, he was treated with EEN.

His symptoms and general wellbeing improved rapidly. Oral azathioprine was added in an attempt to maintain remission so that his growth and puberty would progress satisfactorily. A few weeks after completing EEN therapy, he relapsed clinically with a mild rise in inflammatory markers. He was commenced on steroid therapy to which he responded quickly.

Colorectal Surgery: Clinical Care and Management, First Edition.
Edited by Bruce George, Richard Guy, Oliver Jones, and Jon Vogel.
© 2016 John Wiley & Sons, Ltd. Published 2016 by John Wiley & Sons, Ltd.

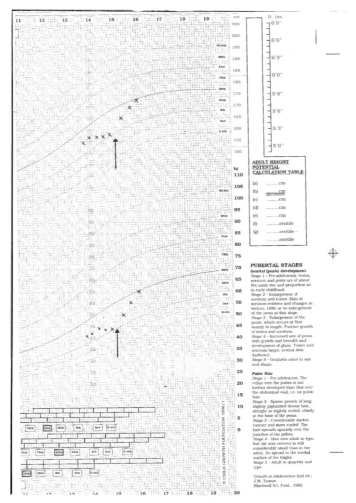

Figure 14.1 Growth chart showing slowing of growth before surgery and improvement after surgery.

As the dose of steroids was reduced, his symptoms recurred. Adherence to azathioprine was confirmed and 6-thioguanine levels were satisfactory. He was nearly 14½ years old, but was prepubertal and his growth velocity had slowed (Figure 14.1). Inflammatory markers were normal. High-frequency ultrasound revealed terminal ileal thickening.

DECISION POINT

Should he have biological therapy or surgical resection?

The boy's parents were influenced by the rare but documented risk of hepatocellular T cell lymphoma with anti-TNF treatment and opted for surgery.

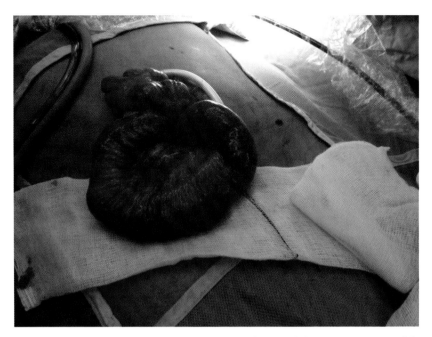

Figure 14.2 Operative photograph showing exteriorized terminal ileum. Fat wrapping of the ileum, normal-looking cecum, and prominent mesenteric lymph nodes may be seen.

At laparoscopy, he was found to have a 17 cm segment of thickened terminal ileum with fat wrapping (Figure 14.2).

There was no abscess or fistula. The rest of the small bowel was "run" and confirmed to be normal. An ileocecal resection with primary anastomosis was performed and postoperative recovery was uneventful. He remained on azathioprine therapy. Within months, he had a growth spurt as can be seen on his growth chart (see Figure 14.1).

At follow-up 24 months post surgery, he is in clinical and biochemical remission.

LEARNING POINTS

- In paediatric IBD practice, gastroscopy and biopsy are routinely undertaken in addition to colonoscopy. Microscopic inflammation, including granulomas, are seen much more commonly in the stomach than in adult practice and may help to make the diagnosis of Crohn's disease.
- Avoiding ionizing radiation is important in all patients, but especially in younger patients and those with chronic relapsing diseases.
- Monitoring growth and pubertal development in children is important. It is a good indicator of disease remission, especially in Crohn's disease. At every clinic visit, growth parameters should be plotted on a growth chart and pubertal progress documented.

- Enteral nutritional therapy is commonly employed as an alternative to steroids in young patients with Crohn's disease.
- Delayed growth and pubertal development is a relative indication for surgical resection in teenagers.

LETTER FROM AMERICA

The ASCRS clinical practice guidelines for Crohn's disease note that medical, nutritional, and surgical therapy may be required to turn the tide of growth retardation in young patients with Crohn's disease and advocate support surgical therapy in cases with "significant growth retardation despite appropriate medical therapy." The guideline includes the following notice: "Early surgical intervention for growth retardation is only indicated in cases with clearly localized disease because of the risk of recrudescence with more diffuse involvement ... "

Jon Vogel and Massarat Zutshi

CASE 15

Recurrent Crohn's disease with intraabdominal abscess: when to operate?

Bruce George & Mohamed Abdelrahman
Oxford University Hospitals NHS Foundation Trust, Oxford, UK

A 22-year-old man was referred to the gastroenterologists for management of Crohn's disease. He had been diagnosed with Crohn's aged 16 with symptoms of weight loss, anemia, abdominal pain, and erythema nodosum.

He had been initially managed medically but underwent an open ileocecal resection at the age of 19 years. He remained well for 18 months on no medication before developing further abdominal pain and diarrhea. He was initially restarted on azathioprine. Investigations including colonoscopy and MRE showed preanastomotic recurrence and mild small bowel dilatation. The colon was normal. About 5 months later, his symptoms deteriorated with increased abdominal pain and diarrhea up to 10 times per day. He was treated in hospital with IV steroids and then converted to oral prednisolone. He was referred to the gastroenterology unit for consideration of treatment with anti-TNF biological therapy.

At presentation in Oxford, he was complaining of constant abdominal pain, mainly in the RIF, slight diarrhea, and severe fatigue. On examination, he was slightly overweight (100 kg, BMI 33), apyrexial but with RIF tenderness. No mass was palpable.

DECISION POINT

What would you recommend as next treatment: medical therapy, possibly with anti-TNF therapy, or surgical resection?

He was seen in the joint clinic by a gastroenterologist and IBD surgeon. Review of the radiology suggested that the disease proximal to the previous anastomosis was mainly inflammatory and might respond to escalation of medical therapy. Treatment with adalimumab was planned.

Ten days after the clinic appointment (and before receiving adalimumab), he presented acutely with worsening symptoms. His abdominal pain was more severe, constant, and not manageable at home. He had had a fever with rigor. He was

---

Colorectal Surgery: Clinical Care and Management, First Edition.
Edited by Bruce George, Richard Guy, Oliver Jones, and Jon Vogel.
© 2016 John Wiley & Sons, Ltd. Published 2016 by John Wiley & Sons, Ltd.

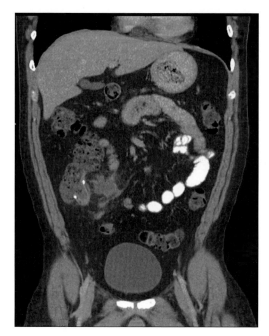

Figure 15.1 CT scan showing abscess within the small bowel mesentery.

taking azathioprine and 20 mg prednisolone. CT scan shortly after admission showed an abscess probably within the small bowel mesentery, just proximal to the previous anastomosis (Figure 15.1).

DECISION POINT

What would you do now: immediate surgery or medical treatment to cool off the acute problem, followed by semi-elective surgery?

It was felt that surgery in the presence of an intraabdominal abscess and steroids would necessitate stoma formation. The alternative approach was to treat with antibiotics and radiological drainage and wean off steroids. After discussion with the patient, the latter approach was adopted.

He was treated with IV antibiotics. The radiologists did not feel that the abscess could be drained. His general condition improved and he went home after 4 days on oral antibiotics. At review in clinic 2 weeks later, he was feeling generally better, but still had abdominal pain requiring tramadol. His steroids had been reduced to 5 mg daily. It was decided to continue oral antibiotics and to schedule surgery 2 weeks later.

At operation, a preanastomotic phlegmonous area of disease was found, but with no detectable abscess. There was mild dilatation of the small bowel proximal to the inflamed area. The rest of the small bowel appeared normal.

DECISION POINT

What would you do next?

The options considered were:
- not resect and close up the abdomen

- resect and bring out a stoma

- resect and anastomose the bowel.

It was decided that he should have a resection and an anastomosis on the grounds that the sepsis had settled, nutrition was satisfactory, and his steroid dose was down to 5 mg daily. Whilst he had been on steroids for 11 weeks, he had been on 10 mg or less for the previous 4 weeks.

He underwent primary anastomosis with an end-side hand-sewn anastomosis. He made a slow but satisfactory recovery. He had a CT scan on day 5 post-op which showed an ileus and some basal atelectasis but no evidence of anastomotic leakage. He was discharged 12 days postoperatively.

DECISION POINT

What postoperative measures should be taken to reduced the risk of future Crohn's disease?

He was continued on azathioprine in view of the aggressive nature of his Crohn's disease. He underwent a colonoscopy about 8 months later that showed no evidence of recurrent inflammation in the colon or around the ileocolic anastomosis. He remains clinically well on regular azathioprine.

LEARNING POINTS

- Patients should be "optimized" prior to surgery for Crohn's disease. Intraabdominal abscess should be drained if possible, steroids reduced, and nutrition improved.
- Postoperative prophylaxis against future Crohn's disease should be considered in all patients.

LETTER FROM AMERICA

Abdominopelvic abscesses less than 3 cm are often effectively treated with antibiotics alone. In some centers in the USA, the surgical treatment of a patient such as this would include resection, anastomosis, and defunctioning proximal ostomy. At present, and perhaps based in part on the work of investigators at the University of Pittsburgh, anti-TNF alpha therapy for secondary prevention seems to be preferred in aggressive cases such as this one.

Jon Vogel and Massarat Zutshi

CASE 16

Very extensive small bowel stricturing disease

Myles Fleming[1] & Neil Mortensen[2]

[1] Auckland Hospital, Auckland, New Zealand
[2] Oxford University Hospitals NHS Foundation Trust, Oxford, UK

A 27-year-old man was referred by the gastroenterologists for surgical management of multiple small bowel strictures (Figure 16.1). He had been diagnosed with Crohn's disease at the age of 22 and had had a laparoscopically assisted resection of 80 cm of jejunum when 23. He had no other medical problems and was a nonsmoker.

He had been well following his first resection, maintained on adalimumab and azathioprine. Over the previous year, however, he started to develop obstructive symptoms, principally colicky abdominal pain and intermittent diarrhea. He had been treated with several courses of steroids but had had no steroids in the 4 months prior to referral. Two months previously, he developed breathlessness and dizziness and was found to have a hemoglobin of 4.9 g/dL (low iron stores, normal B12, and folate). An MRE demonstrated multiple proximal small bowel strictures. Colonoscopy was normal.

DECISION POINT

Is surgery indicated and if so, how should he be prepared for this?

A further increase in medical therapy, checking azathioprine dosage was optimal, and increasing adalimumab to weekly were all considered. However, it was decided that surgery was clearly indicated: multiple tight strictures and anemia despite maximum medical therapy. The MRE suggested multiple strictures and that there was no obvious inflammatory component to these.

He was given an iron infusion. He was reviewed with the nutrition team who estimated that he had lost about 6 kg in the previous 4 months and calculated his BMI to be 24.7. He was given supplementary enteral nutrition for 3 weeks prior to surgery. Contingency plans were made for him to receive TPN postoperatively if required. He was admitted the day before surgery for insertion of a PICC line.

Colorectal Surgery: Clinical Care and Management, First Edition.
Edited by Bruce George, Richard Guy, Oliver Jones, and Jon Vogel.
© 2016 John Wiley & Sons, Ltd. Published 2016 by John Wiley & Sons, Ltd.

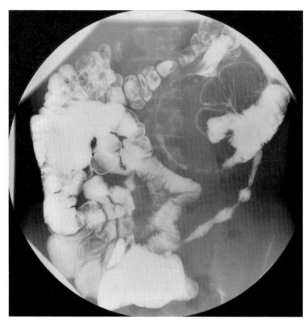

Figure 16.1 Small bowel enema showing extensive jejunal stricturing prior to first surgery age 23.

At laparotomy, his small bowel was characterized on balloon trawl, using a Foley catheter with the balloon inflated to a 2 cm diameter, from the duode-nojejunal flexure to the cecum. He was found to have more than 20 strictures that were impassable by the balloon. The majority of these were in one 120 cm segment (Figure 16.2, Figure 16.3).

DECISION POINT

Which operation should be undertaken?

The following options were considered.

- Resection of 120 cm with multiple tight strictures. This would leave 100–110 cm of small bowel plus colon. This length of bowel would put him at risk of short bowel syndrome and the need for long-term nutritional support.

- Multiple stricturoplasties or a Michelassi type side-to-side isoperistaltic stricturoplasty. After discussion between three consultants, the decision to undertake a "Michelassi" procedure was made, with the two most proximal strictures treated by conventional Heineke–Mikulicz stricturoplasties.

The 120 cm segment was divided at the midpoint and opened longitudinally along the complete length (Figure 16.4). All anastomoses were hand sewn in two layers with interrupted 3/0 vicryl. Prior to final closure of the small bowel, a leak test was performed which confirmed all anastomotic lines were intact. The bowel was measured at the end and showed 70 cm of normal small bowel from

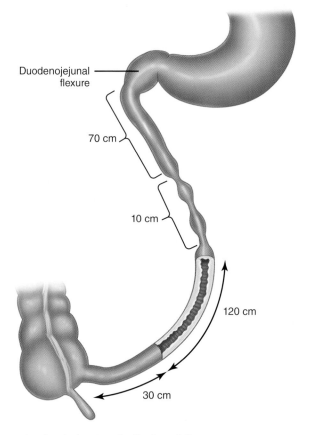

Figure 16.2 Operative sketch showing distribution of disease.

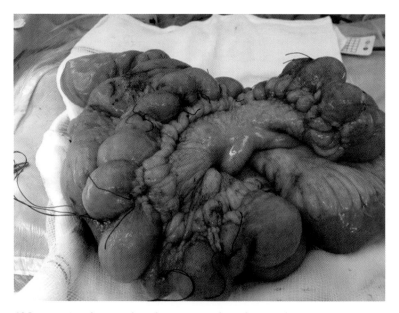

Figure 16.3 Operative photograph with sutures marking the site of strictures.

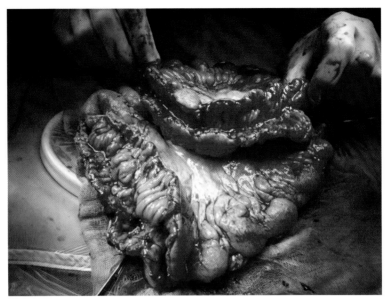

Figure 16.4 Operative photograph showing the strictures in the small bowel after it has been opened along its length.

the duodenojejunal flexure to a 10 cm length of small bowel containing two stricturoplasties. This was followed by a 60 cm Michelassi stricturoplasty (Figure 16.5) and after that there was 30 cm to the terminal ileum. This left a measured length of 170 cm plus colon. In total, 5 cm of small bowel was excised at the ends of the Michelassi stricturoplasty, with histology of this showing severe active Crohn's disease.

DECISION POINT

Should the postoperative management of this patient be different from standard protocols given the number and size of his anastomoses?

It was decided to give a 5-day course of IV antibiotics, to start TPN the day after surgery and to undertake a relook laparotomy at 48 hours to visualize the suture lines even if his general condition was good. It has to be acknowledged that our decision making regarding his postoperative management was not evidence based. However, this was clearly a high-risk procedure.

At 48 hours, he had a planned relook laparotomy during which all anastomoses were found to be intact and there was no contamination seen. His bowels initially tended to diarrhea. This was managed successfully with loperamide and his TPN was stopped on day 11. He was discharged on day 14. He was discharged on azathioprine, adalimumab, lansoprazole, and 3-monthly B12 injections.

At clinic review at 6 months, he reported no recurrence of his symptoms. He had no pain, was gaining weight, and had a good bowel function. Sadly, at

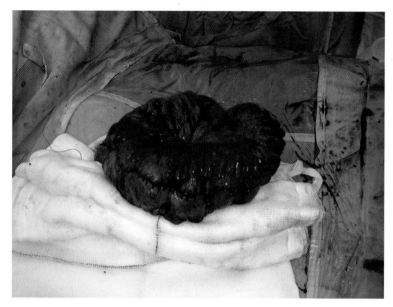

Figure 16.5 Operative photograph showing the appearance after the Michelassi stricturoplasty.

latest follow-up, 18 months postoperatively, he has developed further obstructive symptoms and anemia with evidence of further strictures on MR enterography and he is awaiting further surgery.

LEARNING POINTS

- Anemia is common in patients with IBD. Recent evidence suggests that oral iron is not only poorly tolerated but may compound intestinal inflammation [1]. Newer intravenous iron preparations are well tolerated and achieve rapid resolution of iron deficiency anemia.
- Patients with very extensive small bowel disease are at risk of short bowel syndrome. Principles of gut length preservation include minimal resections and appropriate use of stricturoplasty.

LETTER FROM AMERICA

The perfect case for the Michelassi stricturoplasty!

Jon Vogel and Massarat Zutshi

Reference

1 Gomollon F, Gisbert JP. Current management of iron deficiency anemia in inflammatory bowel diseases: a practical guide. *Drugs* 2013; **73**(16):1761–70.

CASE 17

Long-standing Crohn's colitis and enterocutaneous fistula

Richard Lovegrove

Mount Sinai Hospital, University of Toronto, Toronto, Canada

A 51-year-old woman was referred as an emergency with features of peritonitis following endoscopic dilatation of a stricture at an ileorectal anastomosis (IRA). She had a long history of complex Crohn's disease.

- Age 5 – diagnosed with colonic Crohn's disease. Managed medically throughout childhood.
- Age 16 – diagnosed with primary sclerosing cholangitis.
- Age 17 – colectomy and ileorectal anastomosis. Generally well with good bowel function and stable liver function until age 46.
- Age 46 – anal stenosis and transsphincteric anal fistula, managed by gentle dilatation and loose seton drain.
- Age 49 – deterioration in bowel function. Stricture at IRA identified. Biopsies benign, stricture dilated endoscopically.
- Age 49–51– three further endoscopic dilatations with good effect until emergency presentation with peritonitis following dilatation.

The patient was admitted acutely with signs of peritonitis. She was tachycardic on admission with elevated inflammatory markers. A CT scan of her abdomen and pelvis showed the presence of free air, which was tracking in her retroperitoneal tissues (Figure 17.1).

The patient was consented for a laparotomy, but would not give consent to her ileorectal anastomosis being taken down or for her rectum to be removed. She was keen to avoid a permanent stoma. During what proved to be a challenging laparotomy, an iatrogenic perforation was confirmed at the level of the ileorectal anastomosis and there was free enteric content within the abdomen. As a compromise, a defunctioning loop ileostomy was raised and large-caliber drains placed in the pelvis.

She recovered rapidly from this procedure. At outpatient review 3 months later, she was keen to explore the option of having her ileostomy reversed and bowel continuity restored. Flexible sigmoidoscopy showed a mild anorectal stricture as well as stricturing of the ileorectal anastomosis (Figure 17.2), which was balloon dilated. Biopsies were not taken at this time. A subsequent contrast

Colorectal Surgery: Clinical Care and Management, First Edition.
Edited by Bruce George, Richard Guy, Oliver Jones, and Jon Vogel.
© 2016 John Wiley & Sons, Ltd. Published 2016 by John Wiley & Sons, Ltd.

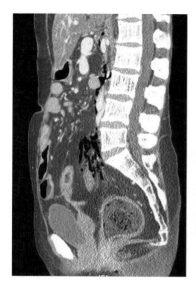
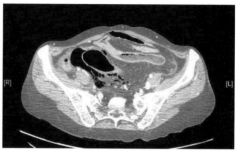

Figure 17.1 CT scan of abdomen and pelvis demonstrating free air in the retroperitoneum and abdomen following iatrogenic perforation of an anastomotic stricture.

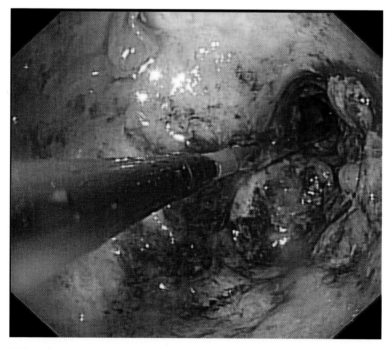

Figure 17.2 Endoscopic picture of anastomotic stricture during a dilatation.

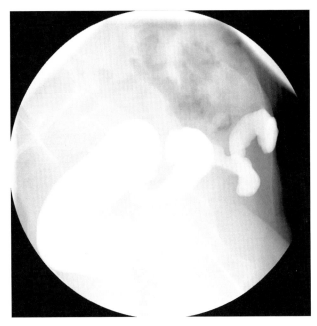

Figure 17.3 Contrast enema demonstrating free passage of contrast through the ileorectal anastomosis following dilatation of stricture.

enema demonstrated free flow of contrast through the rectum and ileorectal anastomosis up to the defunctioning ileostomy (Figure 17.3).

At outpatient review following these investigations, the patient was keen to have the ileostomy reversed. We were extremely reluctant to reverse the stoma because of likely poor function related to persisting narrowing at the IRA and the risk of increasing disease in the anal area. She was advised to wait for at least 12 months to allow "softening" of peritoneal adhesions and to experience life with a stoma before making a final decision regarding reversal.

Several months later (now 11 months post laparotomy), when attending a routine appointment with the gastroenterologists, she complained of lower abdominal pain and weight loss. On examination, it was found that she had a fullness in her lower abdomen and a CT scan of her abdomen and pelvis was arranged. In the interval between her clinic appointment and CT scan, she developed an enteric fluid discharge through her anterior abdominal wall at the lower end of her previous laparotomy incision. The CT demonstrated a large intraabdominal inflammatory mass involving the rectum and small bowel proximal to the IRA (Figure 17.4). The mass extended to the anterior abdominal wall and a fistulous connection was evident. The bladder and uterus appeared thickened.

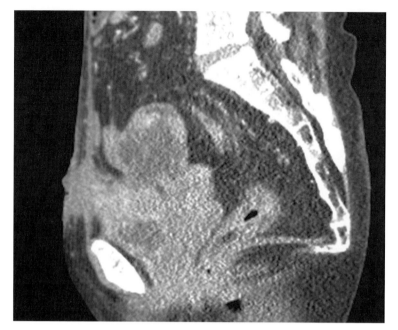

Figure 17.4 Inflammatory mass arising out of pelvis with enterocutaneous fistula.

The CT findings were thought to be in keeping with a complex Crohn's-related mass. She was admitted acutely to the gastroenterology ward. On examination, she looked generally well. She was apyrexial and nontachycardic. Abdominal examination showed a soft nontender upper abdomen but a diffuse indurated swelling in the lower abdomen with a fistulous opening. The volumes passing through the fistula were low (100–200 mL/day).

DECISION POINT

How would you manage the patient now?

It was felt that the patient had a complex inflammatory mass in the pelvis, almost certainly related to the iatrogenic perforation at the IRA. Her general condition and nutritional status were satisfactory, probably as the inflammatory/fistulating area was defunctioned by the loop ileostomy. It was felt that surgical intervention with a view to proctectomy and permanent ileostomy was required. The patient who had been extremely averse to a permanent stoma was now accepting of this plan, even conceding that she should have had it earlier. Although she had lost some weight, she was thought to be well enough to proceed to surgery. TPN was started preoperatively mainly as a "contingency plan" so that it would be up and running if she had a slow postoperative course.

At laparotomy, she was found to have dense adhesions throughout the abdomen. In the lower abdomen, there was a large phlegmon, through which passed the efferent loop of bowel from the ileostomy to the ileorectal anastomosis. The mass was adherent to the back of the bladder, and a cystotomy made when trying to dissect this free. The pelvis was not accessible ("frozen"), and the bowel was divided at the level of the ileorectal anastomosis. The ileostomy was converted to an end stoma. It was not possible to close the top of the rectal stump due to dense fibrosis, and a 30 Fr Robinson's drain was inserted through the left iliac fossa and the tip placed into the top of the stump to create a mucus fistula.

Her postoperative recovery was expectedly slow, and complicated by an intraabdominal fluid collection which discharged spontaneously through the midline wound. Histology of the resected bowel and phlegmon demonstrated a moderately differentiated mucinous adenocarcinoma with tumor present at the site of the enterocutaneous fistula as well as the distal resection margins. The final staging was T4N2 (8/29) M0 L1 V0 R2 Dukes' C1.

Subsequent management was largely palliative. She was never well enough to receive palliative chemotherapy due to grumbling pelvic sepsis. Imaging 8 months post laparotomy showed evidence of liver metastases.

LEARNING POINTS

- Beware of colonic strictures in inflammatory bowel disease. Colonic strictures in Crohn's disease or UC should be considered potentially malignant until proven otherwise by repeat biopsy or excision.
- Important risk factors for malignancy in ulcerative colitis are summarized in Table 17.1.

Table 17.1 Risk factors for colonic malignancy in IBD.

Risk factor	Quantification of risk
Duration of colits	2% at 10 years; 8% at 20 years; 18% at 30 years
Age at diagnosis	Conflicting evidence, but younger onset may be associated with increased risk, independent of disease duration
Extent of colitis	Increased risk with greater extent of disease – RR 1.7 for proctitis, 2.8 for left sided, 14.8 for pancolitis when compared to general population
Severity of inflammation	Increased risk of cancer with increasing severity of inflammation Postinflammatory polyps associated with increased cancer risk
Gender	No significant difference
Family history of sporadic cancer	Increased risk of IBD-related cancer RR 2.5–3.7
Co-existing PSC	Increased risk of IBD-related cancer RR 4.8

IBD, inflammatory bowel disease; PSC, primary sclerosing cholangitis; RR, relative risk.

Could we have done better?

The major criticism of this patient's management is that malignancy was not diagnosed earlier. In hindsight, our index of suspicious should have been much higher.

Although our patient had always had benign biopsies from her anastomotic stricture, when she presented with a lower abdominal mass the risk of neoplasia should have been pursued further. At this time, she had had Crohn's colitis for 47 years and had concurrent primary sclerosing cholangitis, so her individual risk for developing cancer was significant. Although imaging was suggestive of this being a Crohn's-related mass and anastomotic biopsies were benign, radiological guided biopsies may have yielded a malignant diagnosis at an earlier stage.

The second criticism relates to excessive adherence to the patient's wish to avoid a permanent stoma. Perhaps with further involvement of the stoma team and possible involvement of clinical psychologists or psychiatrists, the patient may have come to an earlier decision to accept a permanent ileostomy. If this had been the case, it is possible to postulate that an iatrogenic perforation could have been avoided as well as eliminating the risk of cancer.

LETTER FROM AMERICA

Anastomotic strictures in patients with Crohn's disease may be treated with medical, endoscopic, or surgical techniques. Benign, fibrotic strictures <5 cm and not associated with abscess or fistula are most suitable for endoscopic dilatation. In this patient, with long-standing Crohn's, PSC, and a stricture involving the rectum, histological or cytological biopsies of the IRA stricture may have allowed for an earlier diagnosis of cancer. Biopsy of large bowel strictures in patients with Crohn's disease is a clinical practice guideline of the ASCRS.

Jon Vogel and Massarat Zutshi

CASE 18

Crohn's colitis

Bruce George[1] & Marc Marti-Gallostra[2]

[1] Oxford University Hospitals NHS Foundation Trust, Oxford, UK
[2] University Hospital Vall d'Hebron, Barcelona, Spain

A 25-year-old man was referred by a gastroenterologist because of severe Crohn's colitis resistant to medical therapy. He had been diagnosed with Crohn's colitis aged 16 years. Colonoscopic appearances were typical and histological appearances were diagnostic. He had been managed for about 8 years with azathioprine (200 mg). For the past year, he had had worsening symptoms of diarrhea, up to 10 times per day, weight loss of 8 kg, lethargy, and fear of eating. Adalimumab had been started 6 months previously. After initial improvement, his symptoms were now deteriorating. Adalimumab had been increased from fortnightly to weekly, but with no improvement.

On examination, he looked thin (BMI 22.3). There was a tender fullness in the LIF but no other abnormality. Rectal examination was normal. Rigid sigmoidoscopy in clinic showed minimal rectal inflammation to 15 cm.

Magnetic resonance enterography showed extensive thickening of the distal transverse, descending, and sigmoid colon. The right colon and small bowel were radiologically normal (Figure 18.1). Colonoscopy showed severe left-sided colitis confirmed on biopsy. CMV was negative. Blood tests showed Hb 11.4, CRP 72.

DECISION POINT

Given that the medical approach had failed, an operation was planned. But which operation? The surgical options considered were:
- resection of diseased left colon with transverse to rectal anastomosis +/- defunctioning ileostomy

- subtotal colectomy with ileorectal anastomosis +/- defunctioning ileostomy

- proctocolectomy

- preliminary loop ileostomy with subsequent limited colectomy.
As the patient was systemically unwell with anemia, weight loss, and high inflammatory markers, it was decided to undertake a preliminary defunctioning ileostomy.

He made a good recovery following ileostomy formation. He had a brief readmission to hospital 2 weeks postoperatively with obstructive symptoms that

---

Colorectal Surgery: Clinical Care and Management, First Edition.
Edited by Bruce George, Richard Guy, Oliver Jones, and Jon Vogel.
© 2016 John Wiley & Sons, Ltd. Published 2016 by John Wiley & Sons, Ltd.

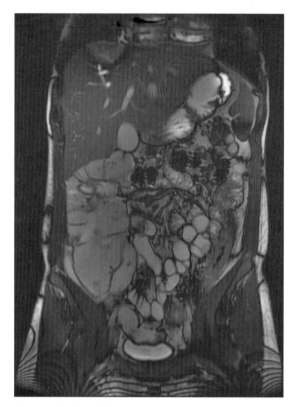

Figure 18.1 MRE showing thickened abnormal left colon.

settled rapidly. At review 6 months later, he was well, had regained weight and energy levels. He was managing the ileostomy without difficulty but was keen to have it reversed if possible.

The defunctioned colon was assessed by contrast enema and colonoscopy. Colonoscopy showed mild defunction changes in the rectum but could not pass into the sigmoid. The contrast study showed normal rectum but a very narrowed sigmoid, descending and most of transverse colon with a normal-looking cecum and ascending colon (Figure 18.2).

As the patient was now systemically well, it was felt reasonable to proceed with reconstruction. It was felt reasonable to preserve the right colon and rectum. It was decided to "double check" the rectum preoperatively.

At flexible sigmoidoscopy, the rectum was found to be noninflamed and compliant. A tattoo was placed at the upper limit of normal compliant rectum at about 15 cm. The patient proceeded to laparotomy. The right colon was normal as far as the proximal transverse and could be preserved. It was decided, however, to undertake a subtotal colectomy with just one anastomosis between ileum (at site of ileostomy) and upper rectum.

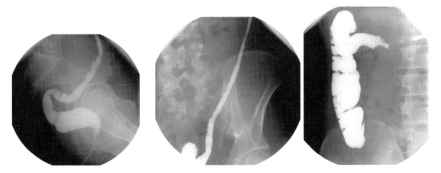

Figure 18.2 Contrast studies showing colonic strictures.

He made a good postoperative recovery. Nine months later, bowel function with regular low-dose loperamide is satisfactory at 4–5 times per day, with no urgency or leakage.

LEARNING POINTS

- The surgical options for large bowel Crohn's disease depend on the exact distribution of inflammation. The presence of significant anal disease or proctitis usually precludes reconstructive surgery.
- A defunctioning stoma is a useful surgical option in patients with severe Crohn's colitis.

LETTER FROM AMERICA

When operative therapy for Crohn's colitis is required, the ASCRS endorses segmental or total colectomy for patients with single-segment disease and total colectomy for multi-segment disease. When the rectum and anus are both usable, total abdominal colectomy with ileorectal anastomosis is often performed.

Jon Vogel and Massarat Zutshi

CASE 19

Fistulating anal Crohn's disease: conservative management

Silvia Silvans[1] & Bruce George[2]

[1] *Hospital del Mar, Barcelona, Spain*
[2] *Oxford University Hospitals NHS Foundation Trust, Oxford, UK*

A 25-year-old female university student presented as an emergency with left buttock pain, which had progressed despite 4 days of co-amoxiclav prescribed by her GP. She was a nonsmoker with no relevant medical or family history. Clinical examination showed a large left ischiorectal abscess.

She underwent examination under anesthetic with incision and drainage of the abscess. No obvious fistula was identified and the rectal mucosa was normal. She was discharged after 24 hours on antibiotic treatment. Three weeks later, she re-presented with pain in the other (right) buttock and a high fever. She started intravenous ceftriaxone and metronidazole.

DECISION POINT

What investigations should be undertaken at this stage?

It was clear that she required another EUA, but in view of the progression of sepsis to the contralateral side and features of systemic toxicity, it was felt that cross-sectional imaging was indicated first. Although an MR would have been preferable, for logistic reasons she had a pelvic CT shortly after admission.

The CT report described a 28×19 mm enhancing wall collection in the right ischiorectal fossa. A tiny residual pocket of fluid and air was identified in the left ischiorectal fossa. At further EUA, no "horse-shoe" communication with the left cavity was detected, nor an obvious fistula to the anal canal. She underwent simple incision and drainage of the right-sided ischiorectal abscess. Rigid sigmoidoscopy showed normal mucosa to 15 cm. She was discharged the following day.

Unfortunately, she was readmitted again 8 days later with further pain and swelling in the perianal region, joint pain, and diarrhea (3–4 times per day) without blood, mucus or pus. A colonoscopy showed normal rectal mucosa. However,

---

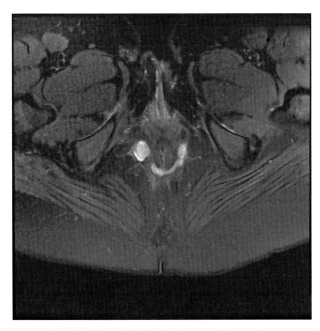

Figure 19.1 MRI scan showing bilateral fluid collections and horse-shoe communication.

from the rectosigmoid junction up to the proximal transverse colon, there were multiple small aphthous ulcers with a preserved background vascular pattern. Deep aphthous ulcers and cobblestoning were seen in the ascending colon. There were a few aphthous ulcers in the terminal ileum. A pelvic MRI (Figure 19.1) showed persisting collections of fluid bilaterally with an obvious horse-shoe connection.

She underwent a further EUA. The bilateral ischiorectal cavities were lavaged via the previous incisions. Gentle probing and hydrogen peroxide injection showed no fistula communications. The colonoscopic biopsies showed chronic inflammation suggestive of Crohn's disease. Rheumatoid factors and ANA were negative. Tests for *Clostridium difficile* and Yersinia were negative.

DECISION POINT

How should she be treated at this stage?

Sepsis seemed to be under control. Medical therapy for Crohn's disease needed to be optimized. She was treated with a short reducing course of steroids and then started on azathioprine and adalimumab.

Over the next few weeks her joint pains and diarrhea settled. At clinic review 3 months later, she was systemically well but had persisting discharge from the abscess drainage incisions. Arrangements for a repeat colonoscopy, MRE, and repeat EUA were made. Colonoscopy showed near complete mucosal healing with just scattered aphthous ulceration in the right colon. MRE showed no evidence of small bowel Crohn's disease. EUA showed a large posterior anal ulcer and two external openings. Hydrogen peroxide into the right fistula opening did not show any communication with the anal canal, but peroxide flowed freely from the right to left external openings.

DECISION POINT

How should this horse-shoe communication without detectable internal communication be managed?

No fistula to the anal canal was easily identified although it was acknowledged that one must exist. Surgical options were considered to be unattractive and a decision made to simply curette and lavage the cavity and to continue with medical therapy.

She remained clinically well, with good energy levels and no symptoms apart from a small amount of discharge from the two fistula openings.

A further EUA 15 months later showed a posterior ulcer in the anal canal (Figure 19.2). There was a scar at the previous left fistula opening that appeared to have healed. On the right side was an external opening which when probed entered a cavity extending to 5–6 cm lateral to anorectum. Injection of hydrogen peroxide confirmed a fistula to the posterior ulcer. There was no proctitis.

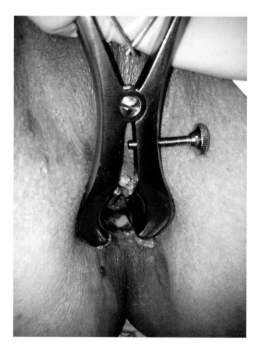

Figure 19.2 Appearances at EUA showing posterior ulcer lined by purulent fluid, healed left-sided scar, and external opening on right. Probing of the external opening showed fistulous communication to posterior ulcer (internal opening).

DECISION POINT

What are the treatment options at this stage?

We are now in the "quality of life" phase (see page 80). The patient is well, on optimum medical therapy, with few fistula symptoms. The option of a loose seton was considered but it was felt it would only prevent any healing with medical therapy. The presence of a persisting ischiorectal cavity and associated induration was felt to make attempted curative surgical options unlikely to be successful. Fistulotomy was considered contraindicated due to the complex and transsphincteric nature of the fistula and the size of the resultant wound and likely very slow healing. The large posterior ulcer was thought to make an advancement flap unlikely to succeed. LIFT was considered but due to the patient's mild symptoms, a decision was made to simply continue current medical therapy with azathioprine 100 mg daily and adalimumab 40 mg every other week.

The patient remains well 2 years after initial presentation. She is maintained on azathioprine and adalimumab. She persists in having a small amount of perianal discharge from the right side, but is content with the current situation.

LEARNING POINTS

- Patients with perianal sepsis who are "not right" after initial incision and drainage should have an MR scan to look for occult/undrained sepsis.
- Management of fistulating anal Crohn's disease may be considered in four phases.
  1. First aid: adequate drainage of perianal sepsis.
  2. Bridging phase: to optimize medical therapy.
  3. Quality of life.
  4. Definitive healing or proctectomy.

LETTER FROM AMERICA

It is pleasantly surprising that this patient got through the acute phase without an ostomy. A primary goal of Crohn's therapy has been achieved: her symptoms are controlled. The pessimist will now rightly question the durability of her disease control and wonder when a permanent ostomy will be required. Hopefully never.

Jon Vogel and Massarat Zutshi

CASE 20

Tail end carnage

Bruce George

Oxford University Hospitals NHS Foundation Trust, Oxford, UK

A 33-year-old man presented as an emergency with perianal pain, swelling, and a fever. He had been diagnosed with Crohn's disease 10 years earlier at a hospital in London but had been lost to follow-up in the interim. At diagnosis a decade ago, he had had a perianal abscess and fistulae, requiring several operations and drains.

At EUA on this occasion, he was found to have very indurated perianal tissues, multiple discharging fistulae, and edematous skin tags. Rigid sigmoidoscopy showed definite proctitis. No obvious large abscess was detected.

The following day, he had an MRI scan, which demonstrated a deep anterior horse-shoe abscess. He underwent a further EUA. Two stab incisions were made anterolaterally (10 and 2 o'clock), resulting in drainage of the horse-shoe abscess. A loose seton drain was placed between the two stab incisions. Flexible sigmoidoscopy confirmed distal proctitis to about 6 cm, but normal-looking mucosa proximally. The pus grew gut organisms and the rectal biopsy showed nonspecific inflammation, with no features to indicate definite inflammatory bowel disease.

Over the next few weeks, a colonoscopy and small bowel enema were arranged. These confirmed limited proctitis, but no other evidence of intestinal inflammation.

DECISION POINT

Should medical treatment for Crohn's disease be started now?

The diagnosis of Crohn's was considered to be robust. Although rectal biopsies were non-diagnostic, the clinical appearances were typical of severe perianal Crohn's disease. Other conditions including hidradenitis suppurativa, tuberculosis, and lymphogranuloma venereum were considered unlikely. It was decided to start azathioprine treatment, but to hold off anti-TNF therapy, as the patient had persisting anal pain despite drainage.

Colorectal Surgery: Clinical Care and Management, First Edition.
Edited by Bruce George, Richard Guy, Oliver Jones, and Jon Vogel.
© 2016 John Wiley & Sons, Ltd. Published 2016 by John Wiley & Sons, Ltd.

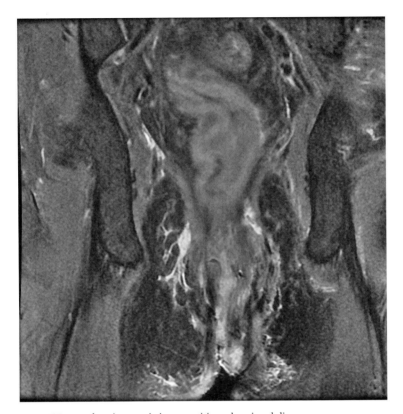

Figure 20.1 MRI scan showing persisting proctitis and perianal disease.

Over the next 4 months the patient required four further EUAs with insertion of multiple drains. Eventually his anal pain settled and MRI scanning showed no undrained sepsis, although persisting severe proctitis (Figure 20.1).

At this stage he started treatment with infliximab. Over the subsequent 6 months, he had regular infusions of infliximab. The clinical situation was just tolerable, with about six loose seton drains in place. A defunctioning stoma was discussed but the patient was very against this.

Unfortunately, over the next few months the situation progressively deteriorated. He presented regularly as an emergency requiring repeated EUAs and some form of drainage. The patient met stomatherapy nurses on several occasions, but initially resisted stoma formation. He eventually agreed to a loop sigmoid colostomy (Figure 20.2). At laparoscopy, there was no evidence of small or large bowel Crohn's disease and no intraperitoneal sepsis. The patient managed the colostomy reasonably well, but continued to present with perianal pain, requiring three further EUAs over the next 8 months.

It became progressively clear to both the patient and doctors that a proctectomy and permanent colostomy were required. Psychologically, he was accepting of a permanent stoma. Nutrition was satisfactory. Infliximab was stopped preoperatively but azathioprine continued.

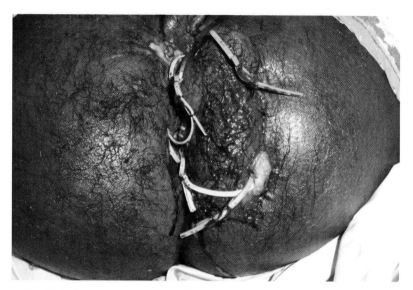

Figure 20.2 Clinical appearance 6 months after defunctioning colostomy formation.

An open proctectomy and myocutaneous flap were undertaken utilizing the rectus abdominis muscle. The abdominal component of the proctectomy was straightforward. The mesorectal plane was used "higher up," avoiding the hypogastric nerves that were easily seen, but coning towards the muscle tube from around the level of peritoneal reflection to reduce the risk of parasympathetic nerve injury. The perineal dissection was more difficult due to induration, multiple fistulae, and cavities in the perianal tissues. A wide dissection to excise sepsis was undertaken from below and the perineal defect was reconstructed with the rectus abdominis myocutaneous flap.

Postoperatively, he made a satisfactory recovery. Six days postoperatively, he developed a fever. A CT scan showed a small collection in the right iliac fossa, which was too small to drain and was treated with intravenous antibiotics. His subsequent recovery was good and he was discharged 15 days postoperatively. Pathology showed features of severe fistulating Crohn's disease.

The patient returned to the ward for wound dressing 2 and 4 weeks postoperatively, but failed to attend subsequent outpatient appointments. He returned to clinic 16 months after the proctectomy with a superficial abscess in the left groin. The perineal flap had healed well and he was managing the colostomy reasonably well. The groin abscess was treated with oral antibiotics.

Sadly, he recently presented with pain in the perineum, just over 3 years after the proctectomy. Examination showed an indurated mass deep to the rectus flap. Investigations including biopsy have shown adenocarcinoma. He is currently undergoing chemoradiotherapy.

Could we have done better?

- Anti-TNF therapy could have been started earlier after initial presentation, with delays occurring due to concerns about undrained sepsis. We could have been "braver" in starting treatment once MRI and EUA findings both suggested no persisting infection.
- The patient underwent a huge number of emergency EUAs, many of which were noncontributory. On these occasions, he was seen by different colorectal and general consultants who each undertook an EUA +/- MRI, without progress towards a proctectomy/stoma.
- The late diagnosis of adenocarcinoma was devastating and unexpected. It is hard to see how this could have been anticipated or prevented but serves as a reminder of the increased risk of malignancy in patients with long-standing Crohn's disease and ulcerative colitis.

LEARNING POINTS

- Deep-seated abscesses may be difficult to detect at EUA, especially when the perianal tissues are indurated from previous inflammation. MRI scanning should be arranged urgently when perianal sepsis is suspected but not detected at EUA.
- Anal Crohn's disease occurs without evidence of intestinal inflammation elsewhere in about 5% of cases.
- Perianal sepsis must be adequately drained before commencing treatment with anti-TNF drugs.
- A defunctioning stoma may be used to control symptoms of severe perianal Crohn's disease.
- Long-standing anal Crohn's disease is associated with an increased risk of anal malignancy and the risk may be exacerbated by immunosuppressive drugs.

LETTER FROM AMERICA

The potential for "malignant degeneration" of a chronically inflamed perineum is demonstrated in this unfortunate case. While pathology review of the resected anorectum did not reveal malignancy, the value of periodic biopsies of the inflamed or unhealed perineum should not be discounted.

Jon Vogel and Massarat Zutshi

CASE 21

Acute severe colitis

Bruce George

Oxford University Hospitals NHS Foundation Trust, Oxford, UK

A 30-year-old woman presented with a 4-week history of bloody diarrhoea, up to 20 times per day. She had friends with diarrhea and vomiting but their symptoms had settled quickly. There was no recent history of travel abroad. Her past medical history was unremarkable. She was treated with a course of ciprofloxacin by her GP, without improvement.

On examination, she looked generally well, pulse rate 104, normotensive, and apyrexial. Abdominal examination showed mild distension but no tenderness. Digital rectal examination was normal. Blood tests showed a hemoglobin 13, white count of 17, CRP of 30, and ESR 45. Initial plain radiology showed mild mucosal edema in the sigmoid and descending colon. Stool cultures were sent and subsequently proved to be negative.

She was admitted under the care of the gastroenterologists. The initial differential diagnosis was of new-onset IBD or postinfective gastroenteritis. As she fulfilled the criteria of ASC, she was treated with high-dose IV and rectal steroids. Flexible sigmoidoscopy the following day showed evidence of continuous inflammation to at least the descending colon (UCEIS V2, M3, E3 = 8/8 *; see page 82) (Figure 21.1).

Over the next 4 days, her general condition remained stable without abdominal tenderness. Stool frequency remained 8/day. Histology from the rectal and colonic biopsies showed severe active ulcerative colitis with evidence of possible superadded infection. There was no evidence of CMV infection. As she had not completely responded, ciclosporin rescue therapy was instituted. Over the next few days, her stool frequency decreased and appetite returned. She was discharged home after 14 days in hospital on oral ciclosporin and a reducing dose of steroids.

One month later when reviewed in clinic, she was feeling well, with normal stools and bowel frequency of once daily. Colonoscopy 2 months after hospital discharge showed minor erythema and loss of vascularity in the rectum but was otherwise macroscopically normal to the terminal ileum. She had

Colorectal Surgery: Clinical Care and Management, First Edition.
Edited by Bruce George, Richard Guy, Oliver Jones, and Jon Vogel.
© 2016 John Wiley & Sons, Ltd. Published 2016 by John Wiley & Sons, Ltd.

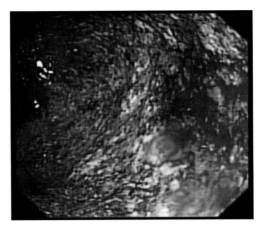

Figure 21.1 Appearances at flexible sigmoidoscopy at presentation.

tailed off steroids at this stage. Maintenance therapy was with ciclosporin and azathioprine.

Two months later, she developed a flare-up of symptoms with urgency, blood, and mucus per rectum and a bowel frequency of 3/day. She was readmitted and treated with intravenous steroids again. Flexible sigmoidoscopy showed active colitis (UCEIS V2, M2, E1 = 5/8). The possibility of colectomy was discussed at this stage, but as she settled so rapidly with steroids, it was considered reasonable to continue medical therapy. Medical treatment was then switched to infliximab, which was started shortly before hospital discharge.

Over the next 5 months she had four further doses of maintenance infliximab. Azathioprine was continued, but not ciclosporin. Unfortunately, by February 2013, her symptoms started to relapse.

DECISION POINT

Should she have further medical treatment or is this refractory to medical treatment?

Initial presentation with ASC is a poor prognostic feature with over 75% of patients coming to surgery with a year. Furthermore, she was already on "near maximal" medical treatment with azathioprine and infliximab. Additional medical approaches such as another immunomodulator (e.g. methotrexate) or more novel treatments (e.g. electrophoresis) were considered, but felt to be unlikely to be successful.

A joint medical and surgical decision was taken to proceed to colectomy and ileostomy with preservation of the rectal stump. An immediate proctocolectomy with pouch reconstruction was considered (+/- loop ileostomy) as the patient was systemically well, not on steroids and had no clinical or pathological features to suggest Crohn's disease.

She underwent a laparoscopically assisted subtotal colectomy. The rectosigmoid junction was stapled closed with an endoGIA. A large (28 Fr) Foley catheter was placed in the rectal stump on free drainage and flushed twice daily for 4 days postoperatively.

The patient made a good postoperative recovery, going home 6 days postoperatively.

The pathology report confirmed features of active severe ulcerative colitis, with no evidence of infection or Crohn's disease. She was keen to proceed with ileoanal pouch reconstruction. The risks of pouch surgery were discussed in detail, including failure, expected bowel frequency, and impact on fertility (see the checklist for pouch surgery, pages 84–85). She met the specialist nurses who run the pouch follow-up clinic and she was given information about the "Kangaroo Club," a patient-led group who support patients who have had or are considering pouch surgery (www.kangarooclub.org.uk).

The patient underwent uncomplicated proctectomy and pouch reconstruction with a covering ileostomy 7 months after colectomy. At operation, there were no adhesions from the prior laparoscopic colectomy. The ileostomy was closed 4 months later. At latest follow-up 5 months later, the patient has returned to work and pouch function is satisfactory (6× per day, 0–1× at night, with no urgency/leakage).

Could we have done better?

The patient relapsed when switched from ciclosporin and steroids to ciclosporin and azathioprine. It is possible in retrospect that the dose of azathioprine was not optimum at this stage. It is now recommended practice to measure activity of enzymes responsible for metabolism of azathioprine (thiopurine metyltransferase [TPMT]) and metabolites (6-thioguanine) to predict clinical response and risk of side-effects.

LEARNING POINTS

- Acute severe colitis is defined by the Truelove and Witts criteria: bloody diarrhoea of 6 or more stools per 24 hours and ONE of the following:
  - fever over 37.8°C
  - pulse rate over 90
  - hemoglobin less than 10.5 g/dL
  - ESR over 30 mm/h.
- Management of acute severe colitis depends on:
  - recognition of condition
  - high-dose IV steroids
  - joint medical and surgical care
  - rescue therapy on day 3 with ciclosporin or anti-TNF
  - prompt surgery if not improving by 5–7 days into treatment.

CASE 22

Snare or pouch? The problem of dysplasia in ulcerative colitis

Gareth Horgan[1] & James East[2]

[1] Naas General Hospital, Dublin, Ireland
[2] Oxford University Hospitals NHS Foundation Trust, Oxford, UK

A 54-year-old woman with long-standing left-sided ulcerative colitis for 21 years was seen in clinic. She was clinically in remission from a colitis viewpoint and was maintained on methotrexate 25 mg weekly, folic acid 5 mg weekly, and mesalazine 2 g daily. She was intolerant to thiopurines and had received multiple short courses of steroids since diagnosis over the years. Her last colonoscopy was 7 years previously. At that examination, there had been mildly active left-sided colitis noted endoscopically and histologically.

> **DECISION POINT**
>
> **Does this patient need further colonoscopic surveillance?**
>
> Current guidelines clearly suggest that this patient requires a high-quality colonoscopy, ideally done when the disease is in remission and by an experienced endoscopist using dye spray to enhance detection of dysplasia.

Colonoscopic surveillance examination with pancolonic indigo carmine dye spray showed a patch of inflammation in the cecum. There was quiescent colitis from the rectum to the mid transverse colon. Biopsies from throughout the colon showed no active inflammation apart from mild-to-moderate inflammation in the cecal pole and rectum. However, in the transverse colon, in the endoscopically quiescent colitis there was a 12 mm flat (Paris classification 0-IIa) well-circumscribed lesion (Figure 22.1).

The lesion was suspicious for a dysplastic lesion with Kudo type IIIL pit pattern, but had no areas suggestive of invasion. The endoscopist performing the colonoscopy was an experienced therapeutic endoscopist and in line with current guidelines, an attempt was made to lift the lesion with submucosal injection with a view to snare resection. Unfortunately, this lesion did not lift well, so biopsies were taken and a small tattoo was placed just distal to the lesion. Histological analysis showed the lesion to be a low-grade tubular adenoma.

Colorectal Surgery: Clinical Care and Management, First Edition.
Edited by Bruce George, Richard Guy, Oliver Jones, and Jon Vogel.
© 2016 John Wiley & Sons, Ltd. Published 2016 by John Wiley & Sons, Ltd.

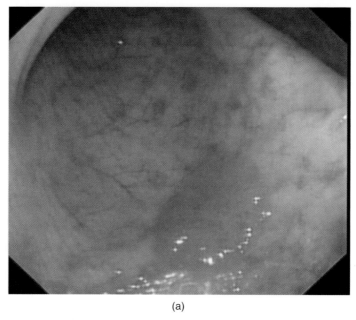

(a)

Figure 22.1 (a) A 12 mm flat (Paris 0-IIa) lesion on a background of quiescent colitis on the transverse colon.

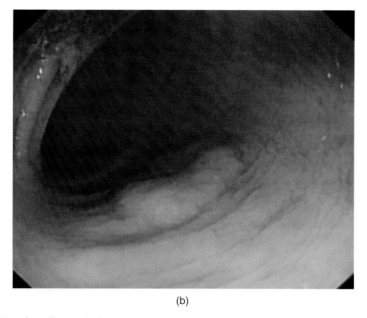

(b)

Figure 22.1 (b) Following indigo carmine dye spray, the edge of the lesion is well seen, suggesting a circumscribed lesion where endoscopic resection may be appropriate.

DECISION POINT

What should you do for this patient following an initially failed endoscopic resection of a circumscribed dysplastic lesion?

Her case was discussed at the MDT meeting. The endoscopic pictures suggested a lesion which "should be" possible to remove colonoscopically. The conclusion was to make a further attempt to resect the polyp endoscopically with further biopsies of the surrounding area to see if there was dysplasia or active inflammation.

A further colonoscopy was performed 6 weeks after the first. Multiple attempts at injection to lift the polyp were tried and attempts were made to grip the polyp with a snare. Even using snare tip diathermy to make an anchor point to improve grip point, it was not possible to grasp the polyp safely and comprehensively. The polyp and surrounding area were biopsied extensively to assess for field change and evidence of colitis. A further tattoo was placed distal to the polyp but it was felt the marking might be suboptimal due to poor lifting, meaning there was limited submucosal space for marking dye. Biopsies again showed this area to be a tubular adenoma with low-grade dysplasia. There was no evidence of endoscopically undetectable dysplasia in the surrounding mucosa but the appearances were of focal active colitis consistent with ulcerative colitis following treatment.

DECISION POINT

What are the options for this patient after a second attempt at endoscopic resection of an isolated dysplastic polyp had failed under optimal conditions?

ECCO guidelines state that if endoscopic resection is not possible or if dysplasia is found in the surrounding flat mucosa, proctocolectomy should be recommended [1]. Following further IBD MDT discussion, a decision was made to recommend surgical resection. The surgical options included proctocolectomy with ileoanal pouch procedure, subtotal colectomy with ileorectal anastomosis, extended right hemi-colectomy or a disk excision. The different options were to be discussed with the patient. As she was in clinical remission with no other areas of dysplasia, a decision was made to perform a laparoscopic disk excision of the area.

She underwent a laparoscopic disk excision of the dysplastic area. The tattooed area was easily identified laparoscopically, mobilized and exteriorized through a small periumbilical incision. She made an uneventful postoperative recovery and was discharged less than 48 hours post resection. Histology confirmed a discrete area of dysplasia with quiescent colitis in the surrounding area. There were no features of high-grade dysplasia or malignancy.

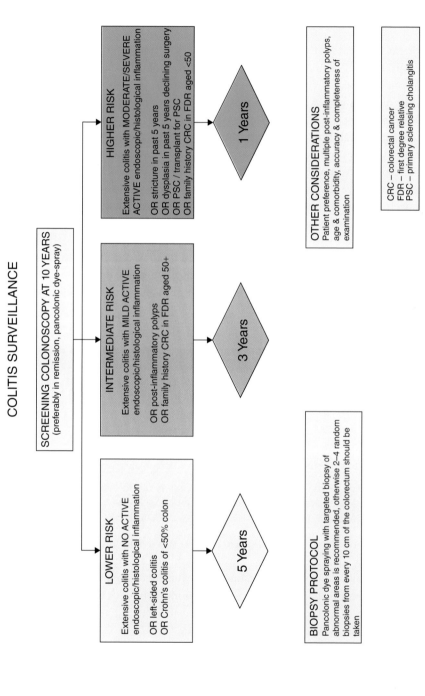

Figure 22.2 Surveillance for colorectal cancer in patients with UC and Crohn's colitis (BSG Guidelines, 2010). *Source:* Cairns [2]. Reproduced with permission of BMJ Publishing Group Ltd.

DECISION POINT

What surveillance should now be offered to this patient?

It is acknowledged that a limited segmental resection for a dysplastic lesion in UC is unorthodox. Our argument was that it seems illogical to accept endoscopic removal, but if not feasible endoscopically then to recommend proctocolectomy. It was decided to keep her under annual colonoscopic follow-up.

She had a repeat dye spray colonoscopy 6 months later and no abnormal areas were detected. Random biopsies from throughout the colon showed normal mucosa. Further dye spray colonoscopy 1 and 2 years later showed mild inflammation in the transverse colon and a cecal patch. No suspicious areas were noted and biopsies showed mild colitis and no dysplasia. She has now had 30 months of surveillance and no further recurrence of dysplasia.

Could we have done better?

This patient should have had colonoscopic surveillance 5 years after her last colonoscopy according to risk stratification by current guidelines (Figure 22.2). Late surveillance may have lead to a more advanced dysplastic lesion that was more difficult to resect endoscopically.

LEARNING POINTS

- Screening colonoscopy should be undertaken in patients with a history of colitis for 10 or more years. Colonoscopy should be undertaken when the disease is in remission, with good bowel preparation and using dye spray techniques. Frequency of screening colonoscopy is determined by risk stratification according to national guidelines.
- In assessing a dysplastic or potentially dysplastic lesion, two key questions are:
  - Is this an isolated area of dysplasia or is there dysplasia adjacent to the lesion or elsewhere in the colon?
  - Is there suspicion or evidence of malignancy (rigidity, fixity, central depression, pit pattern)?
- Discrete dysplastic lesions in colitis may be resected endoscopically, provided there is no evidence of dysplasia elsewhere in the colon and no invasive malignancy. Subsequent close endoscopic follow-up is mandatory.

References

1 Annese V, Daperno M, Rutter MD, *et al*. European evidence based consensus for endoscopy in inflammatory bowel disease. *J Crohn's Colitis* 2013; **7**(12):982–1018.
2 Cairns SR, Scholefield JH, Steele RJ, *et al*. Guidelines for colorectal cancer screening and surveillance in moderate and high risk groups (update from 2002). *Gut* 2010; **59**(5):666–89.

CASE 23

Anal fistula and ulcerative colitis

Richard Guy

Oxford University Hospitals NHS Foundation Trust, Oxford, UK

A previously fit 19-year-old woman with a 4-year history of ulcerative colitis and a 2-year history of ankylosing spondylitis presented with refractory colitis, poorly responsive to corticosteroids and azathioprine. It was not possible to wean her off steroids completely and she had developed osteoporosis.

Urgent laparoscopic subtotal colectomy and end ileostomy was performed with an uneventful recovery and discharge after 7 days. Histopathological examination of the colon confirmed severe total colitis, consistent with ulcerative colitis. The patient was weaned off steroids and was able to return to academic studies. Troublesome proctitis was treated with mesalazine enemas but she remained generally well and counseling took place regarding completion proctectomy and ileoanal pouch surgery (see pages 84–85).

Unfortunately, she then presented with a perianal abscess that required incision and drainage under general anesthesia. A fistula ensued. EUA and endoanal ultrasound with hydrogen peroxide enhancement showed some fissuring at the anterior anal margin and an anterior transsphincteric fistula with a branching track encroaching upon the vagina but without demonstrable connection to the vagina. The tracks were curetted (no granulomas were found on histology) and a silastic seton was inserted.

The patient was keen to be rid of her stoma. Her ankylosing spondylitis was more disabling and she was forced to take a year out from studying. She was treated with methotrexate.

DECISION POINT

What are the surgical options for a patient with histologically proven ulcerative colitis post colectomy but with a recently developed anal fistula?

The case was discussed in the department. There was consensus that ileoanal pouch surgery in the presence of a fistula would be unwise and carry a high risk of failure. The potential for this to be Crohn's disease was high.

Colorectal Surgery: Clinical Care and Management, First Edition.
Edited by Bruce George, Richard Guy, Oliver Jones, and Jon Vogel.
© 2016 John Wiley & Sons, Ltd. Published 2016 by John Wiley & Sons, Ltd.

Whilst the safest option was perhaps proctectomy with permanent ileostomy, the patient was keen to pursue reconstructive options. If fistula healing could be achieved then reconstruction with an ileorectal anastomosis might be an option. It was decided to review the colectomy histology and to undertake flexible sigmoidoscopy and an EUA to assess treatment options for the fistula.

Review of the colectomy pathology was confirmed to be characteristic of UC. Flexible sigmoidoscopy with biopsies showed active chronic indeterminate proctitis. She was commenced on infliximab biological therapy.

At EUA, an anterior transsphincteric fistula was confirmed. A collagen fistula plug was inserted and secured to the internal sphincter at the internal opening and mucosa closed over the top. At 3 months postoperatively, it was clear that the plug had failed and this was confirmed at EUA; again a short track extension to the back of the vagina was demonstrated.

Over the next 6 months, the fistula persisted but she remained generally well. The proctitis and ankylosis spondilitis improved with infliximab therapy. After a further 3 months, EUA showed no active proctitis. The anterior fistula was unchanged but with no evidence of associated sepsis. A ligation of intersphincteric track (LIFT) procedure was carried out in a further attempt to heal the fistula. This time, a single track was identified with no evidence of vaginal encroachment and the procedure was uncomplicated. The fistula healed and this was maintained at 6 months, confirmed on MRI. The patient remained on infliximab for ankylosing spondylitis and was fully active with no joint symptoms.

DECISION POINT

The patient wanted to get rid of her stoma. Is surgery a reasonable option and if so, which operation should be offered?

Following MDT discussion, it was considered that IRA would be a reasonable, if unconventional, option.

Laparoscopic-assisted IRA with an end-to-side circular stapled anastomosis was carried out without complication. Histological examination of the stapler "doughnuts" showed appearances of moderately active UC. At outpatient follow-up after 6 weeks, function was excellent, with bowel frequency of four times daily without antidiarrheal medication and with full continence. There was no anal fistula at 6 months and infliximab had been discontinued.

Could we have done better?

The first attempt to heal the fistula when there was associated proctitis was probably doomed to failure. Surgical healing of fistulae is more likely when proctitis has been controlled.

LEARNING POINTS

- Patients considering ileoanal pouch surgery should be counseled thoroughly before surgery (see pre-op pouch checklist on pages 84–85).
- IRA may be a reasonable option provided that:
  - there is no or minimal proctitis
  - there is no dysplasia
  - close surveillance of the rectum is undertaken.

LETTER FROM AMERICA

The ASCRS ulcerative colitis clinical practice guidelines support the use of ileorectal anastomosis (IRA) in carefully selected UC patients. The ideal patient would accept the risk that up to 53% of patients who choose this option will ultimately require excision or defunctioning of the IRA for refractory proctitis, dysplasia, cancer, or other problems. Further prerequisites for IRA UC include a compliant, relatively disease-free rectum, and a normal anus. In the case described, the occasional disconnect between the appearance and function of the anus and sphincters is illustrated. The appreciation of this disconnect has allowed this patient, for the time being at least, to avoid a permanent ileostomy. Yearly endoscopic (dysplasia) surveillance of the rectal remnant is advocated by the ASCRS.

Jon Vogel and Massarat Zutshi

CASE 24

Poor pouch function

Bruce George
Oxford University Hospitals NHS Foundation Trust, Oxford, UK

A 22-year-old hairdresser presented in 2004 with acute severe ulcerative colitis which did not settle with standard medical therapy including high-dose steroids and ciclosporin (see **Case 21**).

She underwent open subtotal colectomy with ileostomy formation and subcutaneous closure of the rectosigmoid stump. Eleven days post colectomy, she required a further laparotomy and adhesiolysis for persisting obstruction. Subsequent recovery was good. Histology confirmed acute colitis with features of ulcerative colitis. She underwent uncomplicated completion proctectomy and J-pouch reconstruction with a covering loop ileostomy 9 months later. Subsequent pouchogram showed no anastomotic leak and she was planned for ileostomy closure 5 months after the pouch surgery. At EUA, however, the pouch anal anastomosis was found to be stenosed, not even permitting gentle insertion of the little finger. The stenosis was dilated using Hagar's dilators until the index finger could be inserted easily.

DECISION POINT

Is it reasonable to proceed with ileostomy closure?

It is common to find a short membranous stricture at the time of EUA prior to ileostomy closure after pouch surgery, which usually dilates up easily. In such situations, it is reasonable to proceed with closure. On this occasion, the stenosis was felt to be more fibrotic so a decision (perhaps too conservatively) was made to defer ileostomy closure.

She underwent a further EUA 6 weeks later. On this occasion, there was a mild stenosis that dilated easily and the ileostomy closure proceeded uneventfully. She went home after 4 days with satisfactory early pouch function.

Over the next few years, pouch function stabilized at a manageable level. She opened her pouch six times a day, once overnight but with no blood or urgency. In 2009, she developed an acute deterioration in function with increased frequency, blood, and urgency. Flexible pouchoscopy showed a slightly indurated area at the pouch-anal anastomosis, a 1.5 cm noninflamed columnar cuff, and

Colorectal Surgery: Clinical Care and Management, First Edition.
Edited by Bruce George, Richard Guy, Oliver Jones, and Jon Vogel.
© 2016 John Wiley & Sons, Ltd. Published 2016 by John Wiley & Sons, Ltd.

an inflamed pouch with contact bleeding. Biopsies showed chronic inflammatory cells in the mucosa and villous atrophy with focal acute ulceration.

Pouch function improved with a 2-week course of ciprofloxacin. Repeat pouchoscopy showed some improvement in the endoscopic appearances.

Over the next few years, she was treated with cyclical courses of antibiotics and also established on the probiotic VSL-3. Pouch function again stabilized at a satisfactory level, typically 6–8/day and 0–1 at night with no blood or urgency.

Several years later, she presented as an emergency with abdominal pain, distension, and increased frequency. Abdominal examination showed distension and visible loops of distended bowel, but no tenderness. Plain radiology showed markedly distended loops of small bowel. She was managed conservatively initially with fluids and a nasogastric tube. Over the next 24 hours, her pouch stopped working. The working diagnosis was adhesional obstruction. CT scan showed slight dilatation of the pouch, marked dilatation of pre-pouch loops of ileum up to 8 cm diameter with relatively collapsed loops more proximally.

DECISION POINT

How should this be managed?

The CT appearances do not fit with typical adhesional small bowel obstruction. The most distended loops were distal with nondilated loops proximally. A closed loop obstruction was considered but there was no abdominal tenderness, nor fever/raised white count. It was acknowledged that some degree of pre-pouch dilatation is common but not to this extent.

She was managed conservatively, kept "nil by mouth" and given intravenous antibiotics and total parenteral nutrition via a peripheral line. Flexible pouchoscopy showed an area of ulceration in the mid-pouch. The ileum proximal to the pouch was moderately inflamed with aphthous ulceration and contact bleeding. The symptoms of distension gradually settled and her bowels started functioning again at the usual frequency of 6–8/day. She was discharged after 11 days in hospital. Outpatient review at 2 and 5 weeks showed gradual improvement but with persisting distension and poor pouch function.

The biopsies taken during hospital admission showed acute and chronic inflammation in both the pouch and pre-pouch ileum. There were no granulomas or other features suggestive of Crohn's.

DECISION POINT

How should the patient be managed at this point?

It was not clear why there had been a deterioration in pouch function and it was decided to undertake further tests. She underwent pelvic MRI, anorectal physiology with anal ultrasound, and an EUA with further pouchoscopy. Pelvic MRI was normal with no features of peri-pouch inflammation. Anorectal physiology and ultrasound showed intact sphincters with low normal resting and squeeze

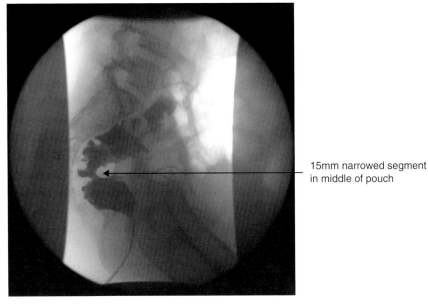

15mm narrowed segment
in middle of pouch

Figure 24.1 Pouchogram showing persistent mild narrowing in mid-section of pouch.

pressures. EUA and pouchoscopy showed no evidence of stenosis at the pouch anal anastomosis. The very short columnar cuff did not look inflamed. The ulceration in the mid portion of the pouch and pre-pouch ileum persisted, however. Pouchoscopy confirmed an area of mild stricturing (15 mm) in the mid section of the pouch (Figure 24.1).

The dominant findings were of mid- and pre-pouch inflammation, but with no definite features to make a diagnosis of Crohn's disease. The gastroenterology team felt it was reasonable to treat with adalimumab. This was followed by a significant improvement in pouch function and general wellbeing.

Pouch function continued at acceptable levels on maintenance adalimumab. She became pregnant in 2014 and delivered a healthy boy in September 2014. Pouch function did not change significantly during or immediately after pregnancy.

LEARNING POINTS

- Assessment of persisting pouch dysfunction. A useful *aide-mémoire* is to consider the pouch to be a box. Investigations should be: in the box, outside the box, above and below the box, and the box must empty normally.
- There is an emerging concept of "Crohn's like" complications in patients with a previous pouch for ulcerative colitis but no histological proof of Crohn's to clinch the diagnosis. Such patients may be managed conservatively with long-term seton drains and anti-TNF therapy.

LETTER FROM AMERICA

The inflammatory changes in the afferent limb (pre-pouch ileum), including ulceration and contact bleeding, do raise the specter of something more sinister than garden variety pouchitis. Is it Crohn's? Hard to know. Lucky for this patient that a trial of Crohn's medical therapy was successful. The alternative would have been an ostomy.

Jon Vogel and Massarat Zutshi

CASE 25

Low rectal cancer in a patient with ulcerative colitis: late reconstruction with continent Kock ileostomy

Par Myrelid[1] & Richard Lovegrove[2]

[1] *University Hospital of Linkoping, Linkoping, Sweden*
[2] *Mount Sinai Hospital, University of Toronto, Toronto, Canada*

A 50-year-old male with a 32-year history of ulcerative colitis presented with rectal bleeding and tenesmus. He was found to have a low rectal cancer just above the dentate line. The colitis was quiescent but extensive. Biopsy of the tumor confirmed adenocarcinoma. Staging by CT and rectal MR suggested a T3N0M0 tumor. He received preoperative chemo-radiotherapy followed by proctocolectomy and permanent end ileostomy. Postoperative recovery was uneventful. The pathology report showed a T3N2M0 tumor and he was offered postoperative adjuvant chemotherapy that he accepted. This was, however, stopped prematurely due to development of severe arthralgia thought to be chemotherapy related.

His arthralgia did not improve and he was put on steroids and later become steroid dependent. He developed a small parastomal hernia. Although the ileostomy functioned normally, the patient struggled to cope with it. Follow-up CT scans at 12 and 24 months postoperatively showed no evidence of recurrent disease.

The patient had heard about continent ileostomy and pushed for a referral for consideration of continent Kock pouch reconstruction.

DECISION POINT

Is it reasonable to consider Kock continent reconstruction in this situation?

The patient was highly motivated and extremely well informed about the option of continent Kock pouch reconstruction. However, we felt that this was inappropriate for several reasons.

Colorectal Surgery: Clinical Care and Management, First Edition.
Edited by Bruce George, Richard Guy, Oliver Jones, and Jon Vogel.
© 2016 John Wiley & Sons, Ltd. Published 2016 by John Wiley & Sons, Ltd.

- He was only 2 years on from treatment for an N2 low rectal carcinoma.
- He was still on steroids for his arthralgia.
- He had unrealistic expectations about the success of Kock pouch surgery.
- He was not coping with his ileostomy. Unclear if this was predominantly because of psychological issues, arthralgia or parastomal hernia.

He agreed to wait until at least a further 12 months. He saw a rheumatologist who diagnosed rheumatoid arthritis. He was treated with hydroxychlorochin. Steroid treatment was gradually weaned.

Two years later, 4 years post cancer treatment, a CT scan of chest and abdomen showed no signs of either local recurrence or distant metastases. The patient remained keen to undergo Kock pouch reconstruction.

DECISION POINT

Is it reasonable to offer Kock pouch reconstruction now?

At this point, it was felt reasonable to proceed with Kock pouch reconstruction. He was cancer free 4 years after diagnosis and was off steroids. He had been counseled repeatedly regarding the risks of Kock pouch surgery. He had coped well with the process of delaying surgery and appeared to be psychologically robust.

He proceeded to laparotomy. At operation, there was no evidence of tumor recurrence and mild soft adhesions. The end ileostomy was mobilized. A Kock pouch was created using approximately 45 cm of the terminal ileum (Figure 25.1). A spherical pouch was made with running sutures and then stapling of the nipple with a bladeless stapler (Figure 25.2). A leak test of the pouch as well as a continence test of the nipple valve were performed (Figure 25.3). The stoma opening

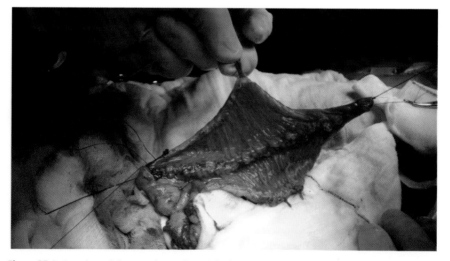

Figure 25.1 Creation of the pouch starting with the opening antemesenterically of 30 cm of distal ileum, leaving the the most distal 15 cm of the ileum untouched.

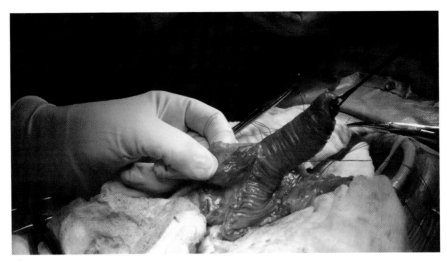

Figure 25.2 The nipple is created from the most proximal part of the remaining terminal ileum using three cartridges and a bladeless stapler.

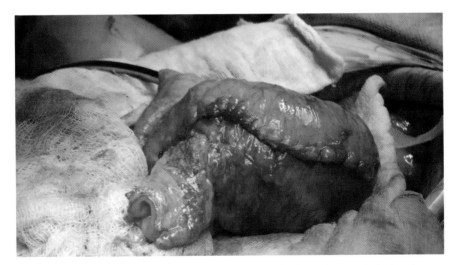

Figure 25.3 Intraoperative filling of pouch with saline to check continence of nipple valve.

in the lower left quadrant was closed after a repair of the parastomal hernia with nonresorbable sutures. The pouch was left intubated with a dwelling and secured Medina catheter for the first 2 weeks and then spigotted during day time and opened during night time for another 2 weeks.

The postoperative period was uneventful and he was brought back to outpatient clinic for removal of the catheter 30 days postoperatively. He now empties his Kock pouch 3–5 times daily using a Medina catheter and it is fully continent.

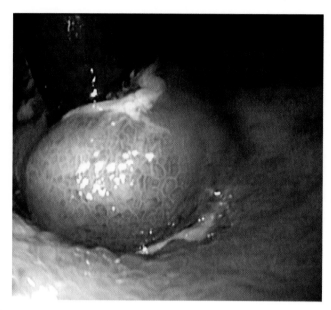

Figure 25.4 One year after formation of the pouch, a pouchoscopy was performed. The nipple valve is quite low but still completely continent.

At 18 months post Kock pouch surgery, he remains well with a continent pouch (Figure 25.4). He has not required any revisional surgery.

LEARNING POINTS

- The continent ileostomy was initially developed by Nils G. Kock of Gothenburg, Sweden, in the 1960s [1]. Since the introduction of ileal pouch anal anastomosis (IPAA), the need for continent ileostomy has diminished drastically. Currently, situations where a continent Kock pouch might be considered are:
  - IPAA not appropriate due to sphincter weakness
  - salvage after failed IPAA
  - previous proctocolectomy and end ileostomy for UC
  - previous proctocolectomy and end ileostomy for exclusively large bowel Crohn's disease with no small bowel disease at long-term follow-up.
- The major problems with Kock pouch surgery are technical, especially related to the nipple valve construction [2, 3]. Revisional surgery is required in approximately one-third of patients. Recognized technical problems include sliding of the nipple valve, nipple base fistula, dislocation of the pouch from the abdominal wall, and stricturing. Pouchitis may also occur and is treated along similar lines to pouchitis after IPAA.

LETTER FROM AMERICA

The ASCRS clinical practice guidelines endorse the use of a continent ileostomy in cases in which an ileal pouch anal anastomosis or a conventional ileostomy is either impractical or undesirable. These guidelines include notation indicating that long-term complications, most often incontinence or obstruction due to valve dysfunction, may occur in up to 60% of cases.

Jon Vogel and Massarat Zutshi

References

1 Kock NG. Intra-abdominal "reservoir" in patients with permanent ileostomy. Preliminary observations on a procedure resulting in fecal "continence" in five ileostomy patients. *Arch Surg* 1969; **99**(2):223–31.

2 Lepisto AH, Jarvinen HJ. Durability of Kock continent ileostomy. *Dis Colon Rectum* 2003; **46**(7):925–8.

3 Wasmuth HH, Trano G, Wibe A, Endreseth BH, Rydning A, Myrvold HE. Failed pelvic pouch substituted by continent ileostomy. *Colorectal Dis* 2010; **12**(7 online):e109–13.

SECTION C
Pelvic floor disorders

Oliver Jones

Oxford University Hospitals NHS Foundation Trust, Oxford, UK

Introduction

The pelvis is often considered to consist of three compartments: the anterior compartment comprising the bladder and urethra, the middle compartment (in females) containing the vagina, uterus, fallopian tubes and ovaries, and the posterior compartment of rectum and anus. The relationship between the three compartments is interdependent as they are bound together by the pelvic fascia and supported on the levator ani muscles. For the purposes of this chapter, we will be focusing predominantly on the posterior compartment, as this is the area of most interest to the colorectal surgeon.

Different anatomical and pathophysiological changes may produce a multitude of simultaneous symptoms, creating a diagnostic challenge for the clinician. Attempting to separate the three pelvic compartments into convenient symptom groups is unrealistic and, ideally, colorectal surgeons with an interest in pelvic floor disorders should be aware of important overlap with gynecological and urological specialists. Indeed, healthy collaboration between these groups and various other clinicians, such as psychiatrists, psychologists, chronic pain specialists and nurses in a true multidisciplinary fashion, is probably essential in dealing with some of these difficult and protracted functional problems. This chapter by necessity will, however, focus on individual conditions even though this is often an oversimplification of the presenting complaints.

External rectal prolapse

Incidence and etiology

Rectal prolapse is the extrusion of the rectal wall and mucosa beyond the anal verge. It will often resolve after an acute presentation in children when it may

Colorectal Surgery: Clinical Care and Management, First Edition.
Edited by Bruce George, Richard Guy, Oliver Jones, and Jon Vogel.
© 2016 John Wiley & Sons, Ltd. Published 2016 by John Wiley & Sons, Ltd.

be associated with an obvious precipitating factor such as diarrhea. However, in general terms, in adults, it tends to recur and most surgeons would advocate repair [1].

External prolapse has been estimated to have an annual incidence of 2.5 per 100,000 population [2].

Clinical assessment

It is important also to ask about constipation and incontinence, either of which may co-exist. Incontinence may occur through perpetual stimulation of the rectoanal inhibitory reflex by the prolapse and resulting internal sphincter inhibition. This appears to recover after surgery [3]. However, whilst improvement in continence is seen in most patients after correction of the prolapse by any method, the abdominal route seems to be more effective [4]. Constipation is seen in one-third to two-thirds of patients [5]. Some surgeons would advocate tailoring the surgical approach to minimize the risk of postoperative constipation.

The patient presenting with rectal prolapse will often be able to demonstrate the prolapse when "bearing down" in clinic.

Treatment

The choice of operation is a contentious issue. There have been many surgical descriptions over the years, reflecting the fact that few operations are suitable for all patients, and "one size doesn't fit all." The surgeon should consider patient fitness and the potential morbidity and mortality of each approach, as well as durability and functional outcome of repair. In broad terms, the surgical approaches can be divided into perineal operations and abdominal operations.

Perineal procedures

The perineal approach entails exteriorization of the rectum with no abdominal incision being made. The most common perineal procedures are perineal rectosigmoidectomy (Altemeier's operation) [6] and mucosectomy with muscle wall plication (Delorme's operation) [7] (see **Case 26**). These operations have the advantage that they can be performed under locoregional anesthesia and so may be advantageous in frail patients. The perineal approach has also previously been advocated for younger patients, on the assumption that there was thought to be a lower risk of sexual nerve dysfunction compared to conventional abdominal procedures such as the posterior rectopexy. A recent randomized trial has suggested no difference between the two perineal approaches in terms of recurrence rates [8], but recurrence rates were surprisingly high for both groups, being seen in 24/102 (24%) patients undergoing Altemeier's versus 31/99 (31%) undergoing Delorme's procedures.

Abdominal procedures

Abdominal procedures involve reduction and fixation of the prolapse (rectopexy). At its simplest, posterior mobilization of the rectum is undertaken followed by fixation of the rectum to the sacral promontory with a suture. Over 40 years ago, Frykman and Goldberg advocated the addition of sigmoid resection in addition to sutured rectopexy to offset the problem of postoperative constipation [9].

Over a number of years, there have been attempts to reduce the risk of recurrent prolapse by use of a mesh to provide a scaffold for scarring and fibrosis. The Ripstein repair involves the use of a mesh as an anterior sling that encircles the rectum [10]. Historically, there were problems with the mesh being too tight with resultant obstructed defecation. The Wells rectopexy involves posterior mobilization and placement of a mesh sling that is attached to the sacrum posteriorly and is partially wrapped around the lateral aspects of the rectum [11]. Yet another operation is the Orr–Loygue procedure that entails lateral fixation of the mesh to the rectum, with fixation of a mesh in turn to the sacral promontory [12].

There are over 100 operations described for rectal prolapse and this, in large part, is because each operation has potential disadvantages. Few surgeons are comfortable performing all operations and many patients are too frail for some operations, particularly open abdominal procedures. Prolapse recurrence is an obvious endpoint to measure when comparing operations, as are morbidity and mortality, but constipation and continence scores and quality of life are also important. Historically, the quality of trials in rectal prolapse has been poor. A Cochrane review of 2008 found only 12 randomized trials and even these were of such poor quality that the authors concluded that it was not possible to use their review to guide practice [13]. For example, only one trial had compared the abdominal and perineal approaches, and that trial randomized only 20 patients [14].

The recently published PROSPER study has attempted to address this [15]. This was a multicenter, factorial (2 × 2) design trial in which patients were randomized between abdominal and perineal surgery, with suture versus resection rectopexy for those having an abdominal procedure, or Altemeier's versus Delorme's for those undergoing a perineal procedure. Some 293 patients were recruited to 340 comparisons. Overall, the high rate of recurrent prolapse was striking. For the resection versus suture rectopexy comparison, recurrence rates were 4/32 (13%) and 9/35 (26%), respectively. Finally, a comparison of perineal versus abdominal approaches yielded recurrence rates of 5/25 (20%) and 5/19 (26%), respectively. Overall, the authors concluded that there was no significant difference between operations and they were unable to recommend one approach over another. Similarly, continence scores and quality of life were significantly improved compared to baseline in all groups, although no differences were seen between the randomized comparisons.

Laparoscopic approach

Many of these operations are now performed laparoscopically. Solomon *et al.* undertook a randomized trial of 40 patients comparing laparoscopic and open posterior mesh rectopexy (without resection) [16]. The trial favored the laparoscopic approach and reported that these patients had less postoperative pain, earlier return to diet and a quicker discharge from hospital, although surgery took longer in the laparoscopic group. There was one recurrence in the open group (median follow-up 24 months).

Laparoscopic ventral mesh rectopexy (VMR) was first described in the literature in its current form by d'Hoore *et al.* [17]. Whilst the patients in this series all had external prolapse, the secondary symptom of incontinence improved in 28 of 31 patients, whilst obstructed defecation improved in 16 of 19 patients. The very limited dissection of laparosopic VMR is said to be responsible for the very low rates of new-onset constipation after surgery [18]. The prolapse recurrence rate has been reported to be between 0% and 5% [19].

Laparoscopic VMR is well tolerated in the elderly. A recent report of laparoscopic VMR in 80 patients over the age of 80, with a mean American Society of Anesthesiology Grade of 2.44, had no mortality and a complication rate of 13%, most of which were minor. The authors argued that this approach had rendered perineal procedures obsolete (see **Case 27**).

The issue of mesh erosion is a new problem that is being increasingly reported. This may occur into the vagina, rectum or bladder and may result in fistulation. Many of these complications require bowel resection in addition to mesh removal [20]. There has been interest in the use of biological or absorbable meshes. It is not known whether this will reduce the mesh infection, nor indeed if the recurrence rate with absorbable meshes is higher [21]. A recent systematic review of short-term recurrence rates after laparoscopic VMR concluded that prolapse recurrence and mesh-related complications were similar in the two groups [22].

Fecal incontinence

Incidence and etiology

Fecal incontinence is a very common problem with the incidence dependent on thresholds for definition and the population under study. However, most studies would put the incidence at around 10% [23].

Sphincter injury has been shown to be associated with a prolonged second stage of labor, instrumental delivery, and episiotomy. Not all obstetric injuries are purely structural injuries of the sphincter complex. For example, neuropraxia of the pudendal nerves may occur during delivery [24] or there may be loss of rectal support resulting in prolapse, leading to loss of continence in the presence of an anatomically intact sphincter.

Clinical assessment and scoring

A detailed history from the patient is paramount, including obstetric background.

Clinical examination should include assessment of the perineum for scars from obstetric tears, episiotomy, and surgery. Asking the patient to bear down allows an evaluation of perineal descent, paradoxical contraction, and even external prolapse. Resting and squeeze pressures may be assessed by digital examination, although this is wholly subjective and notoriously inaccurate.

Investigation

Endoanal ultrasound (EAUS) and anorectal physiology (ARP) are cornerstones in the assessment of the patient with fecal incontinence. EAUS defines the structural integrity of the sphincter, although defects are common in the asymptomatic postpartum female and so images must be interpreted in the light of the patient's symptoms (Figure C.1).

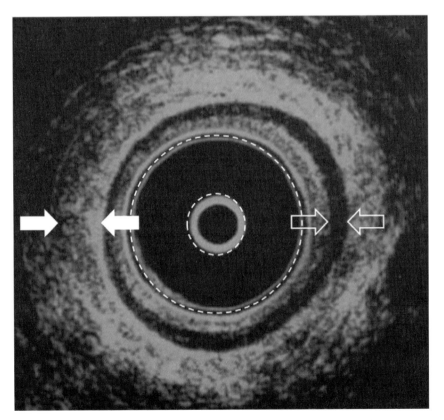

Figure C.1 Endoanal ultrasound appearance of the normal sphincter. The dotted line delineates the probe itself. The internal anal sphincter (delineated by the hollow arrows) appears as a dark circle with the external sphincter (solid arrows) appearing as a lighter structure due to its lower water content.

Anorectal physiology studies measure anal resting pressure (a surrogate for internal anal sphincter function) and squeeze pressure (predominantly external anal sphincter function). Rectal sensory function can be estimated by distension of a balloon in the rectum. With progressive balloon distension, the patient is usually asked to report the first sensation of distension that they detect, when they feel the urge to defecate and the time that they feel they can tolerate distension no longer. These are known as the first sensation, urge volume, and maximum tolerated volume, respectively. Pudendal nerve terminal motor latency (PNTML) is also sometimes measured by use of a St Mark's electrode on the examiner's finger that stimulates the pudendal nerve as it passes over the ischial spine, whilst recording the delay between this and the contraction of the external sphincter. The utility of PNTML in the management and selection of patients with fecal incontinence is controversial.

There is general consensus that these tests are mandatory in the incontinent patient. The utility of these tests has been investigated specifically in a study that showed that a combination of EAUS, ARP, and PNTML changed the surgeon's pretest operative management plan in around 10% of patients [25].

There is a growing consensus that evacuation proctography should also be part of the work-up for patients with fecal incontinence (see **Case 28**).

Treatment

Pelvic floor exercises and biofeedback

There is little standardization either in terminology or in practice with respect to pelvic floor exercises and biofeedback. The former may simply be considered as analogous to strengthening the pelvic floor muscles, whilst the latter is a slightly more specific term based on operant conditioning. Biofeedback utilizes equipment to record and/or amplify the activity of the pelvic floor and then feed this back to the patient. There is no consistent description as to the number of sessions and their duration for either intervention. Either or both may be delivered with more general instruction to the patient about toileting habits, diet, and drug use.

This diversity of definition and practice means that assessing the effectiveness of these interventions is challenging. A recent Cochrane review examined 1525 participants from 21 studies and was unable to conclude whether biofeedback was superior to pelvic floor or anal sphincter exercises alone [26]. It was also difficult to evaluate the value of the individual components of each of the regimens.

Dietary manipulation

The addition or reduction of fiber to the diet to control symptoms of fecal incontinence is contentious. Some authors have proposed high fiber whilst others have proposed a low-fiber diet. Lauti *et al.* conducted a randomized cross-over trial on 63 patients addressing this issue [27]. Patients were given 6 weeks of low-residue diet with placebo fiber supplement and loperamide followed by 6 weeks of fiber supplement, neutral diet, and loperamide, or the reverse order. The baseline Fecal Incontinence Severity Index (FISI) was 31. This fell to 18.4 after low-residue diet and placebo fiber and loperamide compared to 18.8 after fiber supplementation and loperamide (no significant difference). However, the authors reported marked differences in individual responses, with some patients favoring more fiber and others less. It would seem sensible to advise patients to experiment with changing fiber levels to see if this changes their symptoms.

Pharmacological manipulation

Loperamide has long been a mainstay of treatment of fecal incontinence. It is often preferred over codeine phosphate because of its lower side-effect profile, and in particular its tendency to cause less drowsiness and addiction. Apart from its effects as a constipating agent, it has other actions including increasing internal anal sphincter tone, increasing whole gut transit time, and possibly modifying local reflexes such as the rectoanal inhibitory reflex [28].There is good evidence for its effectiveness [29].

There has been some interest in using amitriptyline in patients with incontinence. There have been no randomized studies but an open-label study suggested considerable efficacy [30]. It reduced stool frequency and both the frequency and amplitude of rectal motor complexes.

There has also been interest in topical phenylephrine gel. This is an alpha-adrenergic agonist which has been shown to increase anal sphincter pressures in fecally incontinent patients with structurally normal sphincters. Its clinical effectiveness to date has not been demonstrated in any group other than ileoanal pouch patients [31].

Anal sphincter repair

Anal sphincter disruption is most commonly due to obstetric trauma, though more rarely seen after anorectal surgery and other trauma. Factors associated with anal sphincter obstetric trauma include episiotomy (especially when performed in the midline), third-degree tears, and instrumental delivery [32]. They can be classified into four grades of injury (Table C.1).

The incidence of sphincter injury after childbirth is high but depends on the method used to evaluate the problem, and many patients are asymptomatic. In a metaanalysis of studies assessing primiparous and multiparous women with EAUS, the incidence of sphincter disruption was 26.9% after first delivery, with an 8.5% incidence of new defects in multiparous women [33].

In most countries, colorectal surgeons are involved only in secondary anal sphincter repair some months or years after initial obstetric injury and primary repair. There is a general consensus that overlapping repair is better than end-to-end repair, although there is only a single, randomized trial addressing the subject which, whilst probably underpowered, failed to show any differences

Table C.1 Classification of anal sphincter injuries.

Grade of injury	Anatomical description of injury
I	Laceration of vaginal mucosa
II	Tear of transverse perinei muscles
IIIa IIIb IIIc	Tear of less than 50% of the external anal sphincter
	Tear of greater than 50% of the external anal sphincter
	Tear of the internal anal sphincter
IV	Tear involving the rectal mucosa

in outcome [34]. A single randomized trial of diversion (colostomy formation) versus no diversion for 27 patients undergoing sphincter repair suggests that wound breakdown and functional outcomes do not differ between the groups. However, the stoma itself, and its reversal, may be the source of significant morbidity [35]. Most surgeons would not advocate diversion prior to a secondary repair.

Several large series describe good results from sphincter repair in the short term, with around 60% of patients achieving some benefit [36]. However, there is emerging evidence that the benefit diminishes with time.

Malouf *et al.* reported the St Mark's Hospital experience of long-term outcome in 55 patients after sphincter repair with at least 5 years follow-up [37]. Overall, 47 patients were contactable, although a further nine were excluded as they had undergone further surgery for incontinence (seven patients) or had a stoma (one patient following proctectomy for Crohn's disease, one patient never having had a covering stoma closed after sphincter repair). Of the remaining 38 patients, 20 still wore a pad and 25 patients reported lifestyle restriction. Only 23 patients had had a "successful outcome," defined as no further surgery and urge incontinence less than once a month. The Cleveland Clinic group has described functional outcomes of a cohort of patients following sphincter repair at both 5 [38] and 10 years [39]. There was significant deterioration in function between the two reports, suggesting that there was ongoing deterioration in their cohort between 5 and 10 years. The pathophysiology of this remains unclear.

Younger age and absence of pudendal neuropathy both appear to be predictors for a better outcome from sphincter repair.

Sacral nerve stimulation

In recent years, a number of new therapies have emerged for the treatment of fecal incontinence. Sacral nerve stimulation (SNS) seems the most promising of these, although the mechanism of its action remains rather obscure [40].

Sacral nerve stimulation was initially applied to patients with fecal incontinence with intact or minimally disrupted sphincters [41]. More recently, however, it has been performed in patients with external sphincter defects too, with good results. A study of SNS from Chan and Tjandra included 21 patients who had external sphincter defects [42]. Weekly incontinent episodes decreased from 13.8 to 5 (p<0.0001) for patients with external sphincter defects, a finding replicated in other studies (see **Case 29**)

Long-term follow-up is needed for these patients, with battery changes needed every 6–10 years and troubleshooting of any problems with the device occasionally required (see **Case 30**).

Laparoscopic ventral mesh rectopexy

Although not initally developed as a treatment for fecal incontinence, laparoscopic VMR has also been shown to improve continence in patients with fecal incontinence and internal rectal prolapse [43]. Historically, defecating proctography has not been part of the work-up for the patient with fecal incontinence, yet a study from Oxford has suggested that high-grade intussusception may be a common finding in the patient with "unexplained" fecal incontinence [44].

Obstructed defecation

Incidence and etiology

Obstructed defecation (OD) is a common problem but there is little data on its incidence; a figure of around 10–20% of adults would seem to be a reasonable estimate. It is one of the causes of constipation, and is generally distinguished from impaired colonic transit or slow transit constipation which, although considered separately in this chapter, may often co-exist.

The causes of OD may range from functional causes, most commonly anismus, or anatomical ones including rectal prolapse, enterocele, and rectocele. An enterocele is a downward herniation of the peritoneum into the rectovaginal septum, whilst a rectocele is a failure of the rectovaginal septum, resulting in bulging forward of the rectum into the vagina.

The prime etiology is childbirth though this initial injury may cause few symptoms until aging and the menopause exacerbate the initial obstetric injury. However, it is also noteworthy that many patients may be nulliparous or male. Previous pelvic surgery, in particular hysterectomy, may play an important etiological role [45].

Clinical assessment and scoring

A careful history should include questions on toileting habits. Particularly relevant questions are the number of bowel movements weekly, time spent on the toilet, the number of unsuccessful visits, toilet revisiting and assistance, either through vaginal or anal digitation. Background history should also include obstetric and surgical history.

Clinical assessment of the patient should include an inspection of the perineum for scarring, and digital assessment for resting and squeeze sphincter pressure. During the digital examination, the patient can be asked to bear down and the clinician may make an assessment of appropriate puborectalis relaxation. If contraction is felt, then a diagnosis of anismus should be considered. Rectal examination can also assess for the presence of a rectocele. Rigid sigmoidoscopy is a simple test that looks for intraluminal pathology and, on withdrawal of the scope with the patient bearing down, it may be possible to make an assessment of internal rectal prolapse (rectal intussusception).

Diagnosis

Defecating (evacuation) proctography is the key radiological investigation for OD (Figure C.2). Useful information includes the degree of emptying of rectal contrast and the appropriate, or inappropriate, relaxation of the puborectalis.

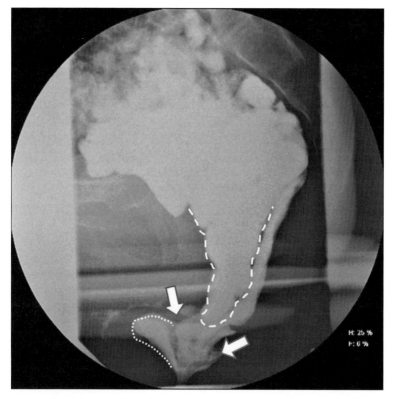

Figure C.2 Still image from a defecating proctogram. The intussusception is shown as an infolding of the rectal wall, delineated by the white arrows. The rectocele bulges forward from the rectum into the vagina (shown in this study with a dotted line; the patient consented to having a contrast-soaked tampon inserted into the vagina). An enterocele is also shown (indicated by the dashed line), the patient having ingested oral contrast 1 hour prior to the start of the study.

Table C.2 Oxford Prolapse Grading System.

Grade	Anatomical description
1	Full-thickness infolding of rectal wall
2	Prolapse of rectal wall to the top of the rectocele
3	Prolapse of the rectal wall to the top of the anal canal
4	Prolapse of the rectal wall into anal canal
5	Prolapse of rectal wall beyond anal verge (external prolapse)

Source: Wijffels *et al*. [46]. Reproduced with permission of Wiley.

Anatomically, the radiologist can report on the size and depth of the rectocele and whether it traps barium. However, it is controversial whether these parameters correlate with symptoms or are predictors of outcome from surgery [47].

One of the principal uses of proctography has been to assess the degree of internal prolapse. There are many ways of reporting this intussusception, but one of the simplest and most widely used systems is the Oxford Prolapse Grade (Table C.2).

The significance of "abnormalities" found at proctography continues to be debated widely. One of the most widely quoted (and misquoted) papers is that of Shorvon *et al.* which analyzed proctographic results in 47 normal volunteers [48]. The headline figures state that rectoceles were seen in 81% of women and 13% of men. However, most of these were small and only one subject had a rectocele more than 2 cm in depth. Few surgeons would consider a rectocele of less than 2 cm to be of any significance. There were no cases of external prolapse seen. However, intussusception was reported as being seen in 50% of men and 50% of women, although the authors include within these figures rectorectal intussusception that many surgeons now regard as insignificant. When one considers only rectoanal intussusception, the figures drop to 21% and 19%, respectively. These figures are still significant and illustrate that proctographic appearances need to be considered carefully in the light of a patient's symptoms and a surgeon's clinical examination findings.

Treatment

Rectocele

Most surgeons would recommend initial conservative treatment of a rectocele. Laxatives, fluid intake, and pelvic floor retraining may help many patients [49]. However, as mentioned above, there are few clues from proctography in terms of which patients are likely to fail conservative measures and, similarly, there are no reliable proctographic predictors of response to surgery. From a symptom perspective, there is no real evidence that the need to digitate vaginally preoperatively predicts a favorable outcome from surgery [50]. However, patients with symptoms suggestive of slow transit constipation and those using regular laxatives seem to be at increased risk of poor outcome from surgery [51].

The options for surgical repair are usually classified into transvaginal, transrectal, and transperineal. Transvaginal repair involves excision of vaginal mucosa from the posterior vaginal wall with plication of the rectovaginal fascial defect, variously done longitudinally or transversely, usually combined with a repair of the perineal body. There are advantages to the vaginal approach: it provides the surgeon with an opportunity to combine the surgery with repair of an enterocele or cystocele, and a vaginal vault prolapse repair may also be undertaken. A wide spectrum of results has been reported in the literature, but around 60–80% report an improvement in symptoms, especially that of vaginal bulge, although symptoms of persistent or new-onset digitation or fecal incontinence are common [52]. One of the concerns with the transvaginal approach is the potential for increased dyspareunia [53].

The problem of dyspareunia was a driver for the development of the transanal approach to rectocele repair. This involves the elevation of mucosal flaps over the rectocele and transverse or longitudinal plication of the muscle and fascia before the mucosal edges are trimmed and closed. The transanal approach has the disadvantage of requiring anal instrumentation and dilatation, and studies suggest that around one-fifth of patients experience some fecal incontinence postoperatively [54]. A reported benefit of the approach is in avoiding a vaginal incision and thus having a lower rate of dyspareunia.

There have been two randomized trials comparing the transvaginal and transrectal approaches. The first of these included 30 patients; there was significant overall improvement with both techniques, although there was a trend towards a reduced need for vaginal digitation in those patients undergoing the vaginal approach. Recurrence rates were significantly higher in the transrectal group (40% versus 7%). There were no reports of *de novo* dyspareunia in either group, with 27% patients overall reporting an improvement in this symptom [55]. Similar results in favor of the transvaginal approach were reported from a second randomized trial [56].

A newer transanal approach to rectocele is the stapled transanal rectal resection (STARR), which involves the firing of two circular staplers placed transanally. The first resects the anterior intussusception and corrects the redundant rectocele, whilst the second firing resects the posterior intussusception. This is considered in more detail below in the section dealing with the surgical treatment of intussusception.

A less common approach to the surgical management of rectocele is the transperineal approach. This may be combined with an anal sphincter repair through the same incision. There is less data available for this approach.

Intussusception

Studies reporting outcomes from pelvic floor retraining often group together patients with very general symptoms or pathology. We have reported on 120 patients with symptoms of fecal incontinence or obstructed defecation, all patients having undergone proctography prior to retraining. There were significant improvements in fecal incontinence, constipation, and quality of life after pelvic floor retraining but only in those without intussusception [57].

Over the years, there have been a number of descriptions of surgical approaches to internal prolapse. One approach has been the internal Delorme's procedure with a circumferential rectal mucosectomy and rectal plication [58].

Stapled transanal rectal resection has also been widely used for the treatment of intussusception, as well as for the treatment of rectocele, as outlined above. A randomized controlled trial has compared STARR to biofeedback in the treatment of OD in patients with intussusception and rectocele. STARR was a more effective treatment for OD, although interestingly there was significant improvement in both groups for this parameter and quality of life relative to baseline. However, dropout rate was high in both groups, with 14% dropout in the surgery group and 50% of those allocated to biofeedback failing to complete their treatment.

The European STARR registry reported the results of 2838 patients undergoing the operation. It reported significant improvements in obstructed defecation and symptom severity scores. However, it reported urgency in 20% of patients. There were two significant complications: rectal necrosis and rectovaginal fistula.

Historically, there had been a feeling that rectopexy was an ineffective treatment for obstructed defecation [59], yet in these historical studies there had generally been an extensive posterior dissection, but the application of laparoscopic VMR has changed this. The initial findings that incontinence and OD in patients with external prolapse improved after rectopexy led to the application of the operation to those with intussusception. This has been controversial because of the common finding of intussusception in asymptomatic patients, and the belief that internal prolapse seldom developed into external prolapse, implying that these are two different conditions, rather than part of a spectrum. This latter hypothesis remains controversial [60].

However, in recent years, a number of centers have reported their experience of treating patients with internal prolapse with laparoscopic VMR. Surgeons in Bristol, UK, reported resolution of OD in 20 of 25 (80%) patients with internal prolapse [61], and this was followed by reports from other centers [62] (See **Case 31**).

Some centers have advocated the use of robotic surgery for rectopexy. This may have advantages in facilitating dissection deep into the rectovaginal septum and also for suturing. A nonrandomized comparison from Nantes, France, has suggested that OD scores may be better in patients undergoing robotic rectopexy compared with those having conventional laparoscopic surgery [63]. Further data are awaited on this subject.

There has been interest in mesh-related morbidity, in particular mesh erosion. This is considered in more detail in the section on external prolapse. Finally, many patients have both an evacuatory and a transit problem. A recent review of experience in Oxford suggests that these patients are equally well served by rectopexy with similar outcomes to those with an isolated evacuatory problem [64].

Enterocele

Symptomatic enteroceles should be managed conservatively in the first instance. For those failing conservative measures, repair may be undertaken via the perineal or abdominal route. Gynecologists more commonly employ a perineal approach for cystocele and rectocele repair. It is noteworthy that STARR in isolation does not correct an enterocele and, indeed, many surgeons consider an enterocele to be a relative contraindication to this procedure [65].

By contrast, many abdominal enterocele repairs are done in combination with rectopexy. It is difficult to establish, therefore, the importance of an enterocele, and its repair, in isolation. It may be that it is little more than a marker of severe pelvic floor weakness and is seen more commonly with more advanced prolapse as the peritoneum of the pouch of Douglas is pulled ever further caudally [66].

Solitary rectal ulcer (see Case 51)

Solitary rectal ulcer is a poorly understood condition which is characterized histologically by mucosal thickening and extension of smooth muscle fibers up between the crypts [67]. It is known to be associated with rectal prolapse, which may be internal (intussusception) or external [68].

Traditional surgical approaches have included local excision of the ulcer, low anterior resection, stoma, and rectopexy. Outcomes are variable and, historically, there has been a high stoma rate [69].

Experience in Oxford of 36 patients with solitary rectal ulcer has recently been published. The underlying pathology was intussusception in 20 patients, external prolapse in 14 patients, and anismus in two patients. Some 29 patients underwent laparoscopic VMR, of whom nine required a further procedure. Full ulcer healing was seen in 90% of patients [70]. Similar success has been published by other centers [71].

Slow transit constipation

Incidence and etiology

Slow transit constipation is a common problem, although incidence is difficult to define owing to variability in its definition [72]. Most now regard the Rome criteria as the best guide (see later).

Slow transit constipation (STC) is due to myopathy or neuropathy of the colon. An abnormality or absence of interstitial cells of Cajal has been postulated to be responsible for constipation in many patients with slow transit. These are the so-called "pacemaker" cells of the colonic wall.

Clinical assessment and scoring

A history of relevant predisposing medical conditions should be sought, including immobility, disability, dementia and neurological disease, as well as endocrine problems, including diabetes and hypothyroidism. Metabolic abnormalities such as hypercalcemia and hypokalemia should be excluded.

The important distinction is from patients with obstructed defecation, and proctography is key to distinguishing the two. Furthermore, constipation-predominant irritable bowel syndrome may be similar in presentation to STC, but is usually characterized by prominent symptoms of bloating and pain, and differs from STC in that colonic transit is normal.

Anorectal physiology may be helpful in assessing the rectoanal inhibitory reflex which is a simple screening test to rule out short-segment Hirschsprung's disease. Colonoscopy – endoscopic or radiological – is rarely helpful, although it is important to rule out luminal pathology.

Diagnosis

The cardinal feature of STC is delayed transit through the colon. The simplest and most widely used method of assessment is that of Hinton, in which radiopaque markers are swallowed and a plain abdominal radiograph obtained after 5 days. Fewer than 20% of the markers should remain in the colon of a patient with normal transit [73]. An alternative test is scintigraphy, for which the patient ingests a radioisotope before abdominal scanning with a gamma camera. The percentage of total radioisotope activity remaining within the colon gives an indication of transit time.

Treatment

Initial treatment of STC should be conservative. A high-fiber diet supplemented with laxatives – osmotic or stimulant – may be helpful. This may be supplemented by enemas or suppositories. A newer laxative is the selective 5-hydroxytryptamine agonist prucalopride. There is good evidence from randomized, placebo-controlled trials that this may be beneficial for some patients in improving bowel function and reducing symptoms [74]. Biofeedback is often advocated for STC, although evidence for its efficacy is weak. In a study of 30 consecutive, unselected patients with constipation, there was significant improvement in bowel frequency and reduction in straining. Transit time improved in eight of nine patients with initially slow transit, whilst it paradoxically lengthened in four of 11 patients in whom it was initially normal [75].

The role of surgery in STC is controversial. Stoma formation is typically done in three scenarios: as definitive treatment, as a treatment prior to colectomy or as a treatment after colectomy as a consequence of poor function. Its value as a prelude to colectomy may be in selecting patients for resection, as it is postulated that those with a high stoma output may be at higher risk of poor function with an ileorectal anastomosis. Furthermore, a significant number of patients undergoing colectomy ultimately have a stoma and, in some series, this stoma rate may be almost as high as one in four patients [76]. Pretreatment with a stoma may help patients weigh up the risks and benefits of colectomy, given that the end stage may mean a stoma.

A recent study from the Cleveland Clinic reported results of subtotal colectomy, with outcomes considered for those patients with isolated slow transit and those with both slow transit and obstructed defecation. In total, their series contained 144 patients, with 44% having laparoscopic and 56% open colectomy with ileorectal anastomosis. Seven patients had had an initial diverting ileostomy. Median follow-up was 43 months in this telephone study, with 5% of patients in each group having a subsequent ileostomy for poor functional outcomes. There were high levels of patient satisfaction in both groups [77].

In a review of a case series of 32 patients undergoing colectomy for STC over almost 20 years, Knowles *et al.* concluded that median satisfaction rate after surgery was 86% [78]. The median number of bowel movements was 2.9 per day. Some 14% of patients reported incontinence and diarrhea, respectively, with 5% having a stoma. There seemed to be a high rate of small bowel obstruction (18%) with 14% requiring reoperation, although this may decrease in the future with increasing use of the laparoscopic approach. The variability of outcomes in the published case series has led to much interest in trying to identify criteria for selection. Much of the focus has been on trying to exclude those patients with delayed small bowel transit, patients with a predominantly evacuatory disorder, and those patients with significant psychological issues. More studies are needed in this area.

Sacral nerve stimulation is also being used increasingly for constipation. In a recent review of 13 studies (10 in adults), success rate with temporary stimulation was found to vary between 42% and 100%. Of those patients given a permanent implant, up to 87% showed improvement at a mean follow-up of 28 months [79].

The use of the antegrade colonic enema (ACE) procedure, first described by Malone [80], in which the appendix is amputated, reversed and then reinserted into the cecal pole for irrigation through a continent conduit, has also been applied in adults. However, although there is a paucity of published information, the results in adults may be inferior to those in the pediatric population [81].

Anismus

Incidence and etiology

Anismus is a functional form of constipation in which there is failure of pelvic floor relaxation during attempts at defecation. It has also been referred to

Table C.3 Rome III criteria for functional constipation. These must have been fulfilled for the previous 3 months with symptom onset at least 6 months prior to diagnosis.

Grade	Criteria
1	Must include two or more of the following:
	(a) Straining during at least 25% of defecations
	(b) Lumpy or hard stools in at least 25% of defecations
	(c) Sensation of incomplete evacuation for at least 25% of defecations
	(d) Sensation of anorectal obstruction/blockage for at least 25% of defecations
	(e) Manual maneuvers to facilitate at least 25% of defecations (e.g. digital evacuation, support of the pelvic floor)
	(f) Fewer than three defecations per week
2	Loose stools are rarely present without the use of laxatives
3	Insufficient criteria for irritable bowel syndrome

variously as puborectalis syndrome, pelvic dyssynergia, and spastic pelvic floor syndrome.

Its classic symptoms are those of straining, incomplete evacuation, and bloating. Many patients employ digitation to facilitate defecation.

Although early definitions of the condition hinged on the ability to expel an inflated rectal balloon and electromyographic (EMG) evidence of nonrelaxation of the pelvic floor during attempts to defecate, there has been a move away from these tests and few centers perform EMG routinely now.

One prerequisite for diagnosis is the Rome III criteria for functional constipation (Table C.3).

Diagnosis

A full pelvic floor examination is imperative. The specific sign for anismus is failure of the external sphincter and/or puborectalis to relax during straining. Practically, this can be a difficult sign to elicit in the outpatient clinic with an anxious patient.

A proctographic study of patients with a clinical and EMG-based diagnosis of anismus and normal controls was published in 1995 [82]. This suggested that incomplete evacuation of rectal contrast after 30 seconds was seen in over 80% patients with anismus, whilst complete evacuation was seen in all 20 control patients. Whether this distinguishes adequately between patients with mechanical and functional constipation is contentious. Indeed, for those patients who fail to respond to conventional treatments for anismus, many would advocate a further look by examination under anesthesia for an undiagnosed alternative diagnosis [83].

Treatment

Biofeedback has traditionally been the mainstay of treatment for anismus. As mentioned elsewhere in this chapter, there is little standardization of technique for biofeedback, and balloon expulsion-based, EMG, and manometry-based techniques have all been described. There have been no randomized trials and most studies are small with short follow-up. One of the larger studies considered 209 patients with anismus, of whom 173 patients had more than one biofeedback session and formed the study group. Interestingly, of these, only 62% completed their treatment and of these, 55% improved [84].

Surgical treatment has fallen out of favor. Historically, there have been reports of division of puborectalis and anal dilatation but these are not widely performed any more.

Botulinum toxin has emerged as a relatively new treatment for anismus. It has been widely used for spastic disorders of skeletal muscle and has an acceptable long-term side-effect profile. The initial report of its use in anismus described seven patients, with reported improvements in four, with 12 months of follow-up [85].Experience in Oxford has recently been reported [86]. In a series of 56 patients, response was seen in 22 (39%), although this effect gradually wore off after 3–6 months. Repeat injection was performed in 21 patients and all but one (95%) had a sustained response at median follow-up of 19 months. All of the 34 nonresponders underwent examination under anesthetic and 31 had a grade 3–5 prolapse, one an internal sphincter myopathy, and one an anal fissure.

Chronic anorectal pain (see Case 32)

Background

The terminology used for considering chronic anorectal pain is confusing. It is a syndrome involving neurological, musculoskeletal, and endocrine systems and some interaction with behavioral and psychological factors. Chronic idiopathic perineal pain is an umbrella term used to describe the subgroups of patients who present with chronic anorectal pain [87]. Chronic proctalgia is a term used traditionally for the most common pain syndromes termed proctalgia fugax, levator ani syndrome, and coccygodynia, although the Rome III system includes only levator ani syndrome and proctalgia fugax in its classification [88].

Pudendal neuralgia is the term used to describe pain secondary to injury to the pudendal nerve, whilst pudendal pain syndrome refers to pain when there is no obvious injury to the nerve.

Proctalgia fugax

Thaysen introduced the term "proctalgia fugax" in the 1950s. It is characterized by sudden, short, intense pain which is anal in distribution [89]. In most patients, it occurs less than five times per year. It tends to occur at night and is self-limiting, affecting 8–18% [90, 91] of the population aged 30–60. It is equally common in men and women. Unlike levator ani syndrome, patients are asymptomatic during examination and no characteristic clinical findings can be found to support the diagnosis.

Chronic idiopathic anal pain or levator ani syndrome

Patients with this condition will describe a dull ache within the rectum. The pain is exacerbated by sitting and lasts for hours to days. The prevalence in the general population is 6–7% between the ages of 30 and 60 years, with a female predilection [92]. There is an association with previous pelvic surgery or injury and psychological stress or anxiety. Clinically, there is tenderness on palpation of the levator ani muscles [93].

Coccygodynia

Coccygodynia refers to severe rectal, perineal, and sacrococcygeal pain which is more commonly seen in women. The key to diagnosis is manipulation of the coccyx that will trigger the pain and thus differentiate it from levator ani syndrome.

Pudendal neuralgia

Pudendal neuralgia is typically perceived in the perineum from anus to clitoris. Classically, it is a burning pain, worse with sitting, and many patients prefer to remain standing for relief [94]. Those with unilateral pain often favor sitting on one buttock. On clinical examination, pain may be elicited by pressure over the course of the pudendal nerve either by rectal or vaginal examination (see **Case 32**).

Etiology

Advanced or high-grade internal rectal prolapse may be associated with chronic idiopathic perineal pain, particularly when symptoms of obstructed defecation are present. Neil and Swash commented on the high prevalence of pelvic floor laxity in patients suffering from chronic rectal pain [95], and the real significance of internal prolapse only began to be addressed seriously much later in the 1990s and 2000s. Chronic anorectal pain is a common symptom in patients with advanced posterior compartment prolapse presenting with defecatory dysfunction. Some 50% of such patients will complain of pain at least some of the time. This pain often responds to antiprolapse surgery [96, 97].

Many patients with pudendal neuralgia will have a clear history of injury. This may be from previous surgery, including a neuropraxia related to positioning during hip surgery, from transvaginal or transobturator tapes (inserted for urinary stress incontinence), and sacrocolpopexy. Other causes include obstetric trauma and rarer infiltrative causes, including tumors. More chronic causes include chronic constipation and straining, bringing about a stretch of the nerves, prolonged sitting and exercise (especially cycling).

Other pathologies and tests for their exclusion

It is crucial to exclude the more simple causes of organic pain. These include the proctological conditions, most commonly anorectal sepsis, fissure or thrombosed hemorrhoids. Intraluminal pathology (typically anal or rectal cancer) can be excluded by endoscopy, whilst extraluminal or presacral pathology may be delineated by MRI scanning.

Investigations

Anorectal physiology and endoanal ultrasound should be standard work-up investigations. A thick, hypertensive internal anal sphincter is indicative of a rare inherited internal sphincter myopathy and should be confirmed following biopsy demonstrating inclusion bodies on electron microscopy. By contrast, a hypotensive, thickened internal sphincter suggests high-grade intussusception. Pudendal nerve latency may also be tested, but in many patients with pudendal neuralgia this will be normal.

Defecating proctography is very helpful when an underlying diagnosis of prolapse is suspected, although proctography may underestimate the presence of posterior compartment prolapse. It is of paramount importance to pursue a potential prolapse disorder in patients with chronic idiopathic perineal pain where there is a high clinical suspicion and inconclusive proctography. This is especially important if an enterocele is seen on proctography. Enterocele causes a feeling of pelvic pressure and pain and is suggestive of a posterior compartment prolapse and general pelvic floor weakness [98]. Examination under anesthesia is an extremely useful diagnostic tool where proctography has failed, as the true grade of prolapse can be assessed with the patient pain free and relaxed.

Treatment

Multimodality assessment and treatment of the patient with chronic pain is imperative. A combined surgical, pharmacological, rehabilitational, and psychological approach is needed.

The pharmacological treatment of chronic pain is well established. Drugs might include tricyclic antidepressants and antiepileptic drugs. Opioids may be useful, although constipation may be exacerbated.

If there is pudendal nerve entrapment, an injection of steroid and local anesthetic, under the guidance of a nerve stimulator to identify the nerve at the ischial spine, may be useful, whilst blocks of other nerves may also be undertaken and where necessary done under radiological guidance. There is increasing interest in nerve decompression, which is usually undertaken via the transgluteal or transperineal route [99].

Many patients with chronic idiopathic perineal pain will have evidence of posterior compartment prolapse. Many, but not all, of these patients have symptoms of obstructed defecation. Published data are awaited, but there is some emerging evidence that with careful case selection, treatment of this prolapse may bring about relief of the pain.

References

1 Jones OM, Cunningham C, Lindsey I. The assessment and management of rectal prolapse, rectal intussusception, rectocoele and enterocoele in adults. *BMJ* 2011; **342**:c7099.
2 Kairaluoma MV, Kellokumpu IH. Epidemiologic aspects of complete rectal prolapsed. *Scand J Surg* 2005; **94**:207–10.
3 Farouk R, Duthie GS, Bartolo DC, MacGregor AB. Restoration of continence following rectopexy for rectal prolapse and recovery of the internal anal sphincter electromyogram. *Br J Surg* 1992; **79**:439–40.
4 Tjandra JJ, Fazio VW, Church JM, Milsom JW, Oakley JR, Lavery IC. Ripstein procedure is an effective treatment for rectal prolapse without constipation. *Dis Colon Rectum* 1993; **36**:501–7.
5 Madoff R, Mellgren A. One hundred years of rectal prolapse surgery. *Dis Colon Rectum* 1999; **42**:441–50.
6 Altemeier WA, Culbertson WR, Schwengerdt C, *et al*. Nineteen years' experience with the one-stage perineal repair of rectal prolapse. *Ann Surg* 1971; **173**;993–1006.
7 Delorme R. Sur le traitment des prolapses du rectum totaux pour l'excision de la muscueuse rectale ou rectocolique. *Bull Mem Soc Chir Paris* 1900; **26**;499–518.
8 Senapati A, Gray RG, Middleton LJ, *et al*. PROSPER: a randomised comparison of surgical treatments for rectal prolapse. *Colorectal Dis* 2013; **15**:858–68.
9 Frykman HM, Goldberg SM. The surgical treatment of rectal procidentia. *Surg Gynecol Obstet* 1969; **129**:1225–30.
10 Ripstein CB. Treatment of massive rectal prolapse. *Am J Surg* 1952; **83**:68–71.
11 Wells C. New operation for rectal prolapse. *J Roy Soc Med* 1959; **52**:602–3.
12 Orr TG. A suspension operation for prolapse of the rectum. *Ann Surg* 1947; **126**:833–40.
13 Tou S, Brown SR, Malik AI, Nelson RL. Surgery for complete rectal prolapse in adults. *Cochrane Database Syst Rev* 2008; **4**:CD001758.
14 Deen KI, Grant E, Billingham C, Keighley MRB. Abdominal resection rectopexy with pelvic floor repair versus perianal rectosigmoidectomy and pelvic floor repair for full-thickness rectal prolapse. *Br J Surg* 1994; **81**:302–4.
15 Senapati A, Gray RG, Middleton LJ, *et al*. PROSPER: a randomised comparison of surgical treatments for rectal prolapse. *Colorectal Dis* 2013; **15**:858–68.
16 Solomon MJ, Young C, Eyers AA, Roberts RA. Laparoscopic versus open abdominal rectopexy for rectal prolapse. *Br J Surg* 2002; **89**:35–9.
17 D'Hoore A, Cadoni R, Penninckx F. Long-term outcomes of laparoscopic ventral rectopexy for total rectal prolapse. *Br J Surg* 2004; **91**:1500–5.
18 D'Hoore A, Penninckx F. Laparoscopic ventral recto(colpo)pexy for rectal prolapsed: surgical technique and outcome for 109 patients. *Surg Endosc* 2006; **20**:1919–23.
19 Slawik S, Soulsby R, Carter H, *et al*. Laparoscopic ventral rectopexy, posterior colporraphy and vaginal sacrocolpopexy for the treatment of recto-genital prolapse and mechanical outlet obstruction. *Colorectal Dis* 2008; **10**:138–43.

20 Badrek-Al Amoudi AH, Greenslade GL, Dixon AR. How to deal with complications after laparoscopic ventral rectopexy: lessons learnt from a tertiary referral centre. *Colorectal Dis* 2013; **15**:707–12.

21 Sileri P, Franceschilli L, de Luca E, *et al*. Laparoscopic ventral rectopexy for internal rectal prolapse using biological mesh: postoperative and short-term functional results. *J Gastrointestinal Surg* 2012; **16**:622–8.

22 Smart NJ, Pathak S, Boorman P, Daniels IR. Synthetic or biological mesh use in laparoscopic ventral rectopexy – a systematic review. *Colorectal Dis* 2013; **15**:650–4.

23 Brown SR, Wadhawan H, Nelson RL. Surgery for faecal incontinence in adults. *Cochrane Database Syst Rev* 2013; **7**:CD001757.

24 Keighley M, Williams N. Faecal incontinence. In: Keighley M, ed. *Surgery of the Anus, Colon and Rectum*, vol. **1**. London: WB Saunders, 2001; 592–700.

25 Liberman H, Faria J, Ternent C, Blatchford GJ, Christensen MA, Thorson AG. A prospective evaluation fo the value of anorectal physiology in the management of fecal incontinence. *Dis Colon Rectum* 2001; **44**:1567–74.

26 Norton C, Cody JD. Biofeedback and/or sphincter exercises for the treatment of faecal incontinence in adults. *Cochrane Database Syst Rev* 2012; **7**:CD002111.

27 Lauti M, Scott D, Thompson-Fawcett MW. Fibre supplementation in addition to loperamide for faecal incontinence in adults: a randomized trial. *Colorectal Dis* 2008; **10**:553–62.

28 Sun MW, Read NW, Verlinden M. Effects of loperamide oxide on gastrointestinal transit time and anorectal function in patients with chronic diarrhoea and faecal incontinence. *Scand J Gastroenterol* 1997; **32**:34–8.

29 Read M, Read NW, Barber DC, Duthie HL. Effects of loperamide on anal sphincter function in patients complaining of chronic diarrhoea with faecal incontinence and urgency. *Dig Dis Sci* 1982; **27**:807–14.

30 Santoro GA, Eitan BZ, Pryde A, Bartolo DC. Open study of low-dose amitriptyline in the treatment of patients with idiopathic fecal incontinence. *Dis Colon Rectum* 2000; **43**:1676–81.

31 Carapeti EA, Kamm MA, Nicholls RJ, Phillips RK. Randomized, controlled trial of topical phenylephrine for fecal incontinence in patients after ileoanal pouch construction. *Dis Colon Rectum* 2000; **43**:1059–63.

32 Sultan AH, Kamm MA, Bartram CI, Hudson CN. Anal sphincter trauma during instrumental delivery. *Int J Gynaecol Obstet* 1993; **43**:263–70.

33 Oberwalder M, Connor J, Wexner SD. Meta-analysis to determine the incidence of obstetric anal sphincter damage. *Br J Surg* 2003; **90**:1333–7.

34 Tjandra JJ, Han WR, Goh J, Carey M, Dwyer P. Direct repair vs. overlapping sphincter repair: a randomized, controlled trial. *Dis Colon Rectum* 2003; **46**:937–42.

35 Hasegawa H, Yoshioka K, Keighley MR. Randomized trial of fecal diversion for sphincter repair. *Dis Colon Rectum* 2000; **43**:961–4.

36 Sangalli MR, Marti MC. Results of sphincter repair in postobstetric fecal incontinence. *J Am Coll Surg* 1994; **179**:583–6.

37 Malouf AF, Norton CS, Engel AF, Nicholls RJ, Kamm MA. Long-term results of overlapping anterior anal sphincter repair for obstetric trauma. *Lancet* 2000; **355**:260–5.

38 Halverson AL, Hull TL. Long-term outcome of overlapping anal sphincter repair. *Dis Colon Rectum* 2002; **45**:345–8.

39 Zutshi M, Tracey TH, Bast J, Halverson A, Na J. Ten-year outcome after anal sphincter repair for fecal incontinence. *Dis Colon Rectum* 2009; **52**:1089–94.

40 Matzel KE, Kamm MA, Stösser M, *et al*. Sacral spinal nerve stimulation for faecal incontinence: multicentre study. *Lancet* 2004; **363**(9417):1270–6.

41 Malouf AJ, Vaizey CJ, Nicholls RJ, Kamm MA. Permanent sacral nerve stimulation for fecal incontinence. *Ann Surg* 2000; **232**:143–8.

42 Chan MK, Tjandra JJ. Sacral nerve stimulation for fecal incontinence: external anal sphincter defect vs. Intact anal sphincter. *Dis Colon Rectum* 2008; **51**:1015–24.

43 Collinson R, Wijffels N, Cunningham C, Lindsey I. Laparoscopic ventral rectopexy for internal rectal prolapse: short-term functional results. *Colorectal Dis* 2010; **12**:97–104.

44 Collinson R, Cunningham C, D'Costa H, Lindsey I. Rectal intussusceptions and unexplained faecal incontinence: findings of a proctographic study. *Colorectal Dis* 2009; **11**:77–83.

45 Clark AL, Gregory T, Smith VJ, Edwards R. Epidemiological evaluation of reoperation for surgically treated pelvic organ prolapse and urinary incontinence. *Am J Obstet Gynecol* 2003; **198**:1261–7.

46 Wijffels NA, Collinson R, Cunningham C, Lindsey I. What is the natural history of internal rectal prolapse? *Colorectal Dis* 2010; **12**(8):822–30. doi: 10.1111/j.1463-1318.2009.01891.x.

47 Halligan S, Bartram CI. Is barium trapping in rectoceles significant? *Dis Colon Rectum* 1995; **38**:764–8.

48 Shorvon PJ, McHugh S, Diamant NE, Somers S, Stevenson GW. Defecography in normal volunteers: results and implications. *Gut* 1989; **30**:1739–49.

49 Mimura T, Roy AJ, Storrie JB, Kamm MA. Treatment of impaired defecation associated with rectocele by behavorial retraining (biofeedback). *Dis Colon Rectum* 2000; **43**:1267–72.

50 Mellgren A, Anzen B, Nilsson BY, *et al.* Results of rectocele repair. A prospective study. *Dis Colon Rectum* 1995; **38**:7–13.

51 Van Dam JH, Hop WC, Schouten WR. Analysis of patients with poor outcome of rectocoele repair. *Dis Colon Rectum* 2000; **43**:1556–60.

52 Kahn MA, Stanton SL. Posterior colporrhaphy: its effects on bowel and sexual function. *Br J Obstet Gynaecol* 1997; **104**:82–6.

53 Arnold MW, Stewart WR, Aguilar PS. Rectocele repair. Four years' experience. *Dis Colon Rectum* 1990; **33**:684–7.

54 Ayabaca SM, Zbar AP, Pescatori M. Anal incontinence after rectocele repair. *Dis Colon Rectum* 2002; **45**:63–9.

55 Nieminen K, Hiltunen KM, Laitinen J, Oksala J, Heinonen PK. Transanal or vaginal approach to rectocele repair: a prospective, randomized pilot study. *Dis Colon Rectum* 2004; **47**:1636–42.

56 Kahn MA, Stanton SL, Kumar D, Fox SD. Posterior colporrhaphy is superior to the transanal repair for treatment of posterior vaginal wall prolapse. *Neurourol Urodynam* 1999; **18**:329–30.

57 Adusumilli S, Gosselink MP, Fourie S, *et al.* Does the presence of a high grade internal rectal prolapsed affect the outcome of pelvic floor retraiing in patients with faecal incontinence or obstructed defaecation? *Colorectal Dis* 2013; **15**:e680–5.

58 Berman IR, Harris MS, Rabeler MB. Delorme's transrectal excision for internal rectal prolapse. Patient selection, technique, and three year follow-up. *Dis Colon Rectum* 1990; **33**:573–80.

59 Orrom WJ, Bartolo DC, Miller R, Mortensen NJ, Roe AM. Rectopexy is an ineffective treatment for obstructed defecation. *Dis Colon Rectum* 1991; **34**:41–6.

60 Wijffels NA, Collinson R, Cunningham C, Lindsey I. What is the natural history of internal rectal prolapse? *Colorectal Dis* 2010; **12**:822–30.

61 Slawik S, Soulsby R, Carter H, Payne H, Dixon AR. Laparoscopic ventral rectopexy, posterior colporrhaphy and vaginal sacrocolpopexy for the treatment of recto-genital prolapsed and mechanical outlet obstruction. *Colorectal Dis* 2008; **10**:138–43.

62 Van den Esschert JW, van Geloven AA, Vermulst N, Groenedijk AG, de Wit LT, Gerhards MF. Laparoscopic ventral rectopexy for obstructed defaecation syndrome. *Surg Endosc* 2008; **22**:2728–32.

63 Mantoo S, Podevin J, Regenet N, Rigaud J, Lehur PA, Meurette G. Is robotic-assisted ventral mesh rectopexy superior to laparoscopic mesh rectopexy in the management of obstructed defaecation? *Colorectal Dis* 2013; **15**:e469–75.

64 Gosselink MP, Adusumilli S, Harmston C, *et al*. Impact of slow transit constipation on the outcome of laparoscopic ventral rectopexy for obstructed defaecation associated with high grade internal rectal prolapse. *Colorectal Dis* 2013; **15**:e749–56.

65 Reibetanz J, Boenicke L, Kim M, Germer CT, Isbert C. Enterocoele is not a contraindication to stapled transanal surgery for outlet obstruction: an analysis of 170 patients. *Colorectal Dis* 2011; **13**:e131–6.

66 Jarrett ME, Wijffels NA, Slater A, Cunningham C, Lindsey I. Enterocoele is a marker of severe pelvic floor weakness. *Colorectal Dis* 2010; **12**:e158–62.

67 Madigan MR, Morson BC. Solitary ulcer of the rectum. *Gut* 1969; **10**:871–81.

68 Schweiger M, Alexander-Williams J. Solitary-ulcer syndrome of the rectum: its association with occult rectal prolapse. *Lancet* 1977; **i**:170–1.

69 Sitzler PJ, Kamm MA, Nicholls RJ, McKee RF. Long-term clinical outcome of surgery for solitary rectal ulcer syndrome. *Br J Surg* 1988; **85**:1246–50.

70 Evans C, Ong E, Jones OM, Cunningham C, Lindsey I. Laparoscopic ventral rectopexy is effective for solitary rectal ulcer syndrome when associated with rectal prolapse. *Colorectal Dis* 2014; **16O**:112–16.

71 Badrek-Amoudi AH, Roe T, Mabey K, Carter H, Mills A, Dixon AR. Laparoscopic ventral mesh rectopexy in the management of solitary rectal ulcer syndrome: a cause for optimism? *Colorectal Dis* 2013; **15**:575–81.

72 Mugie SM, Benninga MA, Di Lorenzo C. Epidemiology of constipation in children and adults: a systematic review. *Best Pract Res Clin Gastroenterol* 2011; **25**:3–18.

73 Hinton JM, Lennard-Jones JE, Young AC. A new method of studying gut transit times using radiopaque markers. *Gut* 1969; **10**:842–7.

74 Camilleri M, Kerstens R, Rykx A, Vandeplassche L. A placebo-controlled trial of prucalopride for severe chronic constipation. *N Engl J Med* 2008; **358**:2344–54.

75 Koutsomanis D, Lennard-Jones JE, Kamm MA. Prospective study of biofeedback treatment for patients with slow and normal transit constipation. *Eur J Gastroenterol Hepatol* 1994; **6**:131–7.

76 Hasegawa H, Radley S, Fatah C, Keighley MRB. Long-term results of colorectal resection for slow transit constipation. *Colorectal Dis* 1999; **1**:141–5.

77 Reshef A, Alves-Ferreira P, Zutshi M, Hull T, Gurland B. Colectomy for slow transit constipation: effective for patients with coexistent obstructed defecation. *Int J Colorectal Dis* 2013; **28**:841–7.

78 Knowles CH, Scott M, Lunniss PJ. Outcome of colectomy for slow transit constipation. *Ann Surg* 1999; **230**:627–38.

79 Thomas GP, Dudding TC, Rahbour G, Nicholls RJ, Vaizey CJ. Sacral nerve stimulation for constipation. *Br J Surg* 2013; **100**:174–81.

80 Malone PS, Ransley PG, Kiely EM. Preliminary report; the antegrade continence enema. *Lancet* 1990; **336**:1217–8.

81 Gerharz EW, Vik V, Webb G, Leaver R, Shah PJ, Woodhouse CR. The value of the MACE (Malone antegrade colonic enema) procedure in adult patients. *J Am Coll Surg* 1997; **185**:544–7.

82 Halligan S, Bartram CI, Park HJ, Kamm MA. Proctographic features of anismus. *Radiology* 1995; **197**:679–82.

83 Hompes R, Harmston C, Wijffels N, Jones OM, Cunningham C, Lindsey I. Excellent response rate of anismus to botulinum toxin if rectal prolapse misdiagnosed as anismus ('pseudoanismus') is excluded. *Colorectal Dis* 2012; **14**:224–30.

84 Lau CW, Heyman S, Alabaz O, Iroatulam AJ, Wexner SD. Prognostic significance of rectocele, intussusception, and abnormal perineal descent in biofeedback treatment for constipated patients with paradoxical puborectalis contraction. *Dis Colon Rectum* 2000; **43**: 478–82.

85 Hallan RI, Williams NS, Melling J, Waldron DJ, Womack NR, Morrison JF. Treatment of anismus in intractable constipation with botulinum A toxin. *Lancet* 1988; **2**:714–17.

86 Hompes R, Harmston C, Wijffels N, Jones OM, Cunningham C, Lindsey I. Excellent response rate of anismus to botulinum toxin if rectal prolapse misdiagnosed as anismus ('pseudoanismus') is excluded. *Colorectal Dis* 2012; **14**:224–30.

87 Gunter J. Chronic pelvic pain: an integrated approach to diagnosis and treatment. *Obstet Gynecol Surg* 2003; **58**:615–23.

88 Andromanakis NP, Kouraklis G, Alkiviadis K. Chronic perineal pain: current pathophysiological aspects, diagnostic approaches and treatment. *Eur J Gastroenterol Hepatol* 2011; **23**:2–7.

89 Thompson WG. Proctalgia fugax. *Dig Dis Sci* 1981; **26**:1121–4.

90 Bharucha AE, Trabuco E. Functional and chronic anorectal and pelvic pain disorders. *Gastroenterol Clin North Am* 2008; **37**:685–96.

91 Mazzo L, Formento E, Fronda G. Anorectal and perineal pain: new pathophysiological hypothesis. *Tech Coloproctol* 2004; **8**:77–83.

92 Patel R, Appannagari A, Whang PG. Coccydynia. *Curr Rev Musculoskelet Med* 2008; **1**:223–6.

93 Hompes R, Jones OM, Cunningham C, Lindsey I. What causes chronic idiopathic perineal pain? *Colorectal Dis* 2011; **13**:1035–9.

94 Everaert K, Devulder J, Muynck M, *et al.* The pain cycle: implications for the diagnosis and treatment of pelvic pain syndromes. *Int Urogynaecol J Pelvic Floor Dysfunct* 2001; **12**:9–14.

95 Neill ME, Swash M. Chronic perianal pain: an unsolved problem. *J R Soc Med* 1982; **75**:96–101.

96 Collinson R, Wjiffels N, Cunningham C, Lindsey I. Laparoscopic ventral rectopexy for internal rectal prolapse: short term functional results. *Colorectal Dis* 2010; **12**:97–104.

97 Hompes R, Lindsey I. Chronic anorectal pain: a pathophysiological approach. In: Lindsey I, Nugent K, Dixon A, eds. *Pelvic Floor Disorders for the Colorectal Surgeon.* Oxford: Oxford University Press, 2011; 67–74.

98 Jarrett ME, Wjiffels NA, Slater A, Cunningham C, Lindsey I. Enterocele is a marker of severe pelvic floor weakness. *Colorectal Dis* 2010; **12**:158–62.

99 Robert R, Labat JJ, Bensignor M, *et al.* Decompression and transposition of the pudendal nerve in pudendal neuralgia: a randomized controlled trial and long-term evaluation. *Eur Urol* 2005; **47**:403–8.

CASE 26

Constrictions of prolapse surgery

Richard Guy

Oxford University Hospitals NHS Foundation Trust, Oxford, UK

A 30-year-old woman was referred with obstructed defecation and a rectal stricture. Six months previously, she had undergone a Delorme's procedure for rectal prolapse at another hospital. A postoperative stricture had occurred, and an attempt was then made at the same hospital to excise this stricture circumferentially, but the stricture recurred. On clinical examination, it was evident that a stricture had developed.

DECISION POINT

What are the potential approaches to this problem?

Self-dilatation could be tried but this can be difficult for patients and is rarely a satisfactory long-term solution. It was felt that establishing the patient on self-dilatation, with the assistance of a specialist nurse, would be worthwhile, whilst discussing potential definitive solutions.

The patient was given some Hagar's dilators to use in an attempt to overcome the stricture but this was unsuccessful. A decision was made to submit the patient to examination under anesthetic. At surgery, it was noted that there was a tight stricture that would admit just the tip of the index finger. It was dilated using Hagar's dilators up to 20 mm. A pediatric rigid sigmoidoscope was passed showing normal rectal mucosa beyond.

Postdilatation evacuation proctography 2 weeks later showed restricturing and the presence of a significant enterocele.

DECISION POINT

As dilatation didn't seem to be working, what would your approach be now?

There had already been an attempt to excise the stricture without success. Simple division (stricturotomy) would not work unless some form of strictureplasty could be performed, perhaps using the transanal endoscopic microsurgery (TEMS) equipment. Defunctioning loop colostomy might need to be discussed with the patient if obstruction were to worsen. Ultra-low anterior resection with coloanal anastomosis, or even proctectomy, might also have to come into the reckoning as possibilities, however difficult this would be for the patient to contemplate, having simply presented with rectal prolapse. As it was such a short stricture, a different method of stricture excision was considered.

Colorectal Surgery: Clinical Care and Management, First Edition.
Edited by Bruce George, Richard Guy, Oliver Jones, and Jon Vogel.
© 2016 John Wiley & Sons, Ltd. Published 2016 by John Wiley & Sons, Ltd.

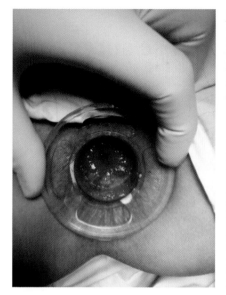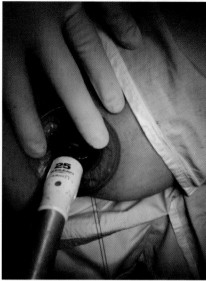

Figure 26.1 Examination under anesthetic with a circular anal dilator (CAD) revealed a stricture 2 cm above the dentate line (*left*). A transanal circular stapler was used to excise a ring of tissue from the stricture.

The patient underwent examination under general anesthetic, which revealed a recurrent short stricture about 2 cm above the dentate line (Figure 26.1).

Dilatation with Hagar's dilators was carried out before inserting a 25 mm circular stapler (EEA, Covidien). A prolene purse-string suture was inserted and the stapler engaged and fired, retrieving a doughnut. The anastomosis was intact and widely patent. The patient was discharged the following day.

At follow-up, the anastomosis remained patent and evacuation unimpaired. She was subsequently investigated for preexisting pelvic floor dysfunction.

Could we have done better?

It is clearly regrettable that the patient experienced a significant post-Delorme's complication. This operation itself seems unusual for such a young person and, undoubtedly, she has pelvic floor dysfunction requiring additional assessment. It may have been that the Delorme's was for a relatively small prolapse and much of the repair was intraanal. The long-term outcome of the stricture excision is yet to be determined but, effectively, the patient has the equivalent of a low stapled anastomosis and this ought to remain patent.

LEARNING POINTS

- Rectal stricture is a recognized complication of Delorme's procedure, and probably results from ischemia and anastomotic breakdown.
- Rectal prolapse in a young woman is unusual and demands a full pelvic floor assessment.
- The use of a circular stapler for low rectal strictures in this way has also been applied to anastomotic strictures after low anterior resection.

LETTER FROM AMERICA

Mild low-lying strictures can be overcome by gentle self-dilatation using the St Marks anal dilators. Moderate strictures may require dilatation in outpatients under sedation or under anesthesia using Hagar's dilators or esophageal dilators. Finally, a strictureplasty may be attempted. Circular stapler may be an option but complications, especially in ischemic tissue, should be expected.

Jon Vogel and Massarat Zutshi

CASE 27

Elderly prolapse dilemma

Koen van Dongen

Maashospital Pantein, Beugen, The Netherlands

A 91-year-old woman was referred to the outpatient clinic with recurrent rectal prolapse following a Delorme's operation 5 years previously. Whilst the recurrent prolapse was initially intermittent, it had become almost permanent and she had virtually no continence. She was housebound and wore pads all the time. Her past medical history included a knee replacement, hypothyroidism, and eyesight problems. She was taking thyroxine and simvastatin.

She was able to walk with a stick but was a little breathless, although able to lie flat without dyspnea. On examination of her abdomen, there was nothing of note. Rectal examination showed a very poor sphincter tone and an obvious external prolapse (Figure 27.1). Rigid sigmoidoscopy was normal.

DECISION POINT

Does this patient need further investigations? Why not just proceed to surgery? Do you think a repeat perineal operation or abdominal operation would be most appropriate?

It was felt that very little needed to be done in this elderly lady other than excluding neoplasia in the left colon, which is an occasional cause of prolapse. In compliant, fit, younger patients with significant symptoms of incontinence, consideration might be given to anorectal physiology and endoanal ultrasound to document sphincter structure and function prior to surgical intervention. If the prolapse had not been evident in clinic, a proctogram might have been worthwhile, but this elderly lady really just needed the prolapse fixing.

The patient underwent flexible sigmoidoscopy which was normal. She went on to have a laparoscopic ventral mesh rectopexy using a three-port technique. Her recovery was unremarkable and she was discharged after 3 days. At 2-month follow-up she was well with no recurrence of the prolapse and had noticed a steady improvement in leakage since her surgery.

Colorectal Surgery: Clinical Care and Management, First Edition.
Edited by Bruce George, Richard Guy, Oliver Jones, and Jon Vogel.
© 2016 John Wiley & Sons, Ltd. Published 2016 by John Wiley & Sons, Ltd.

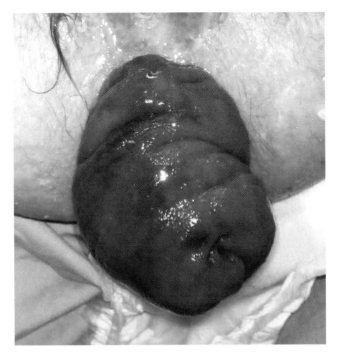

Figure 27.1 External prolapse evident on patient bearing down.

Could we have done better?

Most surgeons in the UK would probably advise a perineal approach for such an elderly lady but repeat perineal surgery can be difficult. She made it through abdominal surgery under general anesthesia uneventfully but this was a calculated risk and might have turned out otherwise. The alternative was to leave her alone. In hindsight, the correct decision was probably made.

LEARNING POINTS

- External rectal prolapse almost always requires surgery – conservative management palliates symptoms poorly and should be used in only the frailest of patients.
- Repeat perineal surgery for prolapse is often difficult and, whilst surgery could have been performed under a spinal anesthetic, scarring from the previous Delorme's operation could easily result in conversion of the procedure to an Altmeier operation, increasing the potential morbidity of the surgery.
- Laparoscopic ventral mesh rectopexy may be tolerated very well by elderly people.

LETTER FROM AMERICA

Most surgeons in the US would also advocate a perineal approach. However, our experience is that a well-done laparoscopic rectopexy in expert hands is a better option in the elderly. However, lax tissues may predispose to recurrence. Continence may be controlled but may still be an issue that can be managed conservatively.

ASCRS guidelines from 2011 in the US indicate that the surgery is dictated by patient co-morbidities and recommend suture rectopexy over a ventral rectopexy.

Jon Vogel and Massarat Zutshi

Chasing incontinence

Oliver Jones
Oxford University Hospitals NHS Foundation Trust, Oxford, UK

A 71-year-old woman was referred from her GP with a history of deteriorating continence over the previous 5 years. She reported that her main symptom was passive fecal incontinence, especially when walking, and exacerbated by loose stools, necessitating use of a pad. She was otherwise fit, without significant past medical history, and took no medications. She had had two previous vaginal deliveries, requiring forceps, an episiotomy, and suture repair after the first of these. On perineal inspection, there was an obvious scar consistent with previous episiotomy. Resting pressure was slightly low on clinical examination but squeeze pressure was reasonable. Rigid sigmoidoscopy was unremarkable.

DECISION POINT

Would you give this lady a trial of conservative treatment and what would that be?

Should you send this lady for tests and, if so, which ones?

Conservative treatment is always to be preferred initially, and this may just be simple dietary alterations, advice on lifestyle changes, reassurance, and prescription of a low dose of an antidiarrheal drug. As a baseline, anorectal physiology and endoanal ultrasound were arranged. These showed normal rectal sensation, slightly low resting pressures but a normal squeeze (Table 28.1). Endoanal ultrasound showed her internal and external sphincters were intact but there was some thickening of her internal anal sphincter (Figure 28.1). She had a colonoscopy and random biopsies, which were normal.

The patient was given loperamide to be used regularly at the lowest effective dose in an effort to firm up stool consistency, and advised to take a low-fiber diet. She was also referred for biofeedback. At clinic review, she reported little change in her symptoms. She had discontinued loperamide as, although it improved her continence, it exposed symptoms of obstructed defecation . There had been some minor benefit from biofeedback.

Colorectal Surgery: Clinical Care and Management, First Edition.
Edited by Bruce George, Richard Guy, Oliver Jones, and Jon Vogel.
© 2016 John Wiley & Sons, Ltd. Published 2016 by John Wiley & Sons, Ltd.

Table 28.1 Results of anorectal physiology.

Parameter	Value	Normal range
Mean resting pressure (mmHg)	40	45–85
Mean squeeze increment (mmHg)	50	50
Balloon volume at first sensation (mL)	15	10–30
Urge to defecate (mL)	150	120–150
Maximum tolerated volume (mL)	300	250–450

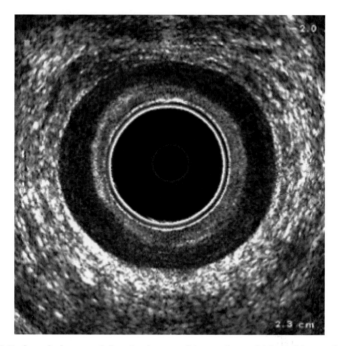

Figure 28.1 Endoanal ultrasound showing intact sphincters but a thickened internal sphincter.

DECISION POINT

Is any further treatment indicated, considering that some improvement had occurred?

Would you consider any further tests?

It might have been reasonable to discharge the patient at this point, with advice on symptom control and reassurance that no serious bowel condition had been found. However, in view of the troublesome obstructed defecation, the patient was keen to explore other options. In this situation, an evacuation proctogram can be very helpful, as internal prolapse should be considered.

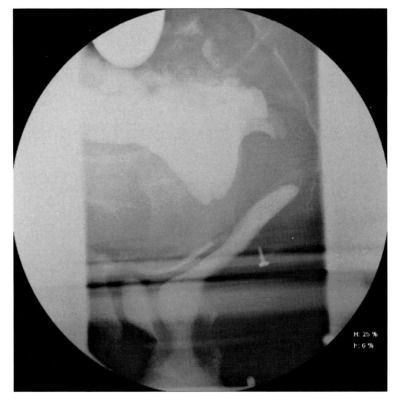

Figure 28.2 Defecating proctography showing a full-thickness rectal prolapse with a moderate anterior rectocele trapping some barium. The pin corresponds to the level of the pelvic floor.

A proctogram was undertaken which, surprisingly, showed a full-thickness rectal prolapse (Figure 28.2).

In view of this obvious prolapse, the patient underwent a laparoscopic ventral mesh rectopexy (Figure 28.3). At follow-up, she reported that evacuation was easier and continence had improved considerably.

Could we have done better?

We were slow to pick up the rectal prolapse which, with careful examination in clinic, should have been evident. If this had been the case, the patient would have proceeded more rapidly to surgery, without the need for all the interim investigations and treatments described.

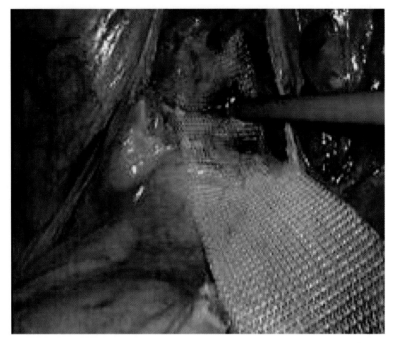

Figure 28.3 Operative photograph from a laparoscopic ventral mesh rectopexy, showing the "hockey stick dissection" into the rectovaginal septum and the mesh being slid into position prior to suture fixation to the rectum and sacral promontory.

LEARNING POINTS

- Rectal prolapse may cause incontinence via several mechanisms.
  - The mechanical consequence of having bowel mucosa exposed beyond the sphincter mechanism.
  - Continual stimulation of the rectoanal inhibitory reflex, resulting in chronic internal anal sphincter relaxation.
  - Repeated dilatation of the sphincter complex by the external prolapse.
- A proctogram should be part of the work-up for the patient with obscure incontinence.

LETTER FROM AMERICA

Solid stool in the rectum when the patient states that she has had a good bowel movement that day is a good sign that a defecatory dysfunction needs to be evaluated. In the US, she would be treated conservatively with fiber supplementation with supplements like magnesium. If symptoms do not improve, she would undergo a defecating proctogram. Ventral rectopexy is not popular in the US for outlet dysfunction constipation, but some centers do perform it.

Jon Vogel and Massarat Zutshi

CASE 29

Sphincter disruption

Kim Gorissen

Oxford University Hospitals NHS Foundation Trust, Oxford, UK

A 61-year-old woman was referred with urge and passive fecal incontinence to solid and liquid stool. She was unable to leave the house for fear of soiling accidents, but was otherwise fit and well. Obstetric history was of four vaginal deliveries, the first complicated by a prolonged second stage followed by a third-degree tear which was repaired by the obstetrician. The second and third deliveries required forceps.

On perineal inspection, a scar corresponding to the previous tear was seen. There was some pelvic floor descent on straining. On digital examination, she had a short anal canal with a very low resting pressure and little increment on squeezing.

Colonoscopy with biopsies was unremarkable. A defecating proctogram showed incontinence to the barium, a moderate rectocele without entrapment of contrast, and no intussusception. Anorectal physiology showed a slightly hypersensitive rectum and confirmed low resting and squeeze pressures (Table 29.1).

On enodanal ultrasound, a short anal canal of 2.8 cm was seen, with a defect from 11 to 2 o'clock of both the internal and external sphincters (Figure 29.1).

The patient was given dietary advice, loperamide, and amitryptiline. Biofeedback was also instituted with both pelvic floor exercises and rectal desensitization training. The interventions reduced the daily leakage considerably, but the patient still had to rush to reach the toilet within 3–5 minutes, causing considerable lifestyle disruption.

DECISION POINT

As conservative management seems to have made little difference, what are the options for treatment now?

Should sphincter repair be carried out?

Anal sphincter repair was considered, as there was a defined sphincter defect, and many patients can really benefit in the shorter term, although repair durability in the longer term is a bit unpredictable. Rectal irrigation would also be an option, flushing out the colon to create "pseudocontinence" and allowing the patient to regain some control over bowel function. Anal bulking agents were also considered, but these tend to be more effective for passive incontinence by augmenting internal sphincter function, and are less useful for patients with urge incontinence. Finally, sacral nerve stimulation (SNS) was thought to be a realistic option for this patient, despite the sphincter defect.

Colorectal Surgery: Clinical Care and Management, First Edition.
Edited by Bruce George, Richard Guy, Oliver Jones, and Jon Vogel.
© 2016 John Wiley & Sons, Ltd. Published 2016 by John Wiley & Sons, Ltd.

Table 29.1 Anorectal physiology results.

Parameter	Value	Normal range
Mean resting pressure	30 mmHg	45–85
Mean squeeze increment	33 mmHg	50
Balloon volume at first sensation (mL)	10	10–30
Urge to defecate (mL)	90	120–150
Maximum tolerated volume (mL)	240	250–450

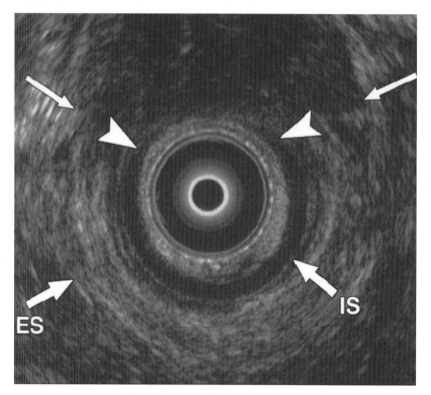

Figure 29.1 Endoanal ultrasound showing a defect (area between arrows) in both the external (ES) and internal anal sphincter (IS).

At clinic review, a trial of SNS was agreed. Under local anesthetic, a temporary electrode was placed through the sacral foramen of S3 and positioned in such a way as to get the best responses of the nerves of the sacral plexus that innervate the rectum (Figure 29.2).

During the 3-week test phase, the patient kept a detailed bowel diary and she was able to report an improvement of 75–80% in passive leakage episodes, and she could hold onto stool for more than 15 minutes, with much reduced urgency. Following the success of the test stimulator, a permanent SNS stimulator

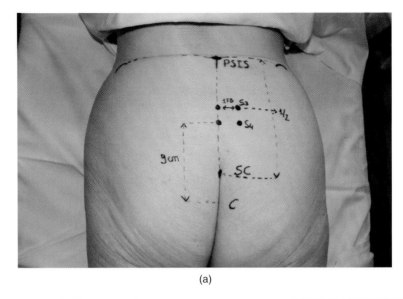

(a)

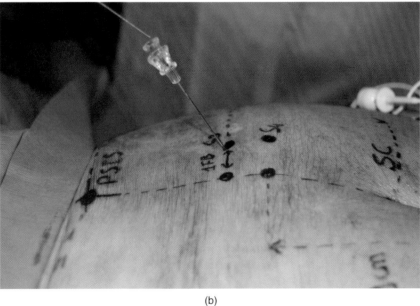

(b)

Figure 29.2 (a) Bony landmarks give an excellent guide to locate the foramen of S3 and S4, negating the need for fluoroscopic guidance. S3 is located halfway between the posterior superior iliac spine (PSIS) and the sacrococcygeal joint (SC). S4 is located 9 cm above the tip of the coccyx (c). (b) To ensure optimal lateral positioning, the needle should be inserted about 1 fingerbreadth (FB) from the midline. The needle is then introduced at a 60° angle.

was implanted under local anesthetic, and 2 weeks later the device was switched on. During the first 6 months, symptom control was very satisfying, but after 1 year the patient was seen back in clinic with recurrence of both urge and passive incontinence.

DECISION POINT

What are the options now? Would you request any investigations? Should sphincter repair now be considered?

The return of symptoms was disappointing, although well recognized, and sphincter repair was considered. In the first instance, however, it was important to ascertain that the SNS device was functioning correctly.

A plain radiograph of the sacrum was obtained in order to assess the position of the lead. This was found still to be in the correct place without signs of migration or fracture. However, when the device itself was checked, it was noticed that the SNS had inadvertently been switched off for several months! This was easily rectified and the patient's symptom control was regained.

Could we have done better?

For this lady, SNS was clearly effective, despite the sphincter injury. She had struggled on after she had inadvertently switched the device off and she should have been instructed to report her clinical deterioration, perhaps with more comprehensive information and support.

LEARNING POINTS

- Sacral nerve stimulation appears to be effective even in the presence of sphincter defects.
- Loss of SNS efficacy may be caused by accidental switching off of the device or deprogramming due to strong electrical fields.

LETTER FROM AMERICA

Based on the degree of incontinence, as per the US guidelines from the ASCRS (2009), the patient would have a trial of conservative treatment and at the next appointment the various available options would be discussed. These would include injectables, anal sphincter repair or SNS. The Secca procedure would not be an option due to the sphincter disruption.

Jon Vogel and Massarat Zutshi

CASE 30

Stimulating complications

Kim Gorissen & Ian Lindsey

Oxford University Hospitals NHS Foundation Trust, Oxford, UK

A 53-year-old woman presented with combined passive and urge fecal incontinence. There was a history of fibromyalgia, chronic fatigue, and low back pain for 7 years, although she was taking no analgesia. A full pelvic floor work-up was undertaken, following which she underwent biofeedback therapy. As this made little difference to her symptoms, she was offered a trial of sacral nerve stimulation (SNS).

Test stimulation under local anesthetic was undertaken. During insertion of the wire, optimal expected sensations in the area innervated by S3 were noted (Table 30.1).

During the 3-week test phase, the patient was asked to keep a detailed bowel diary. On follow-up, she reported an improvement of 90–100% in passive leakage episodes, and she was able to defer defecation for more than 30 minutes. Permanent implantation was therefore undertaken 2 weeks later. Two days later, the patient telephoned to report severe swelling over the device.

DECISION POINT

What could be the cause of the swelling? Would you arrange any investigations?

The thoughts at the time were that this was most likely to be a hematoma and likely to be self-limiting. It seemed a little early for there to be an infection, although this was remotely possible – whilst occurring in only around 2% of cases, it is a potentially major complication often necessitating removal of the device, and insertion should be strictly aseptic with antibiotic cover. Another possibility considered was that there had been tilting of the device so that it might be sitting upright, putting pressure on the skin. This would usually require intervention.

When the patient was reviewed the following day, the swelling and pain were already reducing. On examination, a hematoma was evident but there was no wound redness or tension. The device was difficult to palpate, making tilting of the device less likely. The patient was reassured and sent home with analgesia and 2 days later she reported further improvement. The device was switched on 2 weeks later. After a month, however, she complained of severe pain and was not able to test all four programs for the required 2 weeks each.

Colorectal Surgery: Clinical Care and Management, First Edition.
Edited by Bruce George, Richard Guy, Oliver Jones, and Jon Vogel.
© 2016 John Wiley & Sons, Ltd. Published 2016 by John Wiley & Sons, Ltd.

Table 30.1 Expected responses on test stimulation.

Nerve	Pelvic floor	Leg/ foot	Sensation
S2	May have clamp	Leg/hip rotation, ankle plantarflexion, calf contraction	Generally none
S3	Bellows	Great toe flexion, sometimes other toes	Pulling in rectum, extending forward to scrotum or labia
S4	Bellows	None	Pulling in rectum

DECISION POINT

What could be the cause of the pain now? How would you go about assessing and treating it?

This seemed a little more concerning as infection may well have been the cause. Incorrect sub-fascial placement and device tilting could have also been the problem – plain radiographs can be helpful in evaluating this. Other causes considered at this time related mainly to mechanical and circuitry problems with the device and, in addition to pain over the device, may cause leg pain. These hardware problems include lead damage or short circuit and, if suspected, the device should be switched off to see if the pain disappears, impedance measurements often also being diagnostic.

It was thought that if leg pain was a significant problem, the most likely causes would be incorrect lead placement or lead migration. If incorrect lead placement is suspected, switching off the stimulator should resolve the pain. The advantage of local anesthetic insertion of the device is that leg pain from incorrect placement can be immediately reported by the patient. Lead migration may be prevented by not pushing the dilator too far down the track during insertion. If it becomes a problem, reprogramming and use of leads other than the painful one may be helpful. Again, radiographs can be useful for confirming lead and stimulator position.

On assessment in clinic, it was clear that the pain was located over the device. The patient was prescribed paracetamol, diclofenac, and gabapentin, but was intolerant of the latter and obtained little pain relief. The device was switched off after 2 weeks, leading to recurrence of her incontinence symptoms. Urgent resiting of the device was undertaken and, after a further 2 months, the pain had completely resolved and continence was excellent.

Could we have done better?

There were clearly problems from the outset, which must have been related to some degree of device malplacement, although it is known that patients with chronic pain have a somewhat higher risk for developing pain over the device, leading to a 2.4 times relative risk for secondary intervention. Once the device was moved, the patient was asymptomatic.

LEARNING POINTS

- There may be an advantage to inserting SNS devices under local anesthesia, as the clinician can be guided by sensory responses and patients are able to report leg pain, although motor responses are often only provoked at higher currents which, in conscious patients, might be painful.
- Pain over SNS devices may be easily resolved by resiting.
- Leg pain is most often resolved by reprogramming of the device.

LETTER FROM AMERICA

In the US, there is a low tolerance to device-related issues. Re-siting the device is an option especially in thin patients, or when a seroma/hematoma is suspected or found on exploration of the wound. Leg pain is a frequent complaint which is easily treated with reprogramming. Patients with chronic pain issues, however, can pose problems which may not be easily relieved and may need a preoperative discussion to define expectations.

Jon Vogel and Massarat Zutshi

CASE 31

Crohn's evacuation trouble

Heman Joshi

St Helens and Knowsley NHS Trust, Merseyside, UK

A 41-year-old woman presented with incomplete evacuation. Whilst she was able to open her bowels every day, she rarely felt as if she had emptied completely and would typically revisit the toilet 4–5 times over the course of a morning, usually inserting a finger into the anus to facilitate evacuation. She also reported minor fecal incontinence, mainly to liquid stool, around twice a month.

Seven years previously, she had been diagnosed with terminal ileal Crohn's disease. After failing medical management, she underwent open ileocecal resection from which she made an uneventful recovery and had been well since. Four years ago, she had endured a difficult vaginal delivery, requiring a generous episiotomy. She felt that all of her current symptoms resulted from the time of childbirth. A symptom questionnaire revealed a Wexner constipation score of 23 and a Vaizey incontinence score of 22.

On digital rectal examination, she had slightly diminished anal resting tone and squeeze pressure. She had a moderate anterior rectocele and probable rectal intussusception on rigid sigmoidoscopy.

DECISION POINT

What would your management priorities be? What investigations might be useful?

Whilst there was a clear obstetric history, incontinence was not a major problem but obstructed defecation was worsening. With the history of ileocecal resection, and generally looser stools which tend to follow this, it was thought unusual that there should be an evacuation problem. It was felt that, with the history of Crohn's disease, there was a priority to make sure, in the first instance, that the patient didn't have rectal Crohn's. If that was excluded then further evaluation of the functional problems could go ahead.

Colonoscopy with neoterminal ileal intubation was normal, and multiple random biopsies were unremarkable. A colonic transit study was also normal. Biofeedback was commenced but was of little benefit. Anorectal physiology showed slightly diminished pressures and endoanal ultrasound revealed

Colorectal Surgery: Clinical Care and Management, First Edition.
Edited by Bruce George, Richard Guy, Oliver Jones, and Jon Vogel.
© 2016 John Wiley & Sons, Ltd. Published 2016 by John Wiley & Sons, Ltd.

some scarring within intact internal and external sphincters. An evacuation proctogram showed incontinence to barium at rest, but complete evacuation, with a 1 cm rectocele but no significant intussusception or enterocele.

DECISION POINT

With essentially normal investigations, is there any indication to do anything else?

It might have been reasonable to discharge the patient at this point with firm reassurance. The only real objective abnormalities found had been low sphincter pressures, but the patient's seemingly reliable history was of obstructed defecation, and so further discussion seemed appropriate.

In clinic, a trial of sacral nerve stimulation was suggested, but she was reluctant to try this as she was adamant that her main problem was obstructed defecation. A decision was made to undertake an examination under anesthetic.

With the patient in the lithotomy position, 20 mL of bupivacaine was injected either side of the anal canal towards the ischial spines, to block the pudendal nerves. A circular anal dilator (CAD) was inserted in the anal canal and very gentle traction applied to the lower rectal wall. This showed an obvious unexpected intussusception of the lower rectum into the lower anal canal (Figure 31.1).

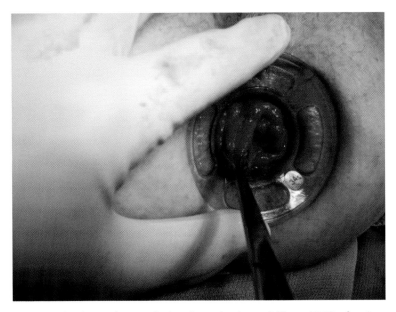

Figure 31.1 Examination under anesthetic using a circular anal dilator (CAD), showing internal prolapse.

DECISION POINT

Does this finding satisfactorily explain her symptoms? What treatment could you offer the patient?

As this was unexpected, there had been no discussion about proceeding immediately to corrective surgery. The two realistic options for this internal prolapse would be stapled transanal resection of the rectum (STARR) or laparoscopic ventral mesh rectopexy. However, incontinence is a contraindication to STARR, with a 20% incidence of urgency 6 months after surgery.

The patient underwent laparoscopic ventral mesh rectopexy, during which a biological mesh (porcine acellular dermal matrix) was inserted, on account of the theoretical risk of nonabsorbable mesh erosion in a patient with Crohn's disease. Recovery was uneventful. At review 12 months following surgery, the patient reported almost complete (90%) symptom resolution. The Wexner constipation score had reduced from 23 to 1, whilst her Vaizey score had reduced from 22 to 0.

LEARNING POINTS

- Proctography can underestimate prolapse owing to patient anxiety and failure to relax, and the barium paste may not mimic the patient's normal stool consistency.
- A detailed patient history is important when trying to unravel pelvic floor disorders.
- Obstructed defecation may co-exist with incontinence.

CASE 32

Disabling anal pain

Martijn Gosselink[1] & Ian Lindsey[2]

[1] *Erasmus Medical Centre, Rotterdam, The Netherlands*
[2] *Oxford University Hospitals NHS Foundation Trust, Oxford, UK*

A 56-year-old man was referred to clinic with intractable anal pain, which had been present for 9 months. The pain was a dull ache and occasionally throbbing in nature, and was worse on sitting but relieved by standing. The pain was also aggravated by defecation, which was difficult and accompanied by straining, but there was no radiation down his legs or into the penis and scrotum. The pain increased in intensity during the day, restricting normal daily activities, and settled during the night. Perineal inspection revealed significant pelvic floor descent on straining; digital rectal examination was normal.

DECISION POINT

What are the common causes of anal pain? How would you go about investigating this man?

This was a fairly unusual presentation which necessitated further investigation. It was felt important to exclude the more common organic causes of pain, including anorectal sepsis, anal fissure, thrombotic hemorrhoidal disease, and anorectal neoplasia. Retrorectal or presacral tumors and sacrococcygeal neoplastic or degenerative disease should also be considered before functional pelvic floor problems. Proctalgia fugax was considered unlikely in the absence of nocturnal symptoms.

Urgent flexible sigmoidoscopy and a pelvic MRI scan were arranged and these were normal. He went on to have a proctogram which revealed significant (8 cm) perineal descent but no internal rectal prolapse. The pain was consistent with pudendal nerve entrapment, and examination under anesthetic was arranged.

Under general anesthesia, with the patient in the prone position, no anorectal abnormalities were seen. Bilateral pudendal nerve block was performed using the following steps (Figure 32.1).

- Marking of the anatomical boundaries: the posterior superior iliac spine and supertrochanteric plane.
- Insertion of the index finger into the anus to locate the ischial spine.
- Percutaneous insertion of a 10 cm nerve stimulator needle along the ischial spine, guided into the correct position using the nerve stimulator to identify

Colorectal Surgery: Clinical Care and Management, First Edition.
Edited by Bruce George, Richard Guy, Oliver Jones, and Jon Vogel.
© 2016 John Wiley & Sons, Ltd. Published 2016 by John Wiley & Sons, Ltd.

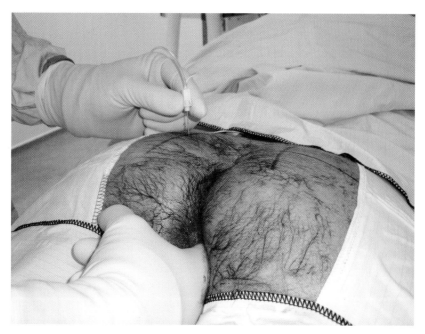

Figure 32.1 Pudendal nerve blockade.

the pudendal nerve (see Figure 32.1), confirmed by the eliciting of twitching on the ipsilateral side of the anus without leg movement at a low current (0.5 mA).

• Injection of 20 mL of 0.5% bupivacaine plus 40 mg Depo-medrone, observing cessation of twitching immediately after infiltration.

• Repeat procedure on the contralateral side.

Immediately after the bilateral pudendal nerve blockade, the patient stated that the pain had disappeared, although he reported a loss of sensation of the genital skin. At 6-week follow-up, the patient reported that the anal pain had reoccurred after 1 day, but that after 2 weeks he had gained marked improvement and relief, which had endured.

Could we have done better?

The diagnosis of pudendal nerve entrapment can be obscure, but there are characteristic symptoms. These were picked up fairly promptly and the treatment, at least in the short term, seems to have been successful. The associated pelvic floor descent is probably significant, as cause or effect, and perhaps the opportunity should have been taken for a more comprehensive pelvic floor work-up. It is likely that the patient will return in the future – work from Oxford shows that relief is maintained long term in around 30% of cases, and repeat injection may be worthwhile for late relapse. Formal pudendal nerve release or decompression (neurolysis) may become necessary, and this may improve symptoms in around two-thirds of patients.

LEARNING POINTS

- Important proctological and sacrococcygeal causes of anorectal pain must be ruled out before attributing symptoms to pelvic floor disorders.
- Pudendal nerve entrapment has characteristic features and may be an underdiagnosed condition.
- Formal pudendal nerve blockade may be diagnostic and therapeutic.

SECTION D

Proctology

Richard Guy
Oxford University Hospitals NHS Trust, Oxford, UK

Hemorrhoids

Epidemiology

Hemorrhoidal disease is common, with a prevalence estimated to be about 4% of the population. The term "hemorrhoids" (Greek "flowing blood") is often used synonymously with "piles" (Latin *pila*, ball), despite their differing derivations.

Pathophysiology

The submucosa of the anal canal comprises numerous arteriovenous channels surrounded by connective tissue. Physiological swellings of this layer are the "anal cushions" which probably have a role in fine control of anal continence. Hemorrhoids are enlarged, prolapsed or symptomatic anal cushions and the causes are probably multifactorial: relaxation of supportive connective tissue, as in pregnancy, or excessive straining, as in chronic constipation, are likely to be involved. High pressure in the internal sphincter has been observed in patients with hemorrhoids, which may contribute to increased shearing forces during defecation, or reduced venous return leading to submucosal vascular engorgement.

Clinical features

The common symptoms are bleeding, prolapse, and discomfort. Bleeding is characteristically bright red on defecation and in the toilet pan or just on the paper. Hemorrhoidal prolapse usually occurs on defecation, although there may ultimately be spontaneous prolapse. Discomfort is nonspecific but there may be an aching sensation or pruritus and irritation. Pain usually only occurs with hemorrhoidal thrombosis.

Colorectal Surgery: Clinical Care and Management, First Edition.
Edited by Bruce George, Richard Guy, Oliver Jones, and Jon Vogel.
© 2016 John Wiley & Sons, Ltd. Published 2016 by John Wiley & Sons, Ltd.

Classification

There is no satisfactory classification but degrees are traditionally reported, although progression through these categories is not necessarily sequential or inevitable.

- First degree – bleed but do not prolapse.
- Second degree – prolapse with straining but reduce spontaneously.
- Third degree – prolapse with straining and require digital reduction.
- Fourth degree – constantly prolapsed.

Examination

Examination in clinic should include inspection of the anus and perineum, digital rectal examination and proctoscopy, with and without straining, to gauge displacement of the anal cushions and degree of pelvic floor descent.

Investigation

Whilst most clinicians carry out rigid sigmoidoscopy in clinic, this is often an unsatisfactory examination and, if there is suspicion of associated or more proximal pathology, flexible sigmoidoscopy following enema administration is probably more useful. It is advisable for patients over the age of 45 years with rectal bleeding to undergo this examination.

Treatment

Treatment of hemorrhoids is based on the patient's symptoms and a tailored approach should be adopted. For patients with minimal symptoms and first-degree hemorrhoids, most will require no treatment at all, other than dietary advice, avoidance of straining, and some reassurance.

Conservative treatment

- Over-the-counter topical preparations are popular but have no proven value, other than a potential lubricant effect.
- Dietary fiber has been demonstrated to have a beneficial effect for symptomatic hemorrhoids [1].
- Oral vasotopic drugs, such as flavonoids, may have some minor benefit.

Outpatient treatments

In the UK, the most common options for outpatient treatment are injection sclerotherapy and rubber band ligation, usually for the treatment of first- and second-degree hemorrhoids, respectively. Other treatments such as infra-red coagulation and cryotherapy are neither widely available nor popular.

Injection sclerotherapy involves injecting 5% oily phenol into the submucous layer proximal to (above) the hemorrohoid as a sclerosant. This must be injected above the dentate line to avoid pain. Serious complications are extremely rare but include prostatitis, rectovaginal fistula, and liver abscess. The oil utilized is usually either peanut (arachis) or almond oil and treatment of patients with nut allergy must be avoided.

Rubber band ligation involves the placement of a small rubber band at the base of the hemorrhoid above the dentate line using a grasper or suction device through a proctoscope, usually at up to three sites. Minor bleeding, discomfort, and sometimes a vasovagal episode can occur. Patients should be warned that minor bleeding after several days is common as the band and mucosa slough away; heavy secondary hemorrhage requiring hospital admission is rare.

Injection sclerotherapy and rubber band ligation should always be performed under direct vision with good lighting, and the use of a bevel-ended proctoscope is to be preferred for this. Of the outpatient treatments, rubber band ligation seems to be the most effective from randomized controlled trial evidence [2].

Surgical treatment

Surgery is usually reserved for patients with persistent hemorrhoidal prolapse, a significant external component, recurrent and excessive bleeding, or sometimes in the case of acute prolapse and thrombosis. The American Gastroenterological Association suggests that hemorrhoidectomy should be recommended only for a small minority of patients with any of the following characteristics [3]:

- failure of medical and nonoperative therapy
- symptomatic third-degree hemorrhoids
- symptomatic hemorrhoids in the presence of a concomitant anorectal condition that requires surgery
- patient preference after discussion of the treatment options with the surgeon.

The main options for surgical treatment include:

- Milligan–Morgan (conventional) hemorrhoidectomy
- stapled hemorrhoidectomy/hemorrhoidopexy
- Doppler-guided hemorrhoidal artery ligation +/- mucopexy.

Conventional hemorrhoidectomy

The most common methods used for excisional hemorrhoidectomy are as follows.

- Open hemorrhoidectomy, described by Milligan and Morgan [4], with excision of the external and internal component of each hemorrhoid, leaving the mucosa and skin open to heal by secondary intention. Excision may be performed with scissors or various energy devices, including electrocautery, Harmonic Scalpel or Ligasure.
- Closed hemorrhoidectomy, described by Ferguson and Heaton [5], which is similar except that the mucosa and anoderm are closed primarily.

In both techniques, it is important to preserve bridges of anoderm between the excised hemorrhoids to reduce the risk of postoperative stenosis. Whilst these two techniques lend themselves to randomized controlled trials, there seems to be little overall difference in terms of healing rates, postoperative pain, and complications. Wound dehiscence following the closed technique simply converts the procedure into an open method. The unhealed hemorrhoidectomy wound can be a particular problem, behaving and appearing like a chronic anal fissure, and treated along similar lines.

Stapled hemorrhoidectomy (syn. hemorrhoidopexy, anopexy, procedure for prolapse and hemorrhoids – PPH)

This procedure involves the use of a specifically designed circular stapling device to remove a cylinder of lower rectal mucosa, thereby achieving a degree of devascularization and "hitching up" the displaced hemorrhoidal cushions into a more anatomical position. As the procedure is performed above the dentate line, it should be relatively painless.

Metaanalyses of RCTs comparing stapled hemorrhoidopexy with conventional hemorrhoidectomy [6] suggest that, whilst stapled hemorrhoidopexy offers some short-term benefits in terms of postoperative pain, overall complication rates are similar. In the longer term, stapled hemorrhoidopexy seems to be associated with higher rates of recurrent hemorrhoidal disease requiring further surgery. The procedure may be most useful for circumferential mucosal prolapse.

Doppler-guided hemorrhoidal artery ligation (DGHAL)

The DGHAL procedure has been adopted enthusiastically, is easily learned and has recently received National Institute for Health and Care Excellence (NICE) approval. The vascular pedicle of the hemorrhoid is identified by Doppler ultrasound and suture-ligated, using commercially available equipment. This devascularization is often combined with anopexy/mucopexy, thereby dealing with the main hemorrhoidal symptoms of bleeding and prolapse. It is relatively painless if sutures are placed above the dentate line, although for a more exaggerated "hitch up," sutures may need to come down lower. A systematic review of 28 studies – of relatively poor overall quality involving 2904 patients – showed a pooled overall recurrence rate of 17.5% (being highest for grade IV hemorrhoids), postoperative bleeding rate of 5% and reintervention rate of 6.4% [7].

Complications

Complicatons of hemorrhoid surgery include:
- urinary retention (5–10%)
- secondary hemorrhage (1–2%)
- fecal incontinence (2–10%)
- stricture (<1%).

In the UK, most surgical procedures for hemorrhoids are now undertaken on an ambulatory (day-case) basis. Adequate analgesia (including generous local anesthesia), stool softeners, and advice are, therefore, essential. Additional pharmacological treatments which may improve postoperative pain include:

- oral metronidazole [8]
- glyceryl trinitrate ointment [9]
- diltiazem ointment [10]
- botulinum toxin injection [11].

Special considerations in the treatment of hemorrhoids

The wide array of reported hemorrhoidal symptoms and spectrum of clinical features make it very difficult to compare surgical treatments. It pays for the surgeon to be familiar with the various surgical techniques as "one size doesn't fit all." Treatment should be tailored according to the predominant abnormality, e.g. stapled hemorrhoidopexy for circumferential prolapse, DGHAL for bleeding second- and third-degree hemorrhoids, excisional hemorrhoidectomy for defined external disease.

Recurrent hemorrhoidal prolapse following surgery should raise suspicion of a more global pelvic floor disorder and relevant investigations, such as evacuation proctography, anorectal physiology and endoanal ultrasound, should be undertaken.

Hemorrhoids in HIV-positive patients may cause some anxiety, in terms of viral transmission during surgery, the potential for poor wound healing, and the consequences of anoreceptive intercourse in homosexual males (see **Case 33**). Perineal sepsis may be more likely if CD4 counts are low, and whilst success is reported in HIV-positive patients, caution needs to be exercised [5].

Anal fistula

Useful position statements and consensus recommendations from the Association of Coloproctology of Great Britain and Ireland [12] and the American Society of Colon and Rectal Surgeons [13] for the treatment of anorectal sepsis and fistula have been published.

Definition and etiology

An anal fistula is an abnormal communication between an internal opening in the anal canal and an external opening in the perineal skin. Most fistulae arise from infection originating in anal glands which lie circumferentially in the intersphincteric (IS) space, draining into the anal canal through the anal valves of Ball at the level of the dentate line.

Acute infection or abscess occurs when an anal crypt gland becomes obstructed with inspissated feces. Fistula formation following an abscess is not inevitable, and in 50% of cases the acute process clears completely following spontaneous or surgical drainage. An anal fistula represents chronic suppuration.

Classification

Anal fistulae are termed cryptogenic or idiopathic and are classified, most conveniently, using Parks' classification [14], according to the relationship between the fistula tract and the anal sphincter muscles (Figure D.1).

By the cryptogenic theory, sepsis originating in the IS space spreads along tissues and planes of least resistance. An IS abscess, therefore, may point in the perianal region as a perianal abscess, and persistence of this track following surgical or spontaneous drainage results in an IS fistula, the most common type of anal fistula.

Pus in the IS space may penetrate the external sphincter, probably doing so by way of fascicles of outer longitudinal smooth muscle, gaining access to the ischiorectal fossa where the looser fat allows for more rapid spread. Pus in the ischiorectal and IS spaces may subsequently spread around the circumference of the anal canal as horse-shoe abscesses. If the connection with the anal canal across the external sphincter (ES) persists following drainage of an ischiorectal abscess, a transsphincteric (TS) fistula may form, the second most common type of anal fistula encountered. The more cephalad the penetration of the ES, the higher and more difficult the TS will be to treat.

By the same token, if a supralevator abscess penetrates the levator plate into the ischiorectal fossa and is drained percutaneously, a suprasphincteric (SS) fistula may result. As the whole of the sphincter complex is incorporated in the fistula track, SS fistulae are particularly challenging to deal with. Fortunately they are relatively rare.

Some extrasphincteric (ES) fistulae may be explained by the cryptogenic theory, but this etiology probably doesn't account for all of them. Supralevator sepsis originating in the IS would need to simultaneously penetrate the rectum and levator plate, which seems unlikely. Some ES fistulae occur as a result of other

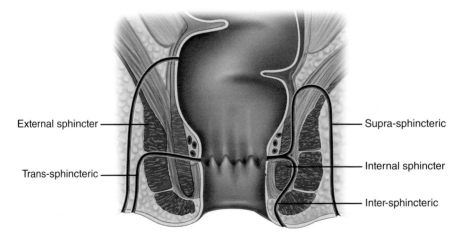

External sphincter — Supra-sphincteric

Internal sphincter

Trans-sphincteric — Inter-sphincteric

Figure D.1 Parks' classification of cryptogenic anal fistulae.

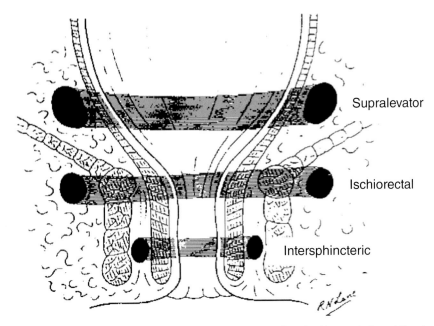

Figure D.2 Horse-shoe abscesses. *Source*: Phillips [15]. Reproduced with permission of Elsevier.

pathology affecting the rectum – such as Crohn's disease or rectal cancer – or abdominal and pelvic viscera – such as appendiceal or diverticular perforation or pelvic inflammatory disease. Some ES fistulae may be iatrogenic, through injudicious probing of a high TS or SS fistula [16].

Pus may also spread around the anorectum within spaces of little resistance, i.e. in the intersphincteric, ischiorectal or supralevator spaces (Figure D.2).

Differential diagnosis

Anal fistulae or sepsis may occur in association with other diseases (Table D.1). In practice, the most common differential diagnoses are Crohn's-related fistulae, infection in adjacent areas (e.g. Bartholin's abscess or pilonidal abscess), and hidradenitis suppurativa.

Clinical features

Perianal and ischiorectal abscesses present with pain and swelling and sometimes systemic upset, and are usually obvious on clinical examination. Submucosal and intersphincteric abscesses present with anal pain and, whilst there may be little to see on external inspection, induration and tenderness may be evident on gentle digital rectal examination. Supralevator sepsis may present with rectal pain and possibly disturbed micturition – if this is suspected, a primary intraabdominal source should be considered.

Table D.1 Differential diagnosis of anal fistulae.

Etiology	Example
Benign anal disease	Cryptogenic/idiopathic
	Secondary to anal fissure
Inflammatory bowel disease	Crohn's (rarely UC)
Adjacent skin sepsis	Sebaceous abscess
	Pilonidal abscess and sinus
Chronic skin infection	Hidradenitis suppurativa
	Tuberculosis
Gynecological	Bartholin's abscess
Malignancy	Anal cancer
	Rectal cancer
Trauma	Penetrating trauma
	Iatrogenic, e.g. hemorrhoid surgery
	Delayed postsurgical, e.g. pouch-perineal fistula

Assessment of an anal fistula in clinic should include the following questions.

Inspection
- What is the location of the external opening(s) (EO) in relation to a clock face, with 12 o'clock in the midline anteriorly?
- What is the distance of the EO from the anal margin in centimeters?
- What is the relationship of the EO to the outside border of the ES (where perianal skin pigmentation changes)?
- Is there any scarring or deformity from previous sepsis or surgery?

Palpation
- Can the track be felt under a lubricated gloved finger?
- Is there any secondary external induration or track?

Rectal examination
- Can an internal opening be felt? This can be difficult but may be felt as a lentil-sized "divot" at the level of the dentate line at the expected site according to Goodsall's rule (Figure D.3).
- Is there any pararectal or supralevator induration? This often has a "woody" feel and there will be asymmetry compared with the other side.
- Are the sphincters intact and does function feel normal?

Internal visualization (usually rigid sigmoidoscopy or proctoscopy)
- Is there any rectal disease, e.g. Crohn's?
- Is there pus coming from an internal opening?

The likely position of the internal opening can sometimes be predicted by Goodsall's rule, which states that anterior fistulae (i.e. anterior to a line drawn between 3 and 9 o'clock on the clock face) pass radially (like the spokes of a wheel) to the internal opening, whereas posterior fistulae pass to an internal opening in the midline posteriorly (see Figure D.3). This is a useful generalization but is less

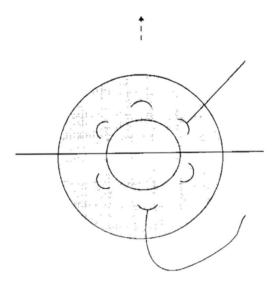

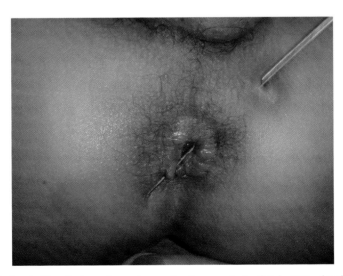

Figure D.3 Goodsall's rule, here shown in practice for an anterior fistula. Note also the clear change in pigmentation which anatomically marks the outer border of the external anal sphincter.

reliable for anterior fistulae, recurrent fistulae, and when the external opening is located more than 3 cm from the anal margin [17].

Investigations

Most simple low fistulae do not need to be investigated, although an exception may be made for an incontinent individual, especially if there is a significant obstetric history, where an assessment of anorectal physiology and sphincter integrity may be helpful. High fistulae, recurrent fistulae, and complex fistulae (i.e. those associated with secondary tracks or sepsis) usually require radiological evaluation.

Suspicion of alternative pathology, such as inflammatory bowel disease or malignancy, may mandate endoscopic or cross-sectional imaging. The most useful radiological tools for anal fistula assessment are MRI and endoanal ultrasound (EAUS). The latter provides an assessment of sphincter integrity as well as primary fistula anatomy, and accuracy is increased by 3D reconstruction and hydrogen peroxide enhancement by injection along the fistula track. Limitations of EAUS are seen in the assessment of secondary tracks and collections, which is best undertaken with MRI.

Anorectal physiology may be helpful in determining treatment options for patients with impaired continence, perhaps through obstetric injury or previous anal surgery, including fistula treatment, and may guide treatment in order to preserve continence [18].

Treatment

Abscesses

Acute perianal abscesses must be treated by adequate drainage of pus. This is likely to require partial deroofing of cavities and locules must be broken down, usually digitally. Where possible, drainage incisions should be curvilinear, in order to minimize sphincter injury, and as close to the anus as possible, in order to reduce the length of any subsequent fistula. For deep cavities, insertion of a mushroom (Malecot) catheter may allow for gentle flushing postoperatively. Horse-shoe abscesses may need additional drainage by counter-incisions on the opposite side, and with complex abscesses such as this, it is often helpful to plan a further examination under anesthetic after 48 hours in order to ensure that adequate drainage has been achieved.

In general, no attempt should be made to treat associated fistulae at the time of acute abscess drainage, and it is better to simply release the pus, as 50% will heal without developing a fistula. Clumsy probing in the acute situation or laying open fistulae may add complexity to a relatively straightforward problem. With horse-shoe abscesses, source control may necessitate use of Penrose or corrugated drains and insertion of a seton (Hanley's procedure), and this should be carried out by an experienced fistula surgeon (Figure D.4).

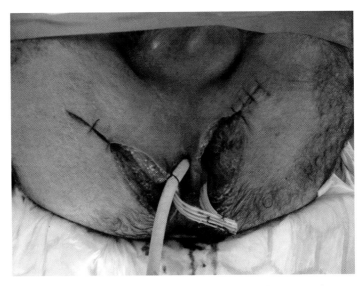

Figure D.4 Drainage of horse-shoe abscess. There has been wide drainage and a corrugated drain has been passed around the horseshoe cavity. Part of the clean wound (at second look) has been closed and a large Foley catheter has been inserted into the anus for irrigation and to reduce wound contamination.

Fistulae

The management of anal fistulae depends critically on the relationship of the fistula to the sphincter muscles. Ultimate outcome will depend upon the desired balance between fistula eradication and maintenance of function (continence), and patient expectations may need to be adjusted accordingly. Patients and surgeons should appreciate that ultimate eradication with preservation of function may take many months and multiple operations, especially with complex and high fistulae.

Simple fistulae

Simple fistulae are usually those which are IS or low TS, i.e. the fistula track crosses a third or less of the lower fibers of the external sphincter. For these fistulae, laying open (fistulotomy) has been the traditional treatment of choice with a low chance of incontinence and a high expectation of complete eradication (Figure D.5).

Wound healing may be faster if the laid-open track is marsupialized (Figure D.6).

Caution should be exercised before undertaking fistulotomy in females who have shorter anal canals, and in those with potential sphincter defects, especially if the fistula is situated anteriorly, where sphincter integrity is anatomically deficient [19]. It should also be appreciated that fistula tracks often run an oblique

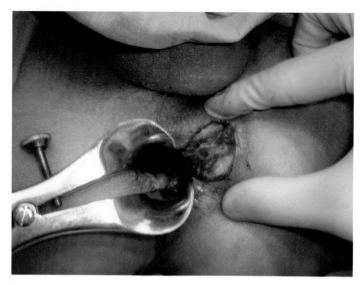

Figure D.5 Fistulotomy wound. Note the distinct fistula track.

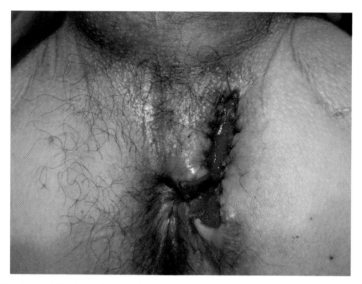

Figure D.6 Marsupialization of transsphincteric fistulotomy wound.

course through the sphincters, resulting in division of more muscle than expected from the level of the internal opening [20].

Despite the success of fistulotomy for low fistulae, there has been a trend in recent years towards sphincter-conserving techniques for even relatively simple fistulae (analogous to the move away from sphincterotomy for anal fissure), largely through fear of incontinence [21].

Complex fistulae

Fistulae which are high, recurrent or complex usually require a staged, sphincter-conserving approach, usually with the placement of a seton as part of this process.

Use of setons (Cases 35, 36)

Setons (Latin "bristle") are invaluable in fistula management. In theory, any suture or similar material can be used, but silastic setons are favored by many surgeons. The seton should be tied loosely in order to allow drainage and patients should be informed that discharge along the track is a normal and desired consequence; indeed, pus may on occasions discharge along this track. A loose seton may also allow the primary track to mature such that subsequent eradication becomes easier, and clinical estimation in the awake patient may be facilitated by the presence of the seton (Figure D.7).

"Tight" or "cutting" setons are placed as an alternative to surgical fistulotomy. By serial tightening of the seton every few weeks, the seton "cheesewires" through the muscle which heals by fibrosis once divided. Unfortunately, long-term studies show no continence advantage compared with fistulotomy and such treatment has been largely abandoned [22]. Interestingly, sequential loose or "snug" setons, if left long enough, may migrate through the muscle, leaving a simple low fistulotomy and success has been reported with this method [23].

Some patients are best advised to accept a long-term loose seton for their complex fistula. Commonly used for Crohn's fistulae, they have an important role in difficult idiopathic fistulae for which surgical treatments have been unsuccessful

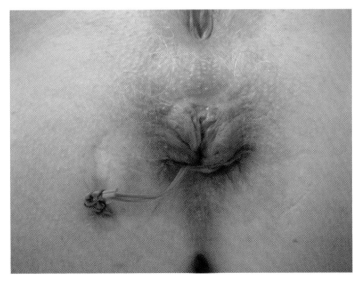

Figure D.7 A loose silastic seton through a transsphincteric fistula in a female.

or abandoned or in incontinent patients. They may be the preferred treatment for suprasphincteric and extrasphincteric fistulae. The setons may need changing at intervals.

Chemical setons, usually impregnated with ayuverdic acid, are most popular on the Indian subcontinent and other parts of Asia. The setons are usually inserted "snug" and gradual fistulotomy occurs, although there are probably no significant advantages over primary fistulotomy [24]. They have not found a place in UK or US practice.

Sphincter-preserving surgical techniques for complex and high fistulae

A variery of sphincter-preserving approaches to anal fistula surgery have been described (Table D.2). The crucial balance remains the preservation of function

Table D.2 Sphincter-preserving procedures for anal fistulae.

Technique	Comments
Endorectal advancement flap	Literature reports approximately 80% success with 13% incontinence, but studies generally small or flawed [25]
LIFT (ligation of intersphincteric fistula track)	Increasingly popular approach (see **Case 36**), recent systematic review and metaanalysis reports 76% success at mean 10-month follow-up, 0% incontinence, 5.5% complications [26]
Anal fistula plug (Surgis AFP, Cook Biotech Inc, US)	Porcine-derived small bowel submucosa. Strong pliable material providing scaffold for fibroblast activity. Overall pooled healing rates from literature 54% [27]
Fibrin glue	Encouraging early reports but long-term results disappointing with wide variation between studies and overall healing rate of 53% [28]
Fistula Tract Laser closure (FiLaC™)	Use of laser to obliterate fistula track, usually combined with internal opening closure. Largest study of 45 patients with median follow-up 30 months, primary healing 71.1% [29]
Video-assisted anal fistula treatment (VAAFT)	Video-assisted endoscopic technique to debride and fulgurate fistula track and close internal opening. Reported 6-month healing rates 70% but longer-term results necessary [30]
OTSC clip	Super-elastic nitinol clip with tooth-like jaws used to close the internal opening [31]
Adipose-derived stem cells	Novel approach using adult mesenchymal stem cells derived from adipose tissue to treat complex fistulae; used in combination with glue. Disappointing long-term healing rates [32]

whilst attempting fistula cure. With these techniques, fistula persistence is more likely than with fistulotomy, which is frustrating for the surgeon and patient, whose expectations may need to be adjusted.

Anal fissure

Anal fissure is common, especially in the second to fourth decades of life, with an estimated lifetime incidence of around 11%. Multiple atypical fissures may represent an underlying pathology such as Crohn's disease, HIV, TB, syphilis or neoplasia. Some primary dermatoses, such as lichen sclerosis, may be associated with fissuring. Nicorandil, a vasodilator used for angina, may also cause anal fissures, which usually heal following cessation of the drug [33].

Pathophysiology

The etiology of fissures is uncertain, but some initiating trauma to the anoderm must occur, possibly with the passage of hard stool. As the posterior midline is a relative watershed, a chronic fissure may represent a relatively ischemic linear ulcer. High resting anal pressure may exacerbate hypoperfusion and cause pain itself through sphincter spasm.

Classification

There is a temporal and clinical classification of chronicity. Acute fissures usually resolve within 6 weeks, and any fissure persisting beyond 6 weeks is termed chronic.

Clinical features

Anal fissures present with severe anal pain during defecation, which may persist for several hours afterwards. Bright red blood is commonly seen on the tissue paper on wiping or as streaking on the stool.

Examination

The anal verge usually needs to be gently separated in order to see an anal fissure. A fissure is seen as a linear ulcer in the anal canal below the dentate line, usually in the midline posteriorly, but occurring anteriorly in 20% of patients, particularly females [34]. Some 8% of fissures occur anteriorly and posteriorly [35]. Internal digital examination may be impossible on account of pain. Associated perianal sepsis should be excluded and examination under anesthetic may be required for this. The cardinal features of a chronic anal fissure include:
- raised fibrous edges
- visible internal sphincter fibers

- presence of a sentinel tag
- a hypertrophied anal papilla.

Management

Most acute fissures will heal spontaneously, with the help of stool softeners and topical analgesics. Chronic fissures may be a challenge and are much less likely to respond to simple medical therapy.

Conservative therapy is directed at lowering resting tone by reducing internal anal sphincter pressure. Surgical therapy includes sphincter-lowering procedures and flaps, sometimes in combination.

Nonsurgical treatment

A number of topical treatments have emerged, each designed to lower internal sphincter pressure by a process of "chemical sphincterotomy." The most commonly prescribed treatments are glyceryl trinitrate and diltiazem. Inducing internal sphincter relaxation may reduce the pain associated with sphincter spasm, whilst also facilitating improved perfusion.

Glyceryl trinitrate (GTN) is a nitric oxide donor and is usually prescribed in a 0.2–0.4% concentration. Application is 2–3 times daily with a gloved finger, in order to reduce absorption through the finger, thereby reducing the risk of headaches. Increasing the dose from 0.2% to 0.4% may not increase efficacy but is likely to increase the incidence of headaches [36].

Diltiazem, prescribed in a 2% strength, is a calcium channel blocker. Headaches are uncommon and so compliance is often better than with GTN.

Glyceryl trinitrate or diltiazem are the usual first-line treatments for fissure, and choice will depend upon local availability and cost in addition to clinical effect and tolerance, particularly headaches [37]. Failure with one preparation may be an indication to switch to the alternative. Patients should be encouraged to persist with treatment for at least 2 months.

Botulinum toxin is a potent and lethal toxin which induces short-term internal sphincter paralysis, by sympathetic noradrenergic blockade rather than a cholinergic effect, which would be seen in skeletal muscle [38]. Its effect typically wears off after about 2–3 months. There is no consensus on the ideal dose, nor the optimum injection site or technique, but most studies report dosages of the equivalent of 20–100 units of Botox as a single dose. Most clinicians inject directly into the internal sphincter and/or the intersphincteric space, in the region of the fissure, and this can be done under local anesthetic. Patients should be warned that paralysis of the internal sphincter may result in reversible minor incontinence. The general acceptance is that fissures which persist after two injections are unlikely to resolve with any more. Interestingly, resolution of fissure symptoms may occur without complete fissure healing.

Overall results of nonsurgical treatment

There seems to be little to choose between the various medical treatments. A recent Cochrane Database review showed similar efficacy between GTN, diltiazem, and Botox. GTN was marginally but significantly better than placebo in healing anal fissure (48.9% vs 35.3%, p<0.0009), but late recurrence was common in the 50% of those initially cured [39]. Incontinence with medical therapy is not a significant issue.

Surgical treatment

For those patients who fail nonoperative treatment, surgical treatment should be considered. Fissurectomy, lateral internal sphincterotomy (see **Case 34**), and anal advancement flaps are the most commonly performed procedures. Anal dilatation has been largely abandoned due to the significant risk of causing fecal incontinence.

Fissurectomy, with excision of the edges of the fissure as well as any sentinel tag and curettage of the base, aims to "freshen" the fissure, effectively converting a chronic fissure to an acute one. It is probably more effective when combined with botulinum toxin injection [40].

Lateral internal sphincterotomy. Division of the lower fibers of the internal sphincter in a controlled fashion under direct vision is a highly effective treatment for chronic fissure (see **Case 34**). This is usually done at the 3 or 9 o'clock positions and not through the fissure itself, which tends to result in a "keyhole" deformity. Whilst traditionally carried out up to the level of the dentate line, a "tailored" sphincterotomy describes division of the internal sphincter up to the level of the top of the fissure, thus reducing the risk of incontinence.

Anal advancement flaps may be particularly useful for "low-pressure" fissures, but may also have a place for normal or high-pressure fissures, particularly if accompanied by pressure-lowering treatment, such as botulinum toxin injection. Various flaps have been described but a small island flap or V-Y advancement flap are most common.

Overall results of surgical treatment

Surgical treatment, particularly lateral sphincterotomy, is far more effective than medical treatment in terms of fissure healing[41] but at the expense of a risk of minor incontinence. Healing rates after sphincterotomy may be around 85%. Long-term continence disturbance is reported in up to 30% of patients following lateral sphincterotomy [42, 43] but with high rates of patient satisfaction.

Pilonidal sinus

Sacrococcygeal pilonidal sinus disease is an acquired, self-limiting condition of recurrent sepsis in the natal cleft. It has an incidence of around 26 per 100,000 population, usually seen most commonly in men between the ages of 18 and 30, and is rare over the age of 45.

Pathophysiology

The exact etiology remains unknown, but the most plausible explanations are that skin debris and hairs enter midline pits, or that stretched hair follicles become infected, and the resulting folliculitis becomes chronic, allowing sinus formation.

Clinical features

Presentation is with recurrent abscesses, sinuses, and fistulation in the natal cleft. Symptoms include pain, swelling, and recurrent discharge.

Examination

Severity of pilonidal disease is very variable but examination of the patient may reveal a midline pit or several pits and lateral extensions to one or both sides, usually in a cephalad direction, although occasionally extension may be towards the anus. Hairs may be seen protruding from sinus orifices and there may be associated sepsis. Clinical diagnosis is usually straightforward, and investigations are rarely necessary, but recurrent disease or significant sepsis may warrant MR imaging. This, together with examination under anesthetic, may also be required in order to distinguish pilonidal sinus disease from a complex anal fistula.

Management

Conservative

Attention to natal cleft hygiene, depilation, and occasional courses of antibiotics may suffice for many patients, particularly if symptoms are not too troublesome. Recurrent episodes of sepsis are an indication for surgery.

Surgical

Pilonidal abscesses should be drained by an off-midline incision where possible and for some patients no further treatment is required. Nonradical elective techniques for pilonidal sinus include brushing of tracks, phenolization, laser treatment, and fibrin glue, none of which is likely to lead to long-term cure [44].

Historically, attempts at eradication involved wide excision leaving disabling open wounds, protracted recovery, and high recurrence rates. Wide elliptical excision and midline primary closure are not now recommended. With an appreciation of the superficial epidermal etiology of pilonidal sinus, eradication procedures associated with the highest healing rates involve less radical excisions and simple flaps to create an off-midline wound [45]. The most commonly used and most successful flap techniques are those described by Karydakis [46] – reporting a recurrence rate of only 1% in almost 7000 cases – and Bascom [47]. These procedures are very similar in that an off-midline wound is created; the main differences are that the Karydakis excision is elliptical and the flap is thicker, whilst the Bascom excision is more superficial and eccentric, leaving a fat pad to cover the midline, and achieves a more substantial cleft lift (see **Case 38**). Most cases can be performed as day cases and many under local anesthesia [48].

Rhomboid flap

The Karydakis and Bascom flaps are most suited to midline and unilateral pilonidal sinus disease. Sinuses on both sides of the midline can present more of a challenge as a simple flap may not be sufficient. The Limberg flap is a rhomboid-shaped rotational flap that satisfactorily deals with this problem [49], although cosmetically it results in a more extensive wound (Figure D.8). Healing outcomes seem to be comparable to those for the Karydakis/Bascom flaps.

Even more extensive disease may necessitate wider excision and the use of gluteal advancement flaps (Figure D.9), usually best undertaken by a plastic surgeon.

Topical negative pressure therapy may also be useful for extensive disease, especially when there is significant sepsis (Figure D.10). A randomized trial involving 49 patients comparing topical negative pressure therapy with standard open wound care showed that, whilst the negative pressure therapy group wounds were smaller within 2 weeks, the times to complete healing and patient return to normal activities were similar [50].

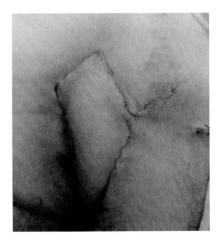

Figure D.8 Postoperative wound following rhomboid (Limberg) flap operation.

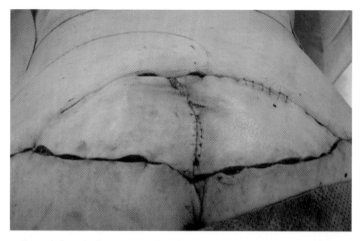

Figure D.9 Bilateral gluteal advancement flaps for extensive sacrococcygeal disease.

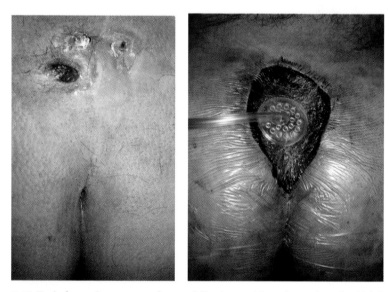

Figure D.10 Topical negative pressure therapy following excision of complex pilonidal disease.

Pruritus ani

Etiology

Pruritus ani is a common symptom of perianal itch and irritation and is usually entirely benign and self-limiting. Around a quarter of cases of pruritus ani are idiopathic and probably related to a minor degree of perianal soiling or poor hygiene, although an obsession with wiping with tissue paper may conversely worsen symptoms, and scratching may exacerbate the problem. Local anorectal causes are common and some systemic conditions may need to be considered (Box D.1) [51].

Box D.1 Causes of pruritus ani.

Infective	Bacterial, e.g. Campylobacter
	Fungal/yeast, e.g. tinea
	Viral, e.g. herpes simplex
	Parasitic, e.g. threadworms
Dermatological	Psoriasis
	Lichen planus, lichen simplex
	Lichen sclerosus et atrophicus
	Contact dermatits and atopic dermatitis
	Bowen's and Paget's disease
Systemic disease	Diabetes mellitus
	Leukemia and lymphoma
	Obstructive jaundice
	Thyroid disorders
Local irritants	Fecal contamination/soiling and moisture
	Perfumed soaps and talcs
	Dietary excess, e.g. alcohol, caffeine
	Topical medications
Anorectal causes	Prolapse (hemorrhoidal, mucosal or full-thickness rectal)
	Fistula in ano
	Fissure in ano
	Incontinence

Diagnosis

Anal inspection, supplemented by proctoscopy and/or rigid sigmoidoscopy, is usually all that is required to make the diagnosis. Excoriation and fecal soiling may be evident and the skin can be inspected for primary dermatoses or fungal infection. Skin tags or hemorrhoidal disease, an anal fissure or fistula may be seen. Digital rectal examination, proctoscopy, and rigid sigmoidoscopy may allow assessment for hemorrhoids, proctitis, neoplasia or threadworms.

Management

Conservative management of idiopathic pruritus ani, including reassurance and advice to achieve a clean, dry perianal skin, including breaking the cycle of scratching and further irritation, will alleviate symptoms in most of cases. Wet cotton wool may be substituted for tissue paper for wiping after defecation. Washing the perianal area with warm water without soap, avoiding medicated or alcohol-impregnated wipes, drying the perianal skin gently or with a hair-dryer and avoiding talcs and perfumed products may also help. For patients with fecal leakage, an antidiarrheal drug such as loperamide may be of benefit, and dietary manipulation, avoiding caffeine, alcohol, and spicy food, may be advisable [52].

Treatment of pathology

Removal of skin tags to enable anal hygiene, and treatment of fissures and fistulae may be necessary. Hemorrhoid treatments and treatment of mucosal prolapse may be effective in alleviating pruritus (see **Case 39**) [53], but counseling patients about the risks of postoperative incontinence, perhaps worsening symptoms of pruritus, is advisable.

Empirical treatment with topical antifungal creams may be worthwhile, but referral to a dermatologist for assessment and treatment of obvious perianal skin disease or in refractory cases of pruritus is often useful.

Management of severe and refractory idiopathic pruritus ani

Topical steroids (1% hydrocortisone) may improve symptoms, but should only be used sparingly for a short period (up to 2 weeks) to avoid skin atrophy. Topical 0.006% capsaicin cream, by producing an intense burning sensation and inhibitory feedback, may eliminate the need to scratch, and has been shown in one randomized trial to improve symptoms in 70% of patients treated [54].

Intradermal methylene blue injection should be reserved for intractable cases as anal tattooing and loss of perianal sensation may persist (see **Case 39**). Whilst some small prospective studies have shown good resolution of symptoms within 1 year (up to 88%) [55], pruritus may recur in the longer term, albeit often less severely, requiring repeat injection.

References

1 Alonso-Coello P, Guyatt G, Heels-Ansdell D, *et al*. Laxatives for the treatment of haemorrhoids. *Cochrane Database Syst Rev* 2005; **4**:CD004649.

2 MacRae HM, McLeod RS. Comparison of hemorrhoidal treatments: a meta-analysis. *Can J Surg* 1997; **40**:14–17.

3 Clinical Practice Committee. American Gastroenterological Association Medical Position Statement: Diagnosis and Treatment of Hemorrhoids. *Gastroenterology* 2004; **126**:1461–2.

4 Milligan ET, Morgan CN, Jones LE, Officer R. Surgical anatomy and operative treatment of haemorrhoids. *Lancet* 1937; **ii**:1119–24.

5 Ferguson JA, Heaton JR. Closed haemorrhoidectomy. *Dis Colon Rectum* 1959; **2**:176–9.

6 Giordano P, Gravante G, Sorge R, Ovens L, Nastro P. Long-term outcomes of stapled hemorrhoidopexy vs conventional hemorrhoidectomy: a meta-analysis of randomized controlled trials. *Arch Surg* 2009; **144**:266–72.

7 Pucher PH, Sodergren MH, Lord AC, Darzi A, Ziprin P. Clinical outcome following Doppler-guided haemorrhoidal artery ligation: a systematic review. *Colorectal Dis* 2013; **15**:e284–94.

8 Carapeti EA, Kamm MA, McDonald PJ, Phillips RK. Double-blind randomized controlled trial of effect of metronidazole on pain after day-case haemorrhoidectomy. *Lancet* 1998; **35**:169–72.

9 Ratnasingham K, Uzzaman M, Andreani SM, Light D, Patel B. Meta-analysis of the use of glyceryl trinitrate ointment after haemorrhoidectomy as an analgesic and in promoting wound healing. *Int J Surg* 2010; **8**:606–11.

10 Sugimoto T, Tsunoda A, Kano N, Kashiwagura Y, Hirose K, Sasaki T. A randomized, prospective, double-blind, placebo-controlled trial of the effect of diltiazem gel on pain after hemorrhoidectomy. *World J Surg* 2013; **37**:2454–7.

11 Patti R, Almasio PL, Muggeo VM, *et al.* Improvement of wound healing after haemorrhoidectomy: a double-blind, randomized study of botulinum toxin injection. *Dis Colon Rectum* 2005; **48**:2173–9.

12 Williams JG, Farrands PA, Williams AB, *et al.* The treatment of anal fistula: ACPGBI Position Statement. *Colorectal Dis* 2007; **9**(Suppl 4):18–50.

13 Steele SR, Kumar R, Feingold D, Rafferty JL, Buie WD. Practice parameters for the management of perianal abscess and fistula in ano. *Dis Colon Rectum* 2011; **54**:1465–74.

14 Parks AG, Gordon PH, Hardcastle JD. A classification of fistula-in-ano. *Br J Surg* 1976; **63**:1–12.

15 Phillips R (ed.). *Colorectal Surgery: A Companion to Specialist Surgical Practice*, 2nd edn. Philadelphia: W. B. Saunders, 2002, p. 302.

16 Seow-Choen F, Phillips RK. Insights gained from the management of problematical anal fistulae at St. Mark's Hospital 1984–88. *Br J Surg* 1991; **78**:539–41.

17 Cirocco WC, Reilly JC. Challenging the predictive accuracy of Goodsall's rule for anal fistulas. *Dis Colon Rectum* 1992; **35**:537–42.

18 Pescatori M, Maria G, Anastasio G, *et al.* Anal manometry improves the outcome of surgery for fistula in ano. *Dis Colon Rectum* 1989; **32**:588–92.

19 Williams AB, Bartram CI, Halligan S, Marshall MM, Nicholls RJ, Kmiot WA. Multiplanar anal endosonography – normal anal canal anatomy. *Colorectal Dis* 2001; **3**:169–74.

20 Buchanan GN, Williams AB, Bartram CI, *et al.* Potential clinical implications of direction of a trans-sphincteric anal fistula track. *Br J Surg* 2003; **90**:1250–5.

21 Blumetti J, Abcarian A, Quinteros F, Chaudhry V, Prasad L, Abcarian H. Evolution of treatment of fistula in ano. *World J Surg* 2012; **36**(5):1162–7.

22 Christensen A, Nilas I, Christansen J. Treatment of transsphincteric anal fistulas by the seton technique. *Dis Colon Rectum* 1986; **29**:793–7.

23 Hammond TM, Knowles CH, Porrett T, Lunniss PJ. The snug seton: short and medium term results of slow fistulotomy for idiopathic anal fistulae. *Colorectal Dis* 2006; **8**:328–37.

24 Ho KS, Tsang C, Seow-Choen F, *et al.* Prospective randomized trial comparing ayurvedic cutting seton and fistulotomy for low fistula-in-ano. *Tech Coloproctol* 2001; **5**:137–41.

25 Soltani A, Kaiser AM. Endorectal advancement flap for cryptoglandular or Crohn's fistula-in-ano. *Dis Colon Rectum* 2010; **53**:486–95.

26 Hong KD, Kang S, Kalaskar S, Wexner SD. Ligation of intersphincteric fistula tract (LIFT) to treat anal fistula: systematic review and meta-analysis. *Tech Coloproctol* 2014; **18**:685–91.

27 O'Riordan JM, Datta I, Johnston C, Baxter NN. A systematic review of the anal fistula plug for patients with Crohn's and non-Crohn's related fistula-in-ano. *Dis Colon Rectum* 2012; **55**:351–8.

28 Swinscoe MT, Ventakasubramaniam AK, Jayne DG. Fibrin glue for fistula-in-ano: the evidence reviewed. *Tech Coloproctol* 2005; **9**:89–94.

29 Giamundo P, Esercizio L, Geraci M, Tibaldi L, Valente M. Fistula-tract Laser Closure (FiLaC™): long-term results and new operative strategies. *Tech Coloproctol* 2015; **19**(8):449–53.

30 Meinero P, Mori L, Gasloli G. Video-assisted anal fistula treatment: a new concept of treating anal fistulas. *Dis Colon Rectum* 2014; **57**:354–9.

31 Prosst RL, Joos AK, Ehni W, Bussen D, Herold A. Prospective pilot study of anorectal fistula closure with the OTSC Proctology. *Colorectal Dis* 2015; **17**:81–6.

32 Guadalajara H, Herreros D, De-La-Quintana P, Trebol J, Garcia-Arranz M, Garcia-Olmo D. Long-term follow-up of patients undergoing adipose-derived adult stem cell administration to treat complex perianal fistulas. *Int J Colorectal Dis* 2012; **27**:595–600.

33 Katory M, Davies B, Kelty C, *et al.* Nicorandil and idiopathic anal ulceration. *Dis Colon Rectum* 2005; **47**:1442–6.

34 Cross KLR, Massey EJD, Fowler AL, Monson JRT. The management of anal fissure: ACPGBI Position Statement. *Colorectal Dis* 2008; **10**(Suppl 3):1–7.

35 Jones OM, Ramalingham T, Lindsey I, Cunningham C, George BD, Mortensen NJ. Digital rectal examination of sphincter pressures in chronic anal fissure is unreliable. *Dis Colon Rectum* 2005; **48**:349–52.

36 Scholefield JH, Bock JU, Marla B, *et al.* A dose finding study with 0.1%, 0.2% and 0.4% glyceryl trinitrate ointment in patients with chronic anal fissure. *Gut* 2003; **52**:264–9.

37 Sajid MS, Whitehouse PA, Sains P, Baig MK. Systematic review of the use of topical diltiazem compared with glyceryl trinitrate for the nonoperative management of chronic anal fissure. *Colorectal Dis* 2013; **15**:19–26.

38 Jones OM, Brading AF, Mortensen NJ. Mechanism of action of botulinum toxin on the internal anal sphincter. *Br J Surg* 2004; **91**:224–8.

39 Nelson RL, Thomas K, Morgan J, Jones A. Non surgical therapy for anal fissure. *Cochrane Database Syst Rev* 2012; **2**:CD003431.

40 Lindsey I, Cunningham C, Jones OM, Francis C, Mortensen NJ. Fissurectomy-botulinum toxin: a novel sphincter-sparing procedure for medically resistant chronic anal fissure. *Dis Colon Rectum* 2004; **47**:1947–52.

41 Nelson RL, Chattopadhyay A, Brooks W, Platt I, Paavana T, Earl S. Operative procedures for fissure in ano. *Cochrane Database Syst Rev* 2011; **11**:CD002199.

42 Garcia-Aguilar J, Belmonte C, Wong WD, *et al.* Open vs closed sphincterotomy for chronic anal fissure: long-term results. *Dis Colon Rectum* 1996; **39**:440–3.

43 Garg P, Garg M, Menon GR. Long-term continence disturbance after lateral internal sphincterotomy for chronic anal fissure: a systematic review and meta-analysis. *Colorectal Dis* 2013; **15**:e104–7.

44 Lee PJ, Raniga S, Biyani DK, Watson AJM, Faragher IG, Frizelle FA. Sacrococcygeal pilonidal disease. *Colorectal Dis* 2008; **10**:639–52.

45 Enriquez-Navascues JM, Emparanza JI, Alkorta M, Placer C. Meta-analysis of randomized controlled trials comparing different techniques with primary closure for chronic pilonidal sinus. *Tech Coloproctol* 2014; **18**:863–72.

46 Karydakis GE. New approach to the problem of pilonidal sinus. *Lancet* 1973; **2**(7843):1414–15.

47 Bascom J, Bascom T. Failed pilonidal surgery: new paradigm and new operation leading to cures. *Arch Surg* 2002; **137**:1146–50.

48 Senapati A, Cripps NP, Flashman K, Thompson MR. Cleft closure for the treatment of pilonidal sinus disease. *Colorectal Dis* 2011; **13**:333–6.

49 Akin M, Gokbayir H, Kilic K, Topgul K, Ozdemir E, Ferahkose Z. Rhomboid excision and Limberg flap for managing pilonidal sinus: long-term results in 411 patients. *Colorectal Dis* 2008; **10**:945–8.

50 Biter LU, Beck GM, Mannaerts GH, Stok MM, van der Ham AC, Grotenhuis BA. The use of negative-pressure wound therapy in pilonidal sinus disease: a randomized controlled trial comparing negative-pressure wound therapy versus standard open wound care after surgical excision. *Dis Colon Rectum* 2014; **57**:1406–11.

51 Markell KW, Billingham RP. Pruritus ani: etiology and management. *Surg Clin North Am* 2010; **90**:125–35.

52 Siddiqui S, Vijay V, Ward M, Mahendran R, Warren S. Pruritus ani. *Ann R Coll Surg Engl* 2008; **90**:457–63.

53 Murie JA, Sim AJW, Mackenzie I. the importance of pain, pruritus ani and soiling as symptoms of haemorrhoids and their response to haemorrhoidectomy or rubber band ligation. *Br J Surg* 1981; **68**:247–9.

54 Lysy J, Sistiery-Ittah M, Israelit Y, *et al*. Topical capsaicin – a novel and effective treatment for idiopathic intractable pruritus ani: a randomised, placebo controlled, crossover study. *Gut* 2003; **52**:1323–6.

55 Samalavicius NE, Poskus T, Gupta RK, Lunevicius R. Long-term results of single 1% methylene blue injection for intractable idiopathic pruritus ani: a prospective study. *Tech Coloproctol* 2012; **16**:295–9.

CASE 33

Hemorrhoids and HIV

Richard Guy

Oxford University Hospitals NHS Foundation Trust, Oxford, UK

A 25-year-old man was referred to the proctology clinic with rectal bleeding, mucus discharge, and sensation of prolapse. He regularly practiced anoreceptive sexual intercourse with his male partner, and was HIV positive but with a normal CD4 count on retroviral therapy. On examination, he was found to have circumferential intero-external hemorrhoids which bled easily. Rigid sigmoidoscopy showed a normal rectum and stool. Resting anal tone was subjectively low. Rubber band ligation (RBL) was undertaken in clinic. On review after 2 months, the patient reported no benefit from RBL and it was recommended that he should undergo Doppler-guided hemorrhoidal artery ligation (DG-HAL) with anopexy procedure. This was carried out uneventfully, but with no benefit in terms of bleeding and prolapse. He was booked for Milligan–Morgan excisional hemorrhoidectomy. At examination under anesthesia, advanced circumferential hemorrhoidal prolapse was evident (Figure 33.1).

DECISION POINT

What operation would you undertake? Would Milligan–Morgan hemorrhoidectomy be appropriate?

It was considered that excisional hemorrhoidectomy was not appropriate as there was circumferential intero-external hemorrhoidal prolapse. This would have created real difficulties with preservation of skin bridges and potential internal sphincter damage in a bloody field, with additional risks of HIV transmission. Stapled anopexy/hemorrhoidectomy (PPH) could be considered, although this can be technically demanding with gross disease. In addition, there are reports of penile trauma from the staple line in homosexuals practicing anal intercourse. The Whitehead operation might have been another option but this is rarely performed, tends to be relatively bloody, and stricturing is a risk. On balance, repeat hemorrhoidal artery ligation procedure with anopexy is probably the most attractive option, combining hemorrhoidal devascularization with mucosal prolapse reduction.

Colorectal Surgery: Clinical Care and Management, First Edition.
Edited by Bruce George, Richard Guy, Oliver Jones, and Jon Vogel.
© 2016 John Wiley & Sons, Ltd. Published 2016 by John Wiley & Sons, Ltd.

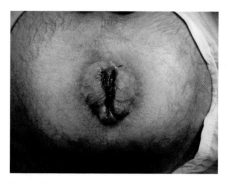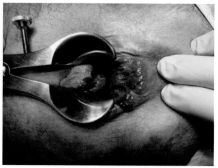

Figure 33.1 Appearance of the anus under anesthesia with obvious circumferential hemorrhoidal prolapse.

Anorectal physiology and endoanal ultrasound examinations were undertaken. These demonstrated low resting pressure but normal squeeze pressure, and intact sphincters. The patient went on to have a repeat DG-HAL and rectoanal repair (RAR), with a good outcome.

Could we have done better?

Whilst examination under anesthetic (EUA) can be useful for planning, it should have been realized that this case was not straightforward, and that Milligan–Morgan hemorrhoidectomy was not ideal. An unnecessary anesthetic could have been avoided.

LEARNING POINTS

- Hemorrhoid treatments should be tailored to individual requirements based upon symptoms, signs, and function – one size does not fit all.
- Low resting anal tone suggests preexisting sphincter injury, known to occur following anal intercourse. Hemorrhoidectomy under these circumstances runs a significant risk of incontinence.
- Hemorrhoid treatments in HIV-positive patients should probably be undertaken in centers frequently dealing with such patients. The risk of sepsis and poor wound healing may be higher, particularly if CD4 counts are subnormal.
- Repeat DG-HAL is feasible and safe.

LETTER FROM AMERICA

The 2013 ASCRS clinical practice guidelines endorse the use of Doppler-guided hemorrhoidal artery ligation (and other types of surgical hemorrhoid treatment) when diet and lifestyle modification and office-based procedures such as rubber band ligation or sclerotherapy fail to control the disease. These guidelines noted that studies of DG-HAL, that include at least 1 year of follow-up, show successful control of hemorrhoidal bleeding, prolapse, and pain in 90% of cases. Aside from the ASCRS guidelines, our experience with PPH is that the staple line will eventually become a minor circumferential scar that should not impede or add danger to the activities of those who undergo the procedure. An office-based digital exam and anoproctoscopy should be performed several months after the procedure to be sure that there are no remaining exposed staples.

Jon Vogel and Massarat Zutshi

CASE 34

Refractory fissure

Richard Guy
Oxford University Hospitals NHS Foundation Trust, Oxford, UK

A 50-year-old woman presented as an emergency with anal pain, which had become worse over 3 months. On examination, she had a chronic posterior fissure and, under local anesthetic with an anal block, she was given a 40 unit Botox injection into the internal anal sphincter (IAS). At clinic review 2 months later, she reported that although her symptoms were less severe, she still had pain and bleeding on defecation. On examination, it appeared that the fissure had almost completely healed and she was prescribed 2% diltiazem gel which further improved her symptoms. However, she re-presented after 6 months with recurrent symptoms and an obvious posterior fissure.

DECISION POINT

What would you advise now? What other aspects in the patient's history might be important?

It is important to make sure that the patient has been fully compliant with the topical treatment. This can be more of a problem with glyceryl trinitrate owing to potentially disabling headaches. A three times daily application rather than twice daily may be worth advising if possible. It was thought in this case that, as there had been some response to the Botox, and only a small dose had been administered, it would be worth trying this again, warning that there was a small risk of minor – usually temporary – incontinence. It is important to document continence and, in females, to take a good obstetric history seeking information on mode of any vaginal deliveries.

The patient proceeded to examination under anesthetic, where an injection of 90 units of Botox was given into the IAS (Figure 34.1). At review 2 months later, her symptoms persisted. She was taking plenty of laxatives but was reluctant to use the toilet, and admitted to pressing on the perineum to assist defecation. Anorectal physiology (ARP) demonstrated normal pressures, and endoanal ultrasound (EAUS) showed intact sphincters.

Colorectal Surgery: Clinical Care and Management, First Edition.
Edited by Bruce George, Richard Guy, Oliver Jones, and Jon Vogel.
© 2016 John Wiley & Sons, Ltd. Published 2016 by John Wiley & Sons, Ltd.

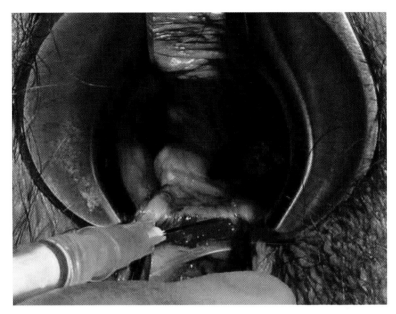

Figure 34.1 Botox injection for posterior fissure. Conventionally, the Botox is injected into the IAS either side of the fissure. The use of a 1 mL insulin syringe allows more accurate dosing.

DECISION POINT

What options are left now? Is surgery now indicated and, if so, what would you suggest?

The refractory fissure is a common problem in proctology clinics. Failure of "chemical sphincterotomy" is frustrating and surgical options far less popular now, despite historically good results in terms of fissure healing, largely on account of purported risks of incontinence. For this patient it was felt that surgery was indicated. Botox is generally not given beyond two doses in view of the risk of permanent IAS paralysis. The apparent evacuation difficulty raised the possibility of a pelvic floor disorder but this might have simply been a reluctance to defecate owing to pain, and further investigations were not considered appropriate. The patient was so fed up that she was very keen to proceed to surgery. The main choice was between lateral internal sphincterotomy and advancement flap. As ARP and EAUS had been normal, sphincterotomy was thought to be the best option, potentially reserving a flap for further recurrence, once anal canal pressures had been lowered.

Following discussion with the patient about risks of minor incontinence, the patient underwent 'tailored' internal sphincterotomy at the 3 o'clock position under direct vision, up to the same level as the top of the fissure (Figure 34.2).

This was uneventful, and at review 2 months later the patient was entirely symptom free. She did report a few episodes of possible flatus incontinence but was not troubled by this.

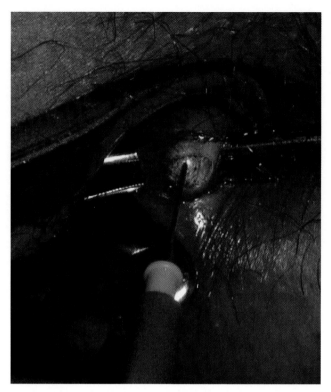

Figure 34.2 Internal sphincterotomy. The IAS should be isolated from the external sphincter laterally and from the mucosa medially, and then divided up to a chosen level under direct vision.

Could we have done better?

There is a tendency to try to keep patients going with intermittent conservative treatment and reassurance. Chemical sphincterotomy is likely to be more successful with more intensive treatment, supervision, and follow-up but this is rarely practical. There was considerable delay between presentation and final solution, and perhaps lateral sphincterotomy could have been performed at an earlier stage.

LEARNING POINTS

- Refractory anal fissures are common and often frustratingly difficult to treat.
- The ideal dosages and frequency of topical "chemical sphincterotomy" treatments and Botox therapy have not been determined.
- Internal sphincterotomy remains a highly effective treatment for chronic fissure, but caution should be exercised, especially in women who generally have shorter anal canals.

CASE 35

Hirschsprung's fistula

Richard Guy

Oxford University Hospitals NHS Foundation Trust, Oxford, Uk

A 30-year-old self-employed man who ran an ice cream company, and was shortly to be married, presented to the emergency service with a 1-week history of left ischiorectal abscess. As a baby, he had undergone coloanal pull-through surgery for Hirschsprung's disease, and had a multiply scarred abdomen, and as an adult his continence was generally poor but he coped with antidiarrheal medication. He was initially managed by a general surgeon who took the patient to theater. A large abscess was drained and deroofed and a silastic seton inserted through a long fistula track. The patient was handed to the colorectal service. Progressive sepsis ensued with a large cavity evident extending out to the left hip joint (Figure 35.1). The internal opening at the level of the old coloanal anastomosis was wide and there was a presacral sinus.

DECISION POINT

What are the options for control of sepsis? Should he have a stoma raised?

Ideally, such a patient with complex anorectal sepsis should be managed by a specialist colorectal surgeon from the outset. This was an unusual set of circumstances and presented particular difficulty in view of the previous Hirschsprung's surgery. Injudicious probing of fistula tracks, where anatomy may not obey the usual rules, may further complicate the issue. The critical decision at this point was whether the sepsis could be controlled without the use of a diverting stoma, and this was an important consideration in relation to the patient's domestic and business circumstances. If a stoma was to be raised, should this be an ileostomy or colostomy? Whilst a colostomy might be more easily managed, the previous coloanal pull-through might make a left-sided colostomy more difficult to raise.

A laparoscopic loop ileostomy was raised uneventfully, and at the same time the colon was irrigated antegradely on-table via the efferent limb of the stoma. Subsequently, serial examinations under anesthetic took place at 4–6-weekly intervals in order to irrigate and curette the wound. Eventually, some wound contraction and maturation was achieved but the cavity was still significant (Figure 35.2).

Colorectal Surgery: Clinical Care and Management, First Edition.
Edited by Bruce George, Richard Guy, Oliver Jones, and Jon Vogel.
© 2016 John Wiley & Sons, Ltd. Published 2016 by John Wiley & Sons, Ltd.

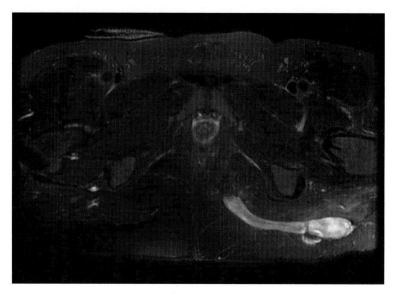

Figure 35.1 MRI scan demonstrating a wide track and abscess cavity extending out towards the left hip.

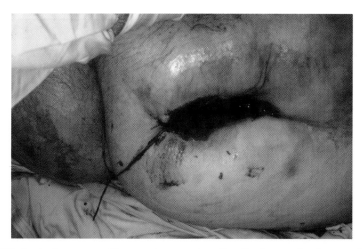

Figure 35.2 Gradual recovery with wound contraction. The silastic seton has been replaced with an Ethibond seton.

DECISION POINT

What plans should now be made? Does he need further investigations? Is fistula eradication a realistic prospect?

Discussion with the patient about the possibilities for long-term eradication took place. The realistic options were:
- endorectal advancement flap (ERAF) with ultimate closure of ileostomy – whilst the circumstances were not ideal, it was considered that "closing the trap door" over the internal opening, whilst ensuring adequate drainage, externally might be feasible
- long-term seton
- long-term diversion (stoma).

Repeat MRI scan was obtained. This showed that the cavity had resolved and a much smaller fistula track existed. A difficult ERAF was undertaken, with vigorous curettage of the external track.

Over the subsequent 3 months, there was a marked improvement in symptoms, with reduction in discharge and requirement for dressings (Figure 35.3). A further MRI still showed persistence of the track but with more fibrosis than active inflammation.

The patient's main concern was a large parastomal hernia, interfering with his ability to work, and he was eager to have the stoma reversed.

DECISION POINT

Would it be possible to simply close the stoma? What about the risk of recurrent sepsis?

Closing the ileostomy would allow much more satisfactory hernia repair and would satisfy the patient's desire to be rid of the stoma. However, whilst the radiological and clinical progress had been marked, there would still be the risk of recurrent fistula and sepsis and it was felt that it was too early to close the stoma. Re-raising of a stoma, should there be troublesome sepsis, would also be a challenge.

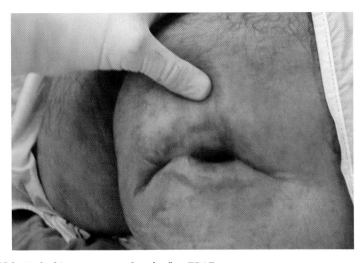

Figure 35.3 Marked improvement after the first ERAF.

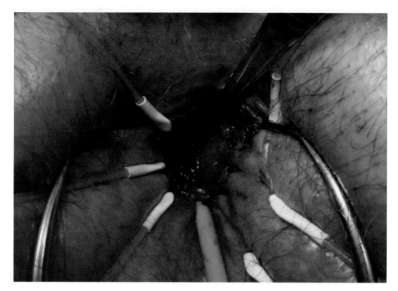

Figure 35.4 Repeat ERAF. A mushroom catheter is evident posteriorly and the curette has been placed in the rectal lumen. Note the use of Lonestar and Gelpey retractors for improved exposure.

Examination under anesthetic (EUA) was undertaken with a view to reversing the ileostomy if healing was considered complete. Gentle probing of the external opening failed to reveal any communication with the anal canal. Anal canal examination revealed that a posterior sinus persisted but this did not seem to communicate with the left ischiorectal fossa. Repeat advancement flap was undertaken, advancing the full thickness of the neorectum to cover this defect, leaving a small mushroom catheter through the posterior suture line, for gentle irrigation over 5 days (Figure 35.4). At the same time, the ileostomy was relocated on the same side of the abdomen, allowing primary repair of the original stomal defect.

After a further 3 months, the fistula had dried up completely. There remained a "divot" posteriorly but MRI appearances were satisfactory. There was a large recurrent parastomal hernia interfering with stoma function and stoma appliance adhesion.

At this point, a calculated risk was undertaken with the patient's informed consent. The ileostomy was closed and hernia repairs undertaken. A month later, the fistula reopened. Averse to further stomas, a seton was reinserted, in the expectation that this would have to remain in place long term.

LEARNING POINTS

- Complex fistulae are time-consuming and best managed by colorectal specialists, especially when there is unusual pathology.
- Defunctioning stomas may be required to allow adequate control of sepsis.
- Long-term setons are often to be preferred for the recalcitrant fistula.

CASE 36

Complex fistula in a young woman

Martijn Gosselink[1] & Richard Guy[2]

[1] Erasmus Medical Centre, Rotterdam, The Netherlands
[2] Oxford University Hospitals NHS Foundation Trust, Oxford, UK

A 35-year-old woman was seen in clinic with a 12-month history of a mucopuru-lent rectal discharge. There was a history of hemorrhoids and she had delivered one baby vaginally, sustaining a perineal tear which was repaired primarily. She reported normal fecal continence. On examination, an anal polyp was seen in the right posterior position and there were second-degree hemorrhoids. Flex-ible sigmoidoscopy was normal and examination under anesthetic (EUA) was arranged with a view to excising the polyp. Whilst waiting for EUA, the patient developed an abscess on the right buttock with a discharging opening close to the natal cleft.

At EUA by a general surgeon, a "low-lying fistula" was reported and an "is-chiorectal sinus." An anal polyp and tag were removed, an MRI scan arranged and referral made to the colorectal service. The MRI scan demonstrated a com-plex high transsphincteric (TS) fistula and horse-shoe abscess.

DECISION POINT

What would be your plan for this fistula? What would you explain to the patient?

It was felt that a further EUA was required in order to delineate the anatomy and to drain secondary sepsis, allowing the anorectum to settle, leaving a single primary track. This can take several repeat surgical sessions, and it is worth pointing out to the patient at the outset that this process is likely to take many months before fistula eradication can be attempted.

At EUA, a long high TS track was evident with an external opening a long way posterior on the right buttock, and an associated cavity. The external opening was enlarged in order to gain access into the cavity, which was curetted and irri-gated. A loose silastic seton was inserted through the primary track. Over the ensuing few weeks, the patient did not tolerate the seton well and the secondary cavity required three further EUAs for adequate drainage and curettage. Repeat MRI showed little improvement in appearances and further EUA was under-taken. Lockhart-Mummery probes demonstrated a long oblique TS fistula with an internal opening below the dentate line in the posterior midline (Figure 36.1).

Colorectal Surgery: Clinical Care and Management, First Edition.
Edited by Bruce George, Richard Guy, Oliver Jones, and Jon Vogel.
© 2016 John Wiley & Sons, Ltd. Published 2016 by John Wiley & Sons, Ltd.

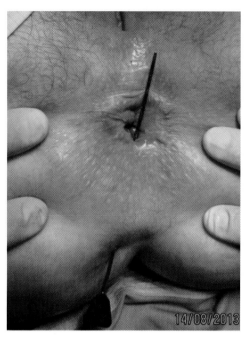

Figure 36.1 Lockhart-Mummery probe within TS fistula. Note the outer border of the external sphincter where there is a subtle pigment change. The external fistula opening clearly lies well outside this.

DECISION POINT

Would you attempt a definitive procedure at this stage? What are the realistic options for eradication?

The realistic options at this point were felt to be as follows.

- Partial fistulotomy, laying open the most peripheral aspect up to the margin of the external sphincter (clearly seen in Figure 36.2 where pigmentation changes), laying open skin and subcutaneous tissue above the track down to muscle and inserting a "snug" seton around the muscle. This would have left her with a substantial wound and an inconvenient seton, which can take a considerable time to migrate through the muscle.

- Fistulectomy and endoanal advancement flap. Fistulectomy for such a long track can be technically difficult, particularly with an associated cavity. An advancement flap to cover such a low internal opening would entail a suture line at the anal margin, risking "ectropion" and mucus leakage.

- Fistulectomy and skin advancement flap into the anal canal. An option for the low internal opening, although function can be a problem.

- Fistula plug. Whilst success of plugs is higher for longer tracks, this was probably too long, and the associated cavity would be a relative contraindication.

- Ligation of intersphincteric fistula track (LIFT). An attractive option if combined with cavity drainage and unlikely to affect function significantly.

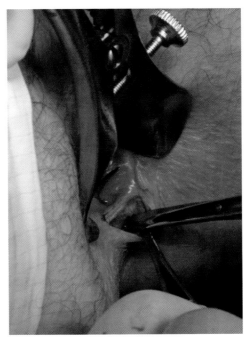

Figure 36.2 Initial dissection of the intersphincteric space via a posterior curvilinear inscision. The probe remains through the track to aid identification.

A LIFT procedure was undertaken (Figures 36.2–36.4). A curvilinear incision was made posteriorly at the anal margin, centered on the fistula track. The intersphincteric (IS) plane was developed and the track identified, thinned down, ligated in continuity and divided, additional sutures being placed to securely obliterate the cut ends of the fistula track, and ensuring by probing that this was the case. The IS space was developed a short way cephalad to ensure that no sepsis had been overlooked. The external opening was then excised and the associated cavity curetted. A Malecot mushroom catheter was inserted via a counter incision on the right buttock in order to allow for gentle irrigation. The LIFT wound was then closed with interrupted absorbable sutures.

Postoperatively, the patient stayed in hospital overnight and was discharged home the following day on a 5-day course of antibiotics. The drain was removed after 1 week. Outpatient review at 3 months revealed complete healing with no evidence of fistula recurrence and good anorectal function.

Could we have done better?

Earlier drainage and control of sepsis and insertion of seton should have occurred, probably at the initial operation at which an anal polyp was removed.

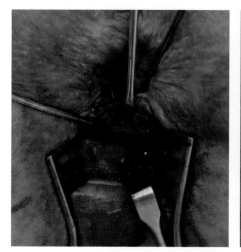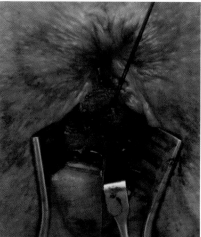

Figure 36.3 (A,B) The intersphincteric space has been developed and the fistula track identified. The "umbrella" Lockhart-Mummery probe is a useful tool for hooking around the track. The track is then thinned down prior to ligation and division.

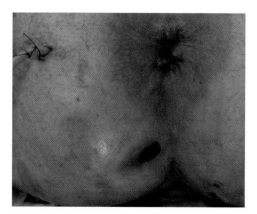

Figure 36.4 The anal wound has been sutured and the external opening excised with curettage of an associated cavity. A Malecot catheter has been inserted via a counter-incision into the cavity to allow for gentle irrigation.

This might have prevented subsequent EUAs. That said, as the horse-shoeing was quite peripheral, an earlier LIFT might have been undertaken in order to prevent further feeding of the cavity.

LEARNING POINTS

- Eradication of a complex fistula whilst trying to maintain sphincter integrity and continence may be a considerable challenge, especially in a female patient with a history of obstetric trauma.

- Ideally, secondary cavities should be dealt with before attempting to eradicate the primary track, but compromise may be needed if there is persistent sepsis.
- The LIFT procedure can be technically difficult, but interruption of the track and eradication of disease in the IS space obeys Parks' recommendations based on the cryptoglandular hypothesis.
- The LIFT procedure is cosmetically acceptable with small wounds, and continence is likely to be maintained.

LETTER FROM AMERICA

The most recent (2011) ASCRS clinical practice guidelines for complex anal fistula not associated with Crohn's disease include a "strong recommendation" for rectal mucosal advancement flap or seton and/or staged fistulotomy, a "weak recommendation" for fibrin glue therapy or anal fistula plug, and "no recommendation" for the LIFT procedure. The authors of this ASCRS guideline noted that the literature at the time of guideline finalization was "too preliminary" for a recommendation to be made. Since 2011, the body of evidence supporting the efficacy of LIFT has grown and the value of this procedure has been appreciated by more practitioners in the USA (Hall JF, Bordeianou L, Hyman N, *et al*. Outcomes after operation for anal fistula: results of a prospective multicenter, regional study. *Dis Colon Rectum* 2014; **57**:1304–8

Jon Vogel and Massarat Zutshi

CASE 37

Recurrent rectovaginal fistula

Bruce George
Oxford University Hospitals NHS Foundation Trust, Oxford, UK

A 43-year-old woman was referred from another hospital with a history of a recurrent rectovaginal fistula. In her obstetric history, she had two vaginal deliveries at term without any tears and had always had good continence. At the age of 40 years, she developed what was thought to be a Bartholin's abscess, although after spontaneous discharge it became clear that she had an anovaginal fistula. This had been repaired by a vaginal advancement flap which became infected and failed. Over the next 2–3 years, she underwent four further attempted repairs and had a defunctioning loop colostomy raised. Examination under anesthetic revealed a large low ano/rectovaginal fistula. The perianal tissues were scarred and indurated, especially anterior and to the right side of the anal canal, as seen in Figure 37.1.

DECISION POINT

What would you do now?

It was felt that to repair the fistula, well-vascularized healthy tissue needed to be placed in the rectovaginal septum. The option of gracilis muscle interposition was discussed in detail. It was emphasized that this was her "last chance" at repair, that success was about 50% and that even if repair was successful and the covering stoma was later closed, future bowel function would be impaired.

The patient decided to proceed with gracilis repair. The rectovaginal plane was developed and a further large vaginal flap raised. The left gracilis was mobilized fully on its proximal vascular pedicle and detached distally (Figure 37.2). The muscle was tunneled subcutaneously to the rectovaginal area (Figure 37.3). The rectal side of the fistula was repaired with interrupted absorbable sutures. The distal part of the gracilis muscle was sutured securely over the rectal repair and then the vaginal flap sutured over the muscle (Figure 37.4).

Postoperatively, the patient recovered well from the procedure. At clinic review, sphincter function was satisfactory. A check EUA 3 months later showed healing of the fistula. She underwent closure of the covering stoma.

Colorectal Surgery: Clinical Care and Management, First Edition.
Edited by Bruce George, Richard Guy, Oliver Jones, and Jon Vogel.
© 2016 John Wiley & Sons, Ltd. Published 2016 by John Wiley & Sons, Ltd.

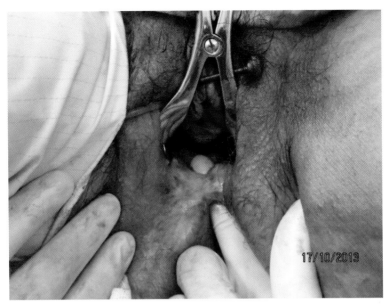

Figure 37.1 Large rectovaginal fistula admitting tip of index finger. Note adjacent scarring.

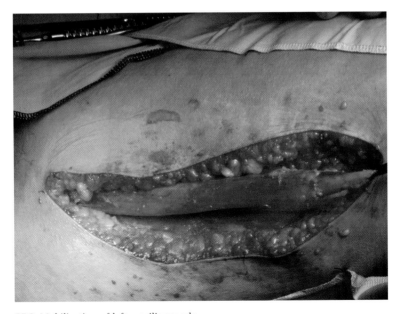

Figure 37.2 Mobilization of left gracilis muscle.

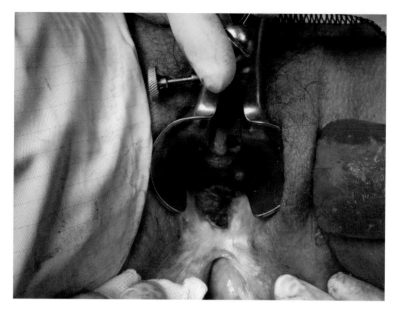

Figure 37.3 Subcutaneous tunneling of muscle to perineum. Note also repair of fistula on anorectal side.

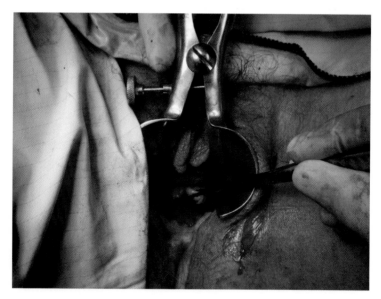

Figure 37.4 Suturing of vaginal flap over interposed gracilis muscle.

At latest follow-up 7 months later, she remains well with no symptoms to suggest recurrent fistulation. Bowel function is frequent with moderate urgency, although adequately controlled with low-dose immodium.

LEARNING POINT

- Gracilis muscle interposition is a reasonable surgical option for recurrent ano- or rectovaginal fistulae.

CASE 38

Adolescent cleft trouble

Richard Guy

Oxford University Hospitals NHS Foundation Trust, Oxford, UK

A 16-year-old schoolboy approaching school examinations presented with a purulent discharging sinus disease in the natal cleft. Four months earlier, he had fallen onto his coccyx, sustaining bruising, and had presented to the Accident and Emergency department. On examination, he was hirsute. There was complex pilonidal sinus disease arising from the midline of the natal cleft with, most notably, a sinus opening 4 cm from the anal margin, a relatively superficial track connecting this to the midline, and a long secondary track cephalad to the left side. Digital rectal examination was unremarkable. An MRI scan was arranged which showed no evidence of coccygeal injury and no evidence of anal fistula. Examination under anesthetic (EUA) was arranged. Rigid sigmoidoscopy and proctoscopy were normal and an anal fistula was excluded. The track close to the anus was superficial to the anal sphincters.

DECISION POINT

How would you approach this problem, considering this young man's commitments but desire to be free of disease as soon as possible? Would you be prepared to undertake radical surgery straight away?

The main problem with this pilonidal sinus was felt to be the track close to the anus, even though superficial. Any resulting wound would have a high chance of infection and breakdown, with difficult management in an adolescent with important commitments. Whilst it was appreciated that radical surgery would ultimately be required for the main sacrococcygeal disease, an attempt at initial conservative treatment was considered worthwhile.

A staged approach was adopted with initial laying open and curettage of the superficial track, which did not involve any external sphincter fibers. A silastic seton was inserted through the main proximal track. After 2 months, the superficial track had healed and a further examination under anesthetic was carried out in order to deal definitively with the main track (Figure 38.1).

Colorectal Surgery: Clinical Care and Management, First Edition.
Edited by Bruce George, Richard Guy, Oliver Jones, and Jon Vogel.
© 2016 John Wiley & Sons, Ltd. Published 2016 by John Wiley & Sons, Ltd.

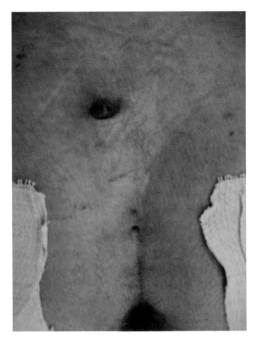

Figure 38.1 Appearance at second EUA (patient prone). The track close to the anus has healed and the main secondary track is seen arising from midline sinuses.

A Bascom excision and cleft closure was performed as a day-case, with an eccentric excision of the midline pits and lateral track, followed by mobilization of the unaffected side and off-midline primary closure over a suction drain. The drain was removed by the district nurse after 3 days and sutures removed after 10 days. At 6 weeks follow-up, there was clearly delayed healing and some overgranulation. Referral was made to a plastic surgeon in anticipation of the requirement for further surgery. However, with regular curettage, silver nitrate application, depilation and dressings over a 6-week period, full healing was eventually achieved (Figure 38.2).

Could we have done better?

This was a difficult problem for an active adolescent. Perhaps a period of conservative treatment, with scrupulous depilation, attention to hygiene and skin toilet might have been worthwhile for a period of several months. This might have allowed continuation of normal activities whilst optimizing local conditions for uncomplicated excision and primary closure.

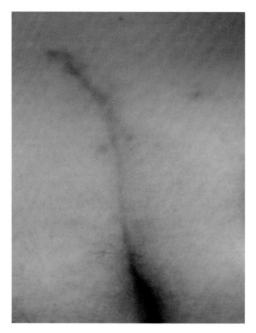

Figure 38.2 Appearance at 6 months showing complete healing.

LEARNING POINTS

- Conservative treatment of sacrococcygeal pilonidal sinus disease is rarely successful but combined excisional and conservative measures may be required.
- Excision and primary closure, with eccentric flap closure, provides the best chance of primary healing for midline and unilateral tracks.

LETTER FROM AMERICA

The 2013 ASCRS guidelines for pilonidal disease include a "strong recommendation based on moderate quality evidence" for the operative management of this condition: excision with primary closure, excision with healing by secondary intention, or excision with wound edge marsupialization. A similar level of recommendation was given for flap-based repairs, particularly for recurrent or complex pilonidal sinus disease when more simple techniques have failed.

Jon Vogel and Massarat Zutshi

CASE 39

Extreme itch

Luana Franceschilli

University of Rome Tor Vergata, Rome, Italy

A 44-year-old male teacher was referred with a 4-year history of hemorrhoids. The predominant symptom reported in clinic was itching, particularly at night. There was occasional bleeding and an anal lump but no pain, and bowel function was unchanged. There was no history of skin disease. Various "over-the-counter" ointments and creams had been tried without lasting benefit. On examination of the perineum, there was perianal excoriation (Figure 39.1), but no evidence of fissure or fistula. Second-degree hemorrhoids were seen on proctoscopy. Resting anal tone was subjectively normal.

DECISION POINT

Would you undertake any investigations? What are the causes of "secondary" pruritus ani? What conservative measures may help this man's symptoms?

Pruritus ani can be fairly unrewarding to treat but it was felt, at the very least, that luminal rectal pathology should be ruled out. The only obvious treatable cause seemed to be some mucosal prolapse so that was considered worth treating.

Flexible sigmoidoscopy was undertaken and this was normal. At the same time, rubber band ligation of hemorrhoids was carried out in an attempt to reduce hemorrhoidal prolapse and mucus discharge. Two months after this treatment, the patient reported a 75% improvement in itching and a resolution of bleeding. However, 3 months later, the patient was re-referred with recurrent symptoms. Further hemorrhoidal banding and also 5% phenol injection were undertaken. Whilst this improved the hemorrhoids, pruritus remained a significant problem, and perianal excoriation worsened. An empirical course of Trimovate (clobetasone butyrate/nystatin/oxytetracycline calcium, GlaxoSmithKline, UK) was prescribed, but this failed to improve the situation.

Colorectal Surgery: Clinical Care and Management, First Edition.
Edited by Bruce George, Richard Guy, Oliver Jones, and Jon Vogel.
© 2016 John Wiley & Sons, Ltd. Published 2016 by John Wiley & Sons, Ltd.

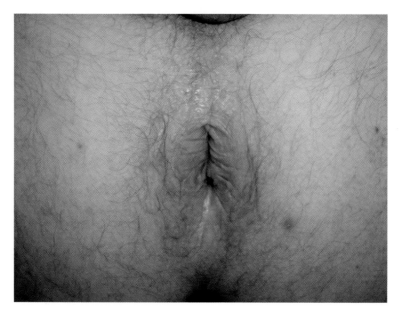

Figure 39.1 Perianal area showing excoriation.

DECISION POINT

What would you offer now? Is there any other worthwhile treatment?

This was considered to be refractory idiopathic pruritus ani, and the patient's condition seemed to be worsening. Rather than discharging the patient to a GP or dermatologist, it was felt that methylene blue injection could be an option.

Under general anesthesia, the patient underwent perianal intradermal injection of a 20 mL solution of methylene blue, comprising 15 mL of 1% lignocaine hydrochloride, 5 mL of 1% methylene blue and 100 mg of hydrocortisone, using a 22 gauge needle, ensuring that all skin furrows were infiltrated (Figure 39.2). At clinic review 6 weeks later, the patient reported complete resolution of symptoms, although permanent tattooing of the perianal skin was noted.

LEARNING POINTS

- Pruritus ani is usually idiopathic and most patients respond to simple measures, a change in toileting and hygiene, and minor lifestyle modifications.
- Local skin conditions and anorectal pathology should be excluded.
- Methylene blue should be reserved for truly intractable cases and patients must be warned about reduction in perianal sensitivity and permanent tattooing.

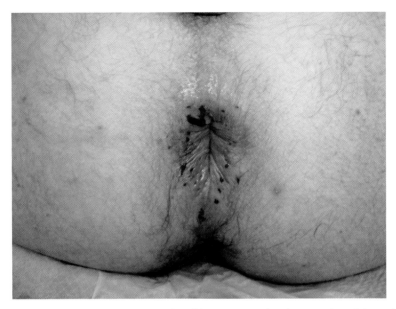

Figure 39.2 Appearance following methylene blue injection, showing tattooing of the perianal skin.

LETTER FROM AMERICA

As stated by Hippocrates, "For extreme diseases, extreme methods of cure, as to restriction, are most suitable" (wiktionary.org, 2015). The Patients Resources section of the ASCRS website notes that injectable methylene blue therapy may be the last line of treatment for refractory cases of pruritus ani.

Jon Vogel and Massarat Zutshi

SECTION E

Emergency colorectal surgery

Richard Guy
Oxford University Hospitals NHS Foundation Trust, Oxford, UK

Abdominal trauma

Initial assessment and diagnosis

Initial resuscitation in trauma should adhere to the widely adopted Advanced Trauma Life Support (ATLS) principles, established by the American College of Surgeons Committee on Trauma [1]. Priority must be given to the airway (with cervical spine control), breathing, and circulation (ABC) in all trauma cases and Accident and Emergency Department management should ideally be delivered by a well-drilled trauma team, including a general surgeon. Treatment priorities must be established and simultaneously implemented at a primary survey and full injury severity and profile ascertained at a secondary survey.

Recognition of patterns of injury is important and comes with experience of managing trauma cases regularly. Where possible, the circumstances of the injury should be obtained from conscious patients, bystanders or on-scene members of the emergency services. This should include information such as vehicular speed, ejection of a person from a vehicle, death of other victims, and observed consciousness of the patient at the scene of the accident.

Blunt injury

Injury usually results from road traffic accidents, pedestrian injury or falls from a height. Blunt abdominal trauma in vehicular accidents is usually caused by deceleration injury, for example from the restraining effects of a seatbelt, or collision with a steering wheel, and vehicular accidents are the most common cause of blunt gastrointestinal injury [2].

Colorectal Surgery: Clinical Care and Management, First Edition.
Edited by Bruce George, Richard Guy, Oliver Jones, and Jon Vogel.
© 2016 John Wiley & Sons, Ltd. Published 2016 by John Wiley & Sons, Ltd.

Assessment

Examination of the abdomen for suspected internal injury should include a careful search for bruising, seatbelt marks (Figure E.1), tyre marks, and any signs of penetrating injury. Assessment for peritonism may be difficult in the presence of abdominal wall or pelvic injury as there may be generalized muscle tenderness or retroperitoneal hematoma, but when true peritonism is present following blunt trauma, the likelihood of perforation is high [3].

A digital rectal examination should be performed following log-rolling, looking for luminal blood and assessing the position of the prostate to exclude urethral injury in the case of a pelvic fracture. Urethral catheterization should be attempted if urethral injury is excluded.

Blast injury (see Case 40)

Blast injury is a specialized form of blunt trauma. Exposure to an explosive device may result in primary, secondary, tertiary or quaternary blast injury as follows.

- Primary – injury caused by the concussive blast wave itself and affecting air-containing organs, especially the ears, sinuses, lungs, and intestine.
- Secondary – injury caused by fragments, e.g. shrapnel.
- Tertiary – injury caused by bodily displacement or falling walls and buildings.
- Quaternary – injury and illness resulting from associated noxious gases, e.g. carbon monoxide, or burns.

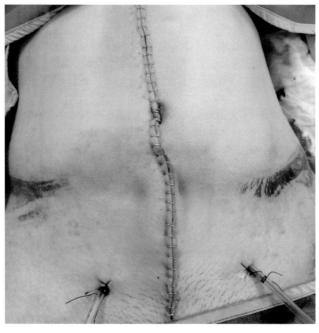

Figure E.1 Seatbelt sign. This is associated with a high chance of visceral injury. This young woman sustained injuries to the jejunum and rectosigmoid.

The main determinant of survival following blast exposure is pulmonary injury, and it is vital that pneumothorax, pulmonary contusion, and airway injury are managed urgently [4]. The principles of surgical management, however, remain the same as for blunt injury from any cause, although surgeons should be aware of the possibility of delayed perforation of intestinal blast contusions, potentially up to 14 days later.

Penetrating abdominal injury occurs with blast when projectiles are energized by the explosion, and fragment injuries are common and unpredictable. The combination of all four types of blast injury results in complex effects and high morbidity and mortality.

Imaging in trauma

Focused assessment with sonography for trauma

Focused assessment with sonography for trauma (FAST) scanning has become increasingly available in Accident and Emergency departments. It may be a useful screening investigation, but is operator dependent and has a significant false-negative rate [5].

Computed tomography (CT)

If the patient is physiologically stable following blunt abdominal trauma, cross-sectional CT imaging of the chest, abdomen, and pelvis should be obtained, and images interpreted carefully in conjunction with an experienced radiologist. Particular radiological attention should be paid to "junctional zones" between body cavities in order, for example, that diaphragmatic injury is dealt with by the most appropriate approach (laparotomy, thoracotomy or thoracoabdominal incision). Presence of free gas and fluid, intestinal ischemia, intestinal rupture, and mesenteric injury can all be determined by CT. In the trauma situation, the sensitivity and specificity of CT are about 80% and 78% respectively [6].

Diagnostic peritoneal lavage (DPL)

The indications for DPL have diminished considerably in recent years as speed of acquisition and quality of cross-sectional imaging have improved. The only realistically reliable indicators of a need for surgery are frank blood in an unstable patient and gross enteric content [7].

Surgical management

Laparoscopy has a limited role in the acute assessment of blunt trauma, although in experienced hands, in the setting of a stable patient with equivocal imaging and localized peritonism, it may have a place in picking up hollow visceral injury, mesenteric injury or diaphragmatic injury. In stab injuries, laparoscopic assessment may be very useful in determining the presence of peritoneal penetration and underlying injury [8].

Physiological instability following abdominal trauma may mandate immediate laparotomy for hemorrhage control, but a negative laparotomy in the presence of chest or pelvic injury may add significant morbidity. Penetrating injury with evisceration also constitutes an absolute indication to proceed to laparotomy. In all other cases, management should be determined following acquisition of detailed imaging.

Damage control surgery (see Cases 40, 43, 46, 47)

The damage control surgery (DCS) approach in abdominal trauma is now well established and effective [9]. The aim is to prevent the "lethal triad" of hypothermia, acidosis, and coagulopathy [10]. DCS involves an initial swift laparotomy, then stabilization on intensive care and then relaparotomy.

Initial abbreviated laparotomy

The emphasis is on hemorrhage control and contamination source control. Techniques to achieve this include abdominal packing, peritoneal lavage, resection of bowel using linear staplers but without reanastomosis and primary repair of simple perforating injuries to small bowel or colon. The abdomen is usually left open as a laparostomy, using one of a variety of available techniques for temporary abdominal closure (TAC). Commonly used methods of TAC include the Bogota bag, "home-made" suction and vacuum methods ("Vac-Pac," Barker or Op-Site sandwich techniques), and commercially available negative pressure therapy systems, such as Abdo-VAC or ABThera, with or without fascial traction. There is some evidence that wound management incorporating negative pressure techniques is associated with improved outcomes compared to alternative methods of temporary abdominal closure [11].

Transfer postoperatively to a critical care environment

The aim is for correction of physiology. Prevention of intraabdominal hypertension (IAH) and abdominal compartment syndrome (ACS) is essential, especially when there is potential concomitant respiratory compromise. Fluid resuscitation, rewarming, and organ support should continue, with correction of acidosis and coagulopathy.

Return to the operating theater

Abdominal reexploration occurs after 24–72 hours, for the purpose of identification of overlooked injuries, definitive bowel repairs, raising of abdominal stomas as appropriate, and abdominal closure if possible. If doubt still remains about feasibility of repairs, or in the presence of intestinal ischemia, further reexploration may need to be planned after another 24–48 hours.

There remains some debate over a blanket policy of DCS for all abdominal injuries. Patients with cardiorespiratory stability and easily definable injury without significant contamination may be suitable for primary repair or reanastomosis and definitive abdominal wall closure, and this must be a team judgment based upon ease of surgery and state of physiology at the time of surgery [12].

Emergency presentations of diverticular disease

Uncomplicated diverticulitis [13]

Acute diverticulitis without abscess formation or perforation is termed uncomplicated. Management depends on accurate diagnosis, often by CT scanning, and tailoring treatment according to severity. It is being increasingly recognized that many patients can be safely treated as an outpatient and without the need for antibiotics [14].

Complicated diverticulitis

Hinchey classified perforating diverticular disease into four groups according to severity (Table E.1) [15].

The management of complicated diverticulitis has been addressed by major guidelines on both sides of the Atlantic recently [13, 16].

Diverticular abscess (Hinchey I and II)

The aim of management of diverticulitis with localized abscess formation is to resolve the sepsis and avoid emergency surgery. Treatment generally relies on intravenous antibiotics and radiological drainage of abscesses.

Follow-up imaging should be undertaken 3–5 days after abscess drainage in order to ensure resolution. Persistent abscess and lack of progress, perhaps with local peritonism, fever, and raised inflammatory markers, may necessitate surgery.

Diverticular peritonitis (Hinchey III and IV)

Patients with generalized peritonitis (Hinchey III and IV) need to proceed to surgical exploration following resuscitation, although cross-sectional imaging should be obtained if possible in order to exclude other pathology, particularly malignancy, as well as confirming the clinical diagnosis.

Table E.1 Hinchey classification.

Hinchey grade	Perforation effect
I	Confined pericolic or mesenteric abscess
II	Pelvic or retroperitoneal abscess
III	Generalized purulent peritonitis
IV	Generalized feculent peritonitis

Source: Hinchey [15]. Reproduced with permission of Elsevier.

Surgical management

Surgical treatment of acute diverticulitis is indicated for generalized peritonitis (Hinchey III and IV) or when nonoperative treatment (of complicated Hinchey I and II) is unsuccessful. The conventional recommendation is to undertake sigmoid resection with colostomy formation (Hartmann's procedure) for most cases requiring surgery in the emergency situation. In recent years, there has been a trend towards the use of laparoscopic wash-out or resection with anastomosis in carefully selected cases.

Laparoscopy and wash-out (see Case 41)

Laparoscopic wash-out for perforated diverticular disease has become popular in recent years in an attempt to avoid emergency resectional surgery and probable stoma [17]. Several key questions related to laparoscopic wash-out remain unanswered:
- which cases are best suited to this approach
- whether an inflammatory phlegmon should be disturbed
- what type and volume of fluid should be used
- whether drains should be left in place.

The long-term results of randomized trials (LapLAND, SCANDIV, DILALA, and LADIES) are awaited with interest [18].

Sigmoid resection

Hinchey IV disease, and most cases of Hinchey III peritonitis, usually demand laparotomy and resection. The most common operation for perforated sigmoid diverticular disease in the UK remains the Hartmann resection. Even in the hands of specialist colorectal surgeons, morbidity and mortality rates are high [19], and a significant proportion of patients never have intestinal continuity restored.

In selected, less unwell patients, usually with less marked peritoneal contamination and fewer co-morbidities, resection and primary anastomosis may be possible with good outcomes in specialist hands [20]. On-table antegrade colonic lavage via the terminal ileum or appendix may be necessary, particularly if there is a plan to defunction the patient with a proximal loop ileostomy.

The place of laparoscopic sigmoid resection for acute complicated diverticulitis remains uncertain but is likely to increase in selected cases [21].

In severely septic cases, the outlook is poor. A DCS approach may be worthwhile, along the same lines as that for trauma [22].

Follow-up after resolution of diverticulitis or diverticular sepsis

In the event of complete resolution of diverticulitis or locally perforated sigmoid disease, it is recommended that patients undergo colonic imaging, by colonoscopy, barium enema or by CT colonography, after an interval of around

6 weeks, in order to confirm the diagnosis of diverticulosis and to exclude other pathology such as colonic cancer or inflammatory bowel disease [13].

There is weak evidence that treatment with fiber or the nonabsorbed antibiotic rifaximin is associated with a reduced risk of recurrent diverticulitis.

Indications for elective resection after nonsurgical management of acute diverticulitis are debatable. There has been a move towards more conservative management in recent years. Generally accepted indications for elective resection are:

- recurrent attacks of proven complicated diverticulitis
- patients who remain symptomatic after proven acute diverticulitis
- patient with fistulae or stricture formation.

Emergency presentations of colorectal cancer

Obstruction
Large bowel obstruction is the most common acute presentation of colorectal malignancy and is discussed in Section A, page 10–11, and Cases 4, 10, and 42.

Perforation
Intestinal perforation in association with colorectal malignancy presents as an emergency and is generally associated with a poor prognosis. Perforation may occur at the site of tumor or remotely such as cecal perforation secondary to distal obstruction.

Predisposing factors for perforation are diverticulitis, chemotherapy-induced colitis, previous radiotherapy, abdominal carcinomatosis, and bowel obstruction. Where perforation of a tumor occurs following chemotherapy, this may be secondary to tumor necrosis. Abdelrazeq and colleagues [23] demonstrated reduced survival in patients with perforated T4 tumors (T4b) compared to those with non-perforated T4 tumors (T4a). The difference, however, was mainly due to reduced 30-day mortality rather than late oncological differences. This emphasizes the importance of optimum emergency surgical management.

Emergency surgery
For perforated colonic cancers in stable patients, resection should follow oncological principles where possible, but there should be a low threshold for stoma formation rather than anastomosis in view of a potentially higher risk of anastomotic leakage.

In the physiologically unstable septic patient, a "damage control" approach may be necessary, with priority being given to control of contamination in the first instance, rather than radical oncological clearance (see Damage control surgery).

Perforated rectal cancer

In rectal cancer perforation, it is usually unwise to attempt resection acutely, and control of contamination with washout, adequate drainage and the raising of a proximal stoma may be more appropriate. Accurate imaging and elective surgical planning should then follow, once sepsis has been controlled.

Colorectal vascular emergencies

Acute mesenteric ischemia (AMI)

This may result from arterial or venous occlusion, low flow states and, very rarely, small vessel disease. The classic presentation of severe abdominal pain "out of proportion to physical signs," a source of embolism and metabolic acidosis, is well known. The condition, however, remains difficult to diagnose early. No clinically useful blood marker exists. The increased availability of high-resolution CT scanning represents the most significant recent advance in the management of AMI [24].

If acute mesenteric ischemia is diagnosed by CT, optimum management depends on joint care involving interventional radiologists, vascular and general surgeons. Critical assessments include the following.
- Has the patient got peritonitis?
- Is the ischemia due to:
  ○ superior mesenteric arterial embolism/thrombosis?
  ○ superior mesenteric venous thrombosis?
  ○ low flow (nonocclusive hypoperfusion)?

Peritonitis (see Case 43)

If the patient has peritonitis then laparotomy is indicated. If ischemic bowel is confirmed, the extent should be carefully assessed. Assessing irreversible ischemia may be difficult even for experienced surgeons. Color and peristalsis should be assessed. Intraoperative perfusion assessment, for example using indocyanine green assessed by near infrared imaging (PinPoint, NOVADAQ, Canada) [25], may be helpful but is rarely available in the emergency setting. The length of remaining small bowel after resection is important to measure. In some situations such as the elderly with less than 50–100 cm of small bowel remaining after resection of ischemic bowel, it may be appropriate to "back off" aggressive treatment.

If aggressive treatment is appropriate, ischemic bowel should be resected and usually the ends stapled as in "damage control surgery." Attention should be given to revascularization of any remaining borderline ischemic bowel. If the ischemia is due to embolism then SMA embolectomy should be considered. If the ischemia is due to thrombosis then radiologically guided stenting may be indicated. If the ischemia is due to venous thrombosis anticoagulation is indicated.

If it is due to "low flow," for example following cardiac surgery, key aspects of management should be directed at improving cardiac output, although the prognosis is poor.

No peritonitis

If the patient does not have peritonitis then intestinal revascularization should be considered. Embolism may be amenable to thrombolysis, endovascular aspiration/mechanical embolectomy or open embolectomy. Arterial thrombosis may be amenable to stenting. Superior mesenteric venous (SMV) thrombosis should be treated by anticoagulation. In low-flow situations, management should again be directed at improving cardiac output.

Superior mesenteric venous thrombosis tends to occur in slightly younger patients than those with arterial occlusions and may arise due to an underlying thrombotic tendency. Patients should be assessed for a primary thrombophilic disorder (such as antithrombin III deficiency, protein C deficiency, protein S deficiency, factor V Leiden mutation, and antiphospholipid syndrome). Venous thrombosis may also be acquired and seen in hypercoagulable states associated with inflammatory and infective conditions such as appendicitis, pancreatitis, diverticulitis, inflammatory bowel disease, trauma, and malignancy.

Prognosis

If massive intestinal resection is undertaken, the metabolic and nutritional consequences in the survivor are considerable. Patients with less than 100 cm of small bowel are likely to require nutritional support, often with long-term parenteral feeding. The presence of colon in circuit, ileocecal valve and normal remaining small bowel increase the chances of maintaining nutritional independence.

Colonic ischemia

Embolic involvement of the inferior mesenteric artery (IMA) occurs less commonly than with the SMA owing to its smaller caliber [26]. Thrombotic or atherosclerotic occlusion, however, may occur in association with infrarenal abdominal aortic aneurysms, although this is often a chronic process allowing revascularization to occur via the collateral circulation. Left colon ischemia and infarction may follow aortic aneurysm surgery when the IMA has been ligated. Whilst some recovery may occur in the presence of adequate collaterals, infarction necessitates colonic resection and is associated with high morbidity and mortality rates under these circumstances.

The "watershed" area of the colon (Griffiths' point), between the SMA and IMA perfusion territories, in the region of the splenic flexure and proximal descending colon, is susceptible to ischemia, particularly if the arc of Riolan is absent or the marginal artery of Drummond poor. It is this area which is vulnerable to ischemic colitis, classically presenting as left-sided abdominal pain and bloody diarrhea in an elderly patient with co-existing cardiovascular or peripheral vascular disease [27].

Management should be supportive, with rehydration, antibiotics and analgesia, in the expectation that spontaneous recovery will occur. Diagnosis should be confirmed by flexible sigmoidoscopy with biopsies, and full colonoscopy 8 weeks after full recovery is advisable. Recovery and healing by fibrosis may result in an ischemic stricture, which may ultimately necessitate resection.

Acute lower gastrointestinal bleeding

Lower gastrointestinal (GI) bleeding usually implies bleeding of colonic, rectal or anal origin.

- Colonic causes: angiodysplasia, diverticular disease, inflammatory bowel disease, malignancy, ischemic colitis.
- Rectal causes: angiodysplasia, malignancy, inflammatory bowel disease, rectal varices.
- Anal causes: hemorrhoids.

Initial management will require either resuscitation or history/examination, depending on the clinic scenario. Initial resuscitation should include administration of oxygen and intravenous fluid. Coagulopathies should be corrected and clotting factors administered as appropriate. The role of procoagulants, such as tranexamic acid, has yet to be determined, particularly in the light of its questionable use for brisk upper gastrointestinal hemorrhage [28].

In the majority of cases of lower GI bleeding, the bleeding subsides spontaneously and investigations, principally colonoscopy, can be undertaken semi-electively.

Patients with continued bleeding, as evidenced by hemodynamic instability, transfusion requirement or falling hemoglobin levels, require urgent investigation and treatment.

Endoscopy

Esophagogastroduodenoscopy (EGD) should be undertaken acutely when brisk rectal bleeding or melena has occurred, in order to exclude a bleeding gastric or duodenal ulcer. Some 10–15% of patients presenting with apparent acute lower GI bleeding will have an upper GI source [29, 30].

Endoscopic examination of the lower GI tract can be challenging in the acute situation, but should include careful evaluation of the anal canal and rectum to exclude hemorrhoids, rectal varices or rectal ulceration. Colonoscopy can identify a definitive source of bleeding in up to 90% of cases [31]. For diverticular hemorrhage, adrenaline injection therapy, clip application or argon plasma coagulation may be useful in skilled hands [32]. Angiodysplasia can usually be managed endoscopically, most successfully using argon plasma coagulation, with sustained benefit [33]. Malignancy, inflammatory bowel disease, and ischemic colitis can all be easily diagnosed by flexible sigmoidoscopy/colonoscopy.

Radiography

Computed tomography angiography has transformed the management of acute gastrointestinal bleeding. A recent metaanalysis reported high levels of diagnostic accuracy for detection and localization of bleeding points [34]. Whilst therapeutic intervention is impossible with CT angiography, localization of a bleeding source allows for targeted therapeutic fluoroscopic angiography. If a site of bleeding is identified, selective transcatheter embolization may be possible, usually using coils. Interventional success rates of about 80% are reported although with a small risk of colonic ischemia [35].

Emergency surgery

Emergency laparotomy for intractable lower gastrointestinal hemorrhage is very rarely required as most bleeding stops either spontaneously or following medical correction of coagulopathy or colonoscopic/angiographic intervention. For those cases of bleeding which do not stop, if the site of bleeding or its cause (e.g. colitis or ischemia) can be determined preoperatively, the surgical plan is usually straightforward. If no bleeding site is identified preoperatively or easily at laparotomy, panendoscopy is required. On-table colonoscopy, small bowel enteroscopy, and EGD are difficult in this situation and should be undertaken by experienced surgeons, assisted if necessary by gastroenterologists.

Volvulus

Cecal volvulus

Cecal volvulus accounts for around 1–3% of all colonic obstructions and around 50% of all cases of colonic volvulus [36]. Patients may present acutely with intractable pain and distension but more often give a history of repeated attacks of intermittent colicky pain, borborygmi, and distension with spontaneous resolution. There may be vomiting if small bowel obstruction is progressive.

Abdominal distension will usually be present on examination with a tympanic abdomen and hyperactive bowel sounds on auscultation in the early stages. Tachycardia, fever, and peritonism indicate probable vascular compromise and potential cecal perforation.

Plain radiography may be diagnostic with the cecum displaced medially and superiorly in the abdomen. Free intraperitoneal gas indicates perforation and CT scanning may be helpful in diagnostic doubt, when the diagnostic "whirl sign" may be seen, as well as allowing for assessment of vascular compromise or to exclude a concomitant neoplasm.

Treatment is usually surgical and in the acute setting, laparotomy is usually undertaken. For the patient with intermittent or resolving symptoms, laparoscopy may be possible if distension is not too extreme. At laparotomy, the right colon will be mobile and, once untwisted, is easily delivered out of the abdomen. Excessive mobility ensures a straightforward right hemicolectomy which should be standard definitive treatment, although if perforation and contamination have occurred, or there is extended vascular compromise involving small bowel, restoring continuity may need to be delayed.

Cecopexy should be avoided, except in the most unstable patients with a viable right colon, as recurrent volvulus is likely.

Sigmoid volvulus (see Case 45)

Sigmoid volvulus occurs when a large redundant sigmoid loop twists around its excessively mobile mesentery, causing obstruction. In contrast to cecal volvulus, sigmoid volvulus is in most cases an acquired disorder. It may be related to colonic dysmotility and chronic constipation causing elongation and dilatation of the sigmoid colon, potentially explaining its higher incidence in older institutionalized adults [37].

Patients present with an insidious onset of abdominal distension, pain, and absolute constipation, which is often recurrent. Patients in institutions may have minimal symptoms and are often referred directly by their carers on account of progressive distension.

Examination usually reveals a grossly distended and tympanic abdomen. Tenderness may indicate ischemia and imminent perforation. The rectum is usually collapsed on digital rectal examination but may be dilated and vacuous if volvulus has occurred on a background of colonic pseudoobstruction and megacolon or megarectum.

A plain supine abdominal radiograph may reveal the grossly dilated sigmoid, with its apex extending into the upper abdomen and its base in the left iliac fossa, creating the pathognomonic "coffee bean" sign. With global gaseous distension, this may be difficult to decipher and cross-sectional CT imaging, ideally with rectal contrast, may be required. This might also allow assessment of colonic viability and perforation and should also distinguish volvulus from acute colonic pseudoobstruction (Ogilvie's syndrome).

Tube decompression

Decompression and untwisting of the sigmoid is achievable at the bedside with insertion of a flatus tube. This can be done by passing a rigid sigmoidoscope up to the level of the twist and then inserting the tube through it, usually with dramatic results. An abdominal radiograph should then be obtained to check for decompression and tube placement, and to exclude perforation.

Decompression is perhaps more satisfactorily achieved by flexible sigmoidoscopy. The twist is overcome under direct vision, the dilated gas- and fluid-filled sigmoid entered and aspirated. Ideally, the examination should be performed with minimal insufflation, preferably using carbon dioxide so as not to exacerbate distension. The advantage of endoscopy is that it allows visualization of the mucosa for assessment of ischemia, usually best achieved after careful washing.

Whilst endoscopic reduction of sigmoid volvulus is almost always successful [38], recurrence occurs in up to 60%, often within a few hours or days.

Surgery

Ischemia or infarction mandates urgent surgical resection unless the patient is moribund. Mortality in patients who have developed infarction may be up to 60%, but only around 10% where progression to infarction has not occurred.

Preincision endoscopic decompression is advisable to assist ventilation and surgical access. Surgery usually involves sigmoid resection, either laparoscopically or open. The common decision relates to anastomosis or exteriorization of the bowel ends. Although primary anastomosis is preferable, many patients will be frail with significant medical co-morbidity and a conservative approach may be necessary.

Percutaneous endoscopic colostomy (PEC) may be feasible but reports of potentially significant morbidity, including leaks and peritonitis, have reduced its popularity [39]. Nevertheless, it may be suitable for the patient considered unfit for anesthesia. Developed along the same lines as percutaneous endoscopic gastrostomy (PEG), it requires at least two points of fixation. A combined endoscopic and laparoscopic technique may be appropriate [40].

Postoperative colorectal complications

A significant part of most colorectal surgeons' working life involves management of postoperative patients. A common problem is the patient who fails to progress as expected and is labeled as "post-op ileus." This and the overlapping issue of management of anastomotic leakage are discussed separately.

Postoperative ileus (see Cases 42, 46, 47)

The problem of the patient who is unable to eat or who has not passed flatus or opened their bowels within 5 days of colorectal surgery is well recognized by colorectal surgeons. The distinction between ileus and obstruction is difficult. The true incidence of this problem is difficult to assess, although a large nationwide American study of almost a million patients between 2006 and 2008 reported that 8.65% developed "early postoperative bowel obstruction," with rates of 5.32% and 13.26% for elective and emergency surgery, respectively [41].

Paralytic ileus is ill defined but generally refers to a period in the first few days after abdominal surgery when small bowel motility ceases, resulting in abdominal distension, nausea, and sometimes vomiting. The duration of expected or "normal" ileus varies with the magnitude of surgery. Associated problems such as hypoalbuminemia, electrolyte disturbance, urinary or chest infections and excess opiate use tend to prolong the duration of ileus.

It is important, but difficult, to distinguish "normal" ileus from mechanical small bowel obstruction and from "abnormal" ileus due to a surgical complication. The aims of assessment of a patient with prolonged postoperative ileus/obstruction picture are to:
- identify "normal" ileus which will resolve with conservative management
- identify "abnormal" ileus due to a complication which needs intervention
- identify mechanical obstruction which needs correction
- avoid unnecessary reoperation, especially in a "hostile" abdomen.

Assessment requires clinical examination, review of observations chart, bloods (white count, CRP, electrolytes, albumin) and radiological assessment, often by contrast CT or a water-soluble Gastrografin follow-through.

If the assessment shows no features of sepsis and no transition point suggestive of mechanical obstruction, the diagnosis sways towards "normal ileus." Treatment is supportive with NG tube and correction of electrolytes, avoiding opiate analgaesics if possible, and possibly parenteral nutritional support.

Assessment may identify mechanical obstruction, for example due to an internal hernia, adhesion or abdominal wall hernia (e.g. port site, incisional or parastomal), which requires surgical intervention (see Case 47). Hold-up at an ileocolic anastomosis is difficult to distinguish from normal ileus although is generally managed conservatively. A water-soluble oral contrast "challenge" may be diagnostic and therapeutic in paralytic ileus [42], in the same way as its beneficial use in adhesional obstruction. If 100 mL of contrast is ingested or put down a nasogastric tube with a syringe, a plain abdominal radiograph after 4 hours gives useful information on the presence of mechanical obstruction and the need for surgery, and the osmotic effect of the contrast agent can stimulate peristalsis.

Assessment may reveal evidence of intraabdominal abscess amenable to radiological drainage or anastomotic leakage (see later).

If reoperation is a possibility, the risk–benefit balance must be carefully considered. Careful early relaparoscopy following a primary laparoscopic procedure is possible in skilled hands, despite the risk of bowel injury if the abdomen is distended. There is usually more reluctance to carry out relaparotomy, in view of its perceived physiological impact and the fear of a negative laparotomy, but procrastination may simply delay the inevitable and worsen the outcome in the presence of genuine pathology. An initial period of conservative management may last at least a week, but surgery beyond the second week becomes increasingly difficult and hazardous, as the bowel loops become "cocooned" and inseparable, with a greater risk of iatrogenic bowel injury and difficult abdominal closure, with the potential for intestinal and abdominal wall failure. A "window of opportunity" seems to exist up to 7–10 days postoperatively.

Anastomotic leak (see Cases 46–48)

The exact incidence of anastomotic leakage in colorectal surgery is unknown due to variations in definition and quality of reporting. What is known is that anastomotic leakage results in major short- and long-term morbidity. Thornton *et al.* reported mean critical care stay of 23 days and hospital stay of 40 days following colorectal anastomotic leakage [43]. Late problems include much higher stoma rates, impaired bowel function, and probably worse oncological outcomes [44].

Risk factors for anastomotic leakage include patient factors, disease-related factors, technical considerations, and institutional factors (Table E.2). Surgeons should avoid anastomosis in high-risk situations but the "tipping point" between anastomosing or not in borderline cases is challenging and often subjective.

Anastomotic leaks may present in numerous ways.
- Obvious: peritonitis, abscess, fistula.
- Subtle: pyrexia, tachycardia, leukocytosis, "ileus" (see earlier).

Table E.2 Risk factors for anastomotic leakage after colorectal surgery.

	Comment	References
Patient-related factors		
Male	Increased risk	[45]
Age	Increased risk	
Obesity	Increased risk	[45, 46]
Co-morbidity	Increased risk	[47]
Drugs		
Steroids	Increased risk	[48]
NSAIDs	? Increased risk	[49]
Anticoagulants	? Increased risk	[45]
Malnutrition	Increased risk	[50]
Disease-related factors		
Emergency surgery	Increased risk	[51]
Level of anastomosis	Lower rectal	[47]
Preoperative	increased risk	[47]
radiotherapy	Increased risk	
Technical factors		
Bowel preparation	? No effect	[52]
Open vs laparoscopic	No difference	[53, 54]
Type of anastomosis	No difference	[55]
Leak testing	Probably beneficial	[56]
Omentoplasty	No difference	[57]
Drains	? No effect	[58]
Epidural	? No effect	[59]
Institutional factors		
Hospital volume	Increased volume	[46]
Surgeon volume	reduced risk	

- Medical: cardiac arrhythmia, respiratory symptoms.
- Late: 42% on readmission and 12% after 30 days in one study [60].
- Incidental: identified by contrast study.

Diagnosis depends on careful clinical assessment and a high index of suspicion. Blood tests may be reassuringly normal and should not be relied upon, although C-reactive protein may be a useful negative predictive marker for leakage [61].

The key investigations are contrast CT, water-soluble contrast studies, and endoscopy [62]. Radiological imaging is usually required once there is a suspicion of anastomotic failure. Early postoperative scanning may be falsely reassuring and pathological radiological features may be difficult to distinguish from expected postoperative findings. Either fluoroscopic water-soluble contrast enema examination or abdominopelvic CT scanning with concurrent administration of rectal contrast will usually be required for diagnosis, unless there is obvious palpable dehiscence on digital rectal examination. The advantage of CT scanning is the additional assessment for the presence of a pelvic or presacral collection or abscess, as well as more global changes such as small bowel obstruction.

Management depends on the clinical situation, the severity of the leak, and the timing of diagnosis. Peritonitis usually demands urgent abdominal exploration, but conservative treatment may be possible if clinical signs are less severe, particularly if the patient already has a defunctioning loop ileostomy.

Nonoperative management demands vigilance and regular review, preferably by the same clinician each time, as early surgical intervention may be necessary if progress is not occurring. Broad-spectrum antibiotics should be given. Examination under anesthetic with gentle flexible sigmoidoscopy permits assessment of rectal or anal anastomosis. Extent of anastomotic separation and bowel vascularity may be assessed and may allow insertion of a drain (such as a Malecot catheter) into the presacral space and into the lumen if necessary. Deficiency of more than 50% of the circumference of the anastomosis is unlikely to be salvageable with conservative treatment.

Percutaneous drainage of infected collections and abscesses may provide dramatic clinical relief, although safe access may be a challenge for the interventional radiologist. Drainage of a pelvic collection via the sciatic notch, for example, may, in addition, be painful for the patient and may result in an enteric fistula but, provided there is no downstream obstruction, this should usually heal uneventfully [63].

Use of negative-pressure therapy applied from the luminal side into the presacral cavity can rapidly reduce and clean up even large presacral cavities, potentially allowing early endoluminal clip closure of defects [64].

Surgical management of an anastomotic leak is challenging. Early laparoscopy, if the index operation was laparoscopic, may allow abdominopelvic wash-out and the raising of a stoma with a high expectation of anastomotic salvage and a satisfactory outcome [65]. At relaparotomy, the critical decision is whether to take down an anastomosis and exteriorize or to attempt anastomotic preservation. The consequences of anastomotic take-down in terms of future gastrointestinal continuity are very different for right-sided compared to low pelvic anastomosis. Nevertheless, the overwhelming priority is control of sepsis and anastomotic disconnection may be necessary, which, in the case of a low anastomosis, is likely to be permanent [66].

As for other abdominal catastrophes described in this chapter, a "damage control" approach may be advisable or necessary, depending upon degree of sepsis, physiological instability, and difficulty with abdominal closure. Ultimate reconstruction and restoration of intestinal continuity will usually need to be delayed for at least 6 months.

References

1 Jayaraman S, Sethi D, Chinnock P, Wong R. Advanced trauma life support training for hospital staff. *Cochrane Database Syst Rev* 2014; **8**:CD004173.

2 Watts DD, Fakhry SM. Incidence of hollow viscus injury in blunt trauma: an analysis from 275,557 trauma admissions from the East multi-institutional trial. *J Trauma* 2003; **54**(2):289–94.

3 Fakhry SM, Watts DD, Luchette FA. Current diagnostic approaches lack sensitivity in the diagnosis of perforated blunt small bowel injury: analysis from 275,557 trauma admissions from the EAST multi-institutional HVI trial. *J Trauma* 2003; **54**(2):295–306.

4 Guy RJ, Kirkman E, Watkins PE, Cooper GJ. Physiologic responses to primary blast. *J Trauma* 1998; **45**(6):983–7.

5 Fleming S, Bird R, Ratnasingham K, Sarker SJ, Walsh M, Patel B. Accuracy of FAST scan in blunt abdominal trauma in a major London trauma centre. *Int J Surg* 2012; **10**(9):470–4.

6 Elton C, Riaz AA, Young N, Schamschula R, Papadopoulos B, Malka V. Accuracy of computed tomography in the detection of blunt bowel and mesenteric injuries. *Br J Surg* 2005; **92**(8):1024–8.

7 Wang YC, Hsieh CH, Fu CY, Yeh CC, Wu SC, Chen RJ. Hollow organ perforation in blunt abdominal trauma: the role of diagnostic peritoneal lavage. *Am J Emerg Med* 2012; **30**(4):570–3.

8 O'Malley E, Boyle E, O'Callaghan A, Coffey JC, Walsh SR. Role of laparoscopy in penetrating abdominal trauma: a systematic review. *World J Surg* 2013; **37**(1):113–22.

9 Loveland JA, Boffard KD. Damage control in the abdomen and beyond. *Br J Surg* 2004; **91**(9):1095–101.

10 Rotondo MF, Zonies DH. The damage control sequence and underlying logic. *Surg Clin North Am* 1997; **77**(4):761–77.

11 Roberts DJ, Zygun DA, Grendar J, *et al.* Negative-pressure wound therapy for critically ill adults with open abdominal wounds: a systematic review. *J Trauma Acute Care Surg* 2012; **73**(3):629–39.

12 Burlew CC, Moore EE, Cuschieri J, *et al.* Sew it up! A Western Trauma Association multi-institutional study of enteric injury management in the postinjury open abdomen. *J Trauma* 2011; **70**(2):273–7.

13 Fozard JB, Armitage NC, Schofield JB, Jones OM. ACPGBI position statement on elective resection for diverticulitis. *Colorectal Dis* 2011; **13**(Suppl 3):1–11.

14 Chabok A, Pahlman L, Hjern F, Haapaniemi S, Smedh K. Randomized clinical trial of antibiotics in acute uncomplicated diverticulitis. *Br J Surg* 2012; **99**(4):532–9.

15 Hinchey EJ, Schaal PG, Richards GK. Treatment of perforated diverticular disease of the colon. *Adv Surg* 1978; **12**:85–109.

16 Feingold D, Steele SR, Lee S, *et al*. Practice parameters for the treatment of sigmoid diverticulitis. *Dis Colon Rectum* 2014; **57**(3):284–94.

17 Myers E, Hurley M, O'Sullivan GC, Kavanagh D, Wilson I, Winter DC. Laparoscopic peritoneal lavage for generalized peritonitis due to perforated diverticulitis. *Br J Surg* 2008; **95**(1):97–101.

18 Angenete E, Thornell A, Burcharth J, *et al*. Laparoscopic lavage is feasible and safe for the treatment of perforated diverticulitis with purulent peritonitis: the first results from the randomized controlled trial DILALA. *Ann Surg* 2014; Dec 8 (epub ahead of print).

19 Constantinides VA, Tekkis PP, Senapati A. Prospective multicentre evaluation of adverse outcomes following treatment for complicated diverticular disease. *Br J Surg* 2006; **93**(12):1503–13.

20 Constantinides VA, Heriot A, Remzi F, *et al*. Operative strategies for diverticular peritonitis: a decision analysis between primary resection and anastomosis versus Hartmann's procedures. *Ann Surg* 2007; **245**(1):94–103.

21 Letarte F, Hallet J, Drolet S, *et al*. Laparoscopic versus open colonic resection for complicated diverticular disease in the emergency setting: a safe choice? A retrospective comparative cohort study. *Am J Surg* 2015; **209**(6):992–8.

22 Kafka-Ritsch R, Birkfellner F, Perathoner A, *et al*. Damage control surgery with abdominal vacuum and delayed bowel reconstruction in patients with perforated diverticulitis Hinchey III/IV. *J Gastrointest Surg* 2012; **16**(10):1915–22.

23 Abdelrazeq AS, Scott N, Thorn C, *et al*. The impact of spontaneous tumour perforation on outcome following colon cancer surgery. *Colorectal Dis* 2008; **10**(8):775–80.

24 Acosta S, Bjorck M. Modern treatment of acute mesenteric ischaemia. *Br J Surg* 2014; **101**(1):e100–8.

25 Ris F, Hompes R, Cunningham C, *et al*. Near-infrared (NIR) perfusion angiography in minimally invasive colorectal surgery. *Surg Endosc* 2014; **28**(7):2221–6.

26 Cappell MS. Intestinal (mesenteric) vasculopathy. II. Ischemic colitis and chronic mesenteric ischemia. *Gastroenterol Clin North Am* 1998; **27**(4):827–60, vi.

27 American Gastroenterological Association. Medical Position Statement: guidelines on intestinal ischemia. *Gastroenterology* 2000; **118**(5):951–3.

28 Gluud LL, Klingenberg SL, Langholz E. Tranexamic acid for upper gastrointestinal bleeding. *Cochrane Database Syst Rev* 2012; **1**:CD006640.

29 Farrell JJ, Friedman LS. Review article: the management of lower gastrointestinal bleeding. *Aliment Pharmacol Therapeut* 2005; **21**(11):1281–98.

30 Laine L, Shah A. Randomized trial of urgent vs. elective colonoscopy in patients hospitalized with lower GI bleeding. *Am J Gastroenterol* 2010; **105**(12):2636–41; quiz 42.

31 Green BT, Rockey DC, Portwood G, *et al*. Urgent colonoscopy for evaluation and management of acute lower gastrointestinal hemorrhage: a randomized controlled trial. *Am J Gastroenterol* 2005; **100**(11):2395–402.

32 Ghassemi KA, Jensen DM. Lower GI bleeding: epidemiology and management. *Curr Gastroenterol Rep* 2013; **15**(7):333.

33 Kwan V, Bourke MJ, Williams SJ, *et al*. Argon plasma coagulation in the management of symptomatic gastrointestinal vascular lesions: experience in 100 consecutive patients with long-term follow-up. *Am J Gastroenterol* 2006; **101**(1):58–63.

34 Garcia-Blazquez V, Vicente-Bartulos A, Olavarria-Delgado A, Plana MN, van der Winden D, Zamora J. Accuracy of CT angiography in the diagnosis of acute gastrointestinal bleeding: systematic review and meta-analysis. *Eur Radiol* 2013; **23**(5):1181–90.

35 Ahmed TM, Cowley JB, Robinson G, *et al*. Long term follow-up of transcatheter coil embolotherapy for major colonic haemorrhage. *Colorectal Dis* 2010; **12**(10):1013–17.

36 Delabrousse E, Sarlieve P, Sailley N, Aubry S, Kastler BA. Cecal volvulus: CT findings and correlation with pathophysiology. *Emerg Radiol* 2007; **14**(6):411–15.

37 Halabi WJ, Jafari MD, Kang CY, *et al.* Colonic volvulus in the United States: trends, outcomes, and predictors of mortality. *Ann Surg* 2014; **259**(2):293–301.

38 Oren D, Atamanalp SS, Aydinli B, *et al.* An algorithm for the management of sigmoid colon volvulus and the safety of primary resection: experience with 827 cases. *Dis Colon Rectum* 2007; **50**(4):489–97.

39 Cowlam S, Watson C, Elltringham M, *et al.* Percutaneous endoscopic colostomy of the left side of the colon. *Gastrointest Endosc* 2007; **65**(7):1007–14.

40 Gordon-Weeks AN, Lorenzi B, Lim J, Cristaldi M. Laparoscopic-assisted endoscopic sigmoidopexy: a new surgical option for sigmoid volvulus. *Dis Colon Rectum* 2011; **54**(5):645–7.

41 Masoomi H, Kang CY, Chaudhry O, *et al.* Predictive factors of early bowel obstruction in colon and rectal surgery: data from the Nationwide Inpatient Sample, 2006–2008. *J Am Coll Surg* 2012; **214**(5):831–7.

42 Khasawneh MA, Ugarte ML, Srvantstian B, Dozois EJ, Bannon MP, Zielinski MD. Role of gastrografin challenge in early postoperative small bowel obstruction. *J Gastrointest Surg* 2014; **18**(2):363–8.

43 Thornton M, Joshi H, Vimalachandran C, *et al.* Management and outcome of colorectal anastomotic leaks. *Int J Colorectal Dis* 2011; **26**(3):313–20.

44 Jung SH, Yu CS, Choi PW, *et al.* Risk factors and oncologic impact of anastomotic leakage after rectal cancer surgery. *Dis Colon Rectum* 2008; **51**(6):902–8.

45 Frasson M, Flor-Lorente B, Ramos Rodriguez JL, *et al.* Risk factors for anastomotic leak after colon resection for cancer: multivariate analysis and nomogram from a multicentric, prospective, national study with 3193 patients. *Ann Surg* 2015; **262**(2):321–30.

46 Manilich E, Vogel JD, Kiran RP, Church JM, Seyidova-Khoshknabi D, Remzi FH. Key factors associated with postoperative complications in patients undergoing colorectal surgery. *Dis Colon Rectum* 2013; **56**(1):64–71.

47 Warschkow R, Steffen T, Thierbach J, Bruckner T, Lange J, Tarantino I. Risk factors for anastomotic leakage after rectal cancer resection and reconstruction with colorectostomy. A retrospective study with bootstrap analysis. *Ann Surg Oncol* 2011; **18**(10):2772–82.

48 Tresallet C, Royer B, Godiris-Petit G, Menegaux F. Effect of systemic corticosteroids on elective left-sided colorectal resection with colorectal anastomosis. *Am J Surg* 2008; **195**(4):447–51.

49 Hakkarainen TW, Steele SR, Bastaworous A, *et al.* Nonsteroidal anti-inflammatory drugs and the risk for anastomotic failure: a report from Washington State's Surgical Care and Outcomes Assessment Program (SCOAP). *JAMA Surg* 2015; **150**(3):223–8.

50 Kwag SJ, Kim JG, Kang WK, Lee JK, Oh ST. The nutritional risk is a independent factor for postoperative morbidity in surgery for colorectal cancer. *Ann Surg Treatment Res* 2014; **86**(4):206–11.

51 Calin MD, Balalau C, Popa F, Voiculescu S, Scaunasu RV. Colic anastomotic leakage risk factors. *J Med Life* 2013; **6**(4):420–3.

52 Guenaga KF, Matos D, Wille-Jorgensen P. Mechanical bowel preparation for elective colorectal surgery. *Cochrane Database Syst Rev* 2011; **9**:CD001544.

53 Weeks JC, Nelson H, Gelber S, Sargent D, Schroeder G. Short-term quality-of-life outcomes following laparoscopic-assisted colectomy vs open colectomy for colon cancer: a randomized trial. *JAMA* 2002; **287**(3):321–8.

54 Guillou PJ, Quirke P, Thorpe H, *et al.* Short-term endpoints of conventional versus laparoscopic-assisted surgery in patients with colorectal cancer (MRC CLASICC trial): multicentre, randomised controlled trial. *Lancet* 2005; **365**(9472):1718–26.

55 Neutzling CB, Lustosa SA, Proenca IM, da Silva EM, Matos D. Stapled versus handsewn methods for colorectal anastomosis surgery. *Cochrane Database Syst Rev* 2012; **2**:CD003144.

56 Beard JD, Nicholson ML, Sayers RD, Lloyd D, Everson NW. Intraoperative air testing of colorectal anastomoses: a prospective, randomized trial. *Br J Surg* 1990; **77**(10):1095–7.

57 Hao XY, Yang KH, Guo TK, Ma B, Tian JH, Li HL. Omentoplasty in the prevention of anastomotic leakage after colorectal resection: a meta-analysis. *Int J Colorectal Dis* 2008; **23**(12):1159–65.

58 Tsujinaka S, Kawamura YJ, Konishi F, Maeda T, Mizokami K. Pelvic drainage for anterior resection revisited: use of drains in anastomotic leaks. *Aust NZ J Surg* 2008; **78**(6):461–5.

59 Lai R, Lu Y, Li Q, Guo J, Chen G, Zeng W. Risk factors for anastomotic leakage following anterior resection for colorectal cancer: the effect of epidural analgesia on occurrence. *Int J Colorectal Dis* 2013; **28**(4):485–92.

60 Hyman N, Manchester TL, Osler T, Burns B, Cataldo PA. Anastomotic leaks after intestinal anastomosis: it's later than you think. *Ann Surg* 2007; **245**(2):254–8.

61 Singh PP, Zeng IS, Srinivasa S, Lemanu DP, Connolly AB, Hill AG. Systematic review and meta-analysis of use of serum C-reactive protein levels to predict anastomotic leak after colorectal surgery. *Br J Surg* 2014; **101**(4):339–46.

62 Hirst NA, Tiernan JP, Millner PA, Jayne DG. Systematic review of methods to predict and detect anastomotic leakage in colorectal surgery. *Colorectal Dis* 2014; **16**(2):95–109.

63 Kirat HT, Remzi FH, Shen B, Kiran RP. Pelvic abscess associated with anastomotic leak in patients with ileal pouch-anal anastomosis (IPAA): transanastomotic or CT-guided drainage? *Int J Colorectal Dis* 2011; **26**(11):1469–74.

64 Verlaan T, Bartels SA, van Berge Henegouwen MI, Tanis PJ, Fockens P, Bemelman WA. Early, minimally invasive closure of anastomotic leaks: a new concept. *Colorectal Dis* 2011; **13**(Suppl 7):18–22.

65 Vennix S, Abegg R, Bakker OJ, *et al.* Surgical re-interventions following colorectal surgery: open versus laparoscopic management of anastomotic leakage. *J Laparosc Adv Surg Tech A* 2013; **23**(9):739–44.

66 Khan AA, Wheeler JM, Cunningham C, George B, Kettlewell M, Mortensen NJ. The management and outcome of anastomotic leaks in colorectal surgery. *Colorectal Dis* 2008; **10**(6):587–92.

CASE 40

Occupational blast disaster

Richard Guy

Oxford University Hospitals NHS Foundation Trust, Oxford, UK

A 47-year-old ordnance expert was admitted to A&E with an abdominal injury sustained when a cluster bomblet exploded in his hand. The bomblet casing was found to have penetrated the abdominal wall and there was evisceration of omentum through a 5 × 5 cm defect. In addition, there was a degloving injury to the right hand and "peppering" injury to the face and corneas. He was conscious, vocalizing, and with no objective evidence of respiratory compromise. Pulse was 92 beats per minute and blood pressure 125/75 mmHg. Following primary and secondary survey, administration of intravenous fluids, antibiotics and analgesia and oxygen by mask, CT imaging was arranged. This showed omental and bowel evisceration with evidence of colonic disruption and the presence of an intraabdominal metallic foreign body (Figure 40.1).

Urgent laparotomy was undertaken through a midline incision. The findings were of a through-and-through injury to the right colon with fecal contamination and a fragment of metal lodged in the retroperitoneum. The right ureter was not damaged. There was no evidence of solid organ injury and no significant hemorrhage.

DECISION POINT

What operation(s) would you perform?

The surgical priorities were to assess the extent of injury, check for additional injuries, and safely remove shrapnel if possible. Regarding the through-and-through injury to the right colon, the options considered included:

- direct repair

- resection of damaged bowel and primary anastomosis

- resection of damaged bowel and stoma formation

- resection of damaged bowel, stapled closure, temporary abdominal closure, and relook at 24–48 hours.

The extent and mechanism of injury meant that simple closure of the colon was clearly inappropriate. Resection and primary anastomosis was considered, particularly as he was hemodynamically stable and peritoneal contamination was recent and minimal. However, it was felt that in view of the mechanism of injury and possibility of associated lung injury, a nonanastomotic approach was safer. It was decided to resect the damaged bowel, staple the ends closed, and relook in 24–48 hours.

Colorectal Surgery: Clinical Care and Management, First Edition.
Edited by Bruce George, Richard Guy, Oliver Jones, and Jon Vogel.
© 2016 John Wiley & Sons, Ltd. Published 2016 by John Wiley & Sons, Ltd.

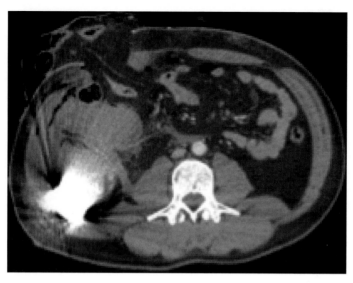

Figure 40.1 Initial CT scan showing evisceration and the projectile in the right retroperitoneum.

Damage control surgery (DCS) was performed with right hemicolectomy, the distal ileum and proximal transverse colon being divided with a linear stapler but not reanastomosed, and left inside the abdomen. Saline lavage and debridement of the entry wound on the anterior abdominal wall completed the procedure and temporary abdominal closure (TAC) was achieved with an Abdo-VAC (KCI) negative-pressure wound therapy (NPWT) dressing (Figure 40.2). Plastic surgeons then proceeded to repair of the hand and the patient was transferred to ICU.

The patient was ventilated, monitored, and supported on ICU prior to a return to theater 48 hours later. Relaparotomy revealed a clean peritoneal cavity with healthy bowel and no other injuries. A side-to-side stapled ileocolic anastomosis was performed and the midline surgical wound and right-sided traumatic wound were both closed. The patient was returned to ICU where he remained ventilated for a further 24 hours. Nasoenteral feeding was commenced on day 1 following relaparotomy. After return to the general ward 2 days later, with physiotherapy and rehabilitation, the patient was finally discharged to outpatient follow-up 17 days after initial injury, where his progress remained satisfactory.

After 6 months, the patient returned to work and follow-up after 2 years revealed that he had resumed duties in explosives research. Mechanical function of the injured hand was unimpaired, with just a small area of sensation loss on the little finger. Abdominal wall function was good, despite a small hernia at the original site of shrapnel entry.

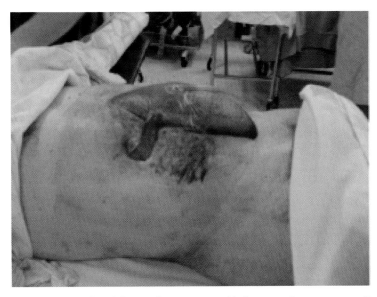

Figure 40.2 AbdoVac in place following laparotomy and before negative pressure application.

Could we have done better?

There remains some debate over a blanket policy of DCS for all abdominal injuries. Patients with cardiorespiratory stability and easily definable injury without significant contamination may be suitable for primary repair or reanastomosis and definitive abdominal wall closure, and this must be a team judgment based upon ease of surgery and state of physiology at the time of surgery. The mechanism of injury with potential lung injury swung the decision in favor of DCS and relook laparotomy, despite relatively localized contamination. The continued need for ventilation following definitive surgery perhaps justified this decision.

> **LEARNING POINTS**
>
> - Abdominal blast injury may be associated with life-threatening pulmonary injury.
> - DCS for penetrating and blunt abdominal trauma with fecal contamination may be a life-saving approach, ensuring rapid transfer to a critical care environment for correction of physiology.
> - Temporary abdominal closure prevents intraabdominal hypertension and abdominal compartment syndrome. Techniques of TAC incorporating negative-pressure systems are probably preferable to alternative techniques.
> - Early fascial closure prevents morbidity associated with laparostomy and improves overall survival.

CASE 41

Wash and go?

Bruce George

Oxford University Hospitals NHS Foundation Trust, Oxford, UK

A 66-year-old woman presented with a 2-week history of left-sided abdominal pain. She had been treated by her GP with broad-spectrum antibiotics for 7 days for a possible urinary infection. She was referred as an emergency due to worsening pain.

On examination, she was mildly pyrexial with a heart rate of 76 beats/min. Abdominal examination revealed tenderness in the left iliac fossa. Urinalysis was normal. Blood tests showed a raised white cell count of 13.6×10^9/L and CRP greater than 156 mg/L.

She was treated with intravenous co-amoxiclav and metronidazole for presumed diverticulitis. Some 36 hours after admission, she complained of worsening abdominal pain and on examination, there were signs of generalized peritonitis. A CT scan showed evidence of free intraperitoneal gas, sigmoid diverticulitis, and an 8 cm pelvic abscess containing gas (Figure 41.1). Systemically, she remained reasonably well, normotensive with a pulse of 80/min, and with a good urine output.

DECISION POINT

What would you do now? Should she proceed straight to surgery?

As the patient had free intraperitoneal gas and clinical features of peritonitis, there was no doubt that surgery was indicated. It was decided to laparoscope her.

At laparoscopy, there was a small amount of fluid visible in the left flank and over the liver. There was some fibrinous exudate in the LIF and over the liver (Figure 41.2). The left upper abdomen looked normal. After mobilization of small bowel loops away from the pelvis and sigmoid, the abscess in the pelvis was easily drained by suction aspiration.

DECISION POINT

What would you do now? Should the diseased sigmoid be resected?

The options considered were: laparoscopic lavage only, sigmoid resection with anastomosis or Hartmann's resection. In view of the relatively mild generalized abdominal findings, it was decided to just drain the pelvic abscess and wash out the peritoneal cavity.

Colorectal Surgery: Clinical Care and Management, First Edition.
Edited by Bruce George, Richard Guy, Oliver Jones, and Jon Vogel.
© 2016 John Wiley & Sons, Ltd. Published 2016 by John Wiley & Sons, Ltd.

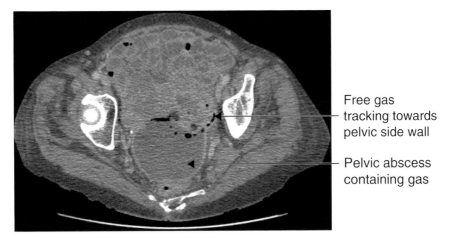

Free gas tracking towards pelvic side wall

Pelvic abscess containing gas

Figure 41.1 CT scan demonstrating pockets of free intraperitoneal gas and abscess anterior to rectum.

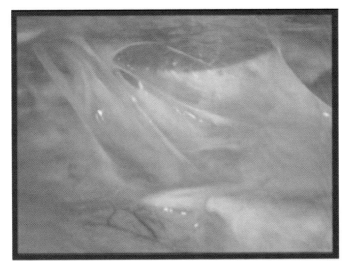

Figure 41.2 Laparoscopic view of fibrin over the liver.

She underwent pelvic abscess drainage and thorough peritoneal lavage with 8 liters of saline, and a nonsuction drain was left in the pelvis. Postoperatively, she remained on broad-spectrum intravenous antibiotics. Three days later, feculent fluid was seen in the pelvic drain. On examination, she was tender with guarding in the left iliac fossa.

DECISION POINT

What would you do now? Should she undergo emergency surgery? What about trying to create a controlled fecal fistula?

The options considered were: continued conservative treatment with antibiotics and fistula care with a view to early elective surgery, or immediate resection. In view of the development of abdominal guarding, a surgical approach was considered most sensible.

She proceeded to relaparoscopy. This revealed the sigmoid colon to be indurated and difficult to mobilize. A decision to convert to midline laparotomy was made early and she underwent a technically difficult Hartmann's procedure. Subsequent postoperative recovery was uneventful and she was discharged home 8 days later. At outpatient review, she was well, and subsequently underwent reversal of Hartmann's.

Could we have done better?

In hindsight, she should have had a Hartmann's procedure at the first operation for Hinchey III perforated diverticulitis.

LEARNING POINTS (SEE PAGES 247–8)

- Perforated diverticulitis with generalized peritonitis (Hinchey III–IV) usually requires sigmoid resection and Hartmann's procedure.
- Laparoscopic peritoneal lavage is becoming increasingly popular in the management of perforated diverticulitis which is not responding to conservative management.
- The challenge is to use laparoscopic lavage appropriately, avoiding its use in milder cases which would respond to antibiotics alone and to avoid undertreating severe cases which really need sigmoid resection.
- Emergency sigmoid resection for complicated diverticulitis may be associated with significant morbidity, and the decision to undertake a Hartmann's procedure or primary anastomosis +/- covering ileostomy is usually made on the basis of surgical intuition rather than evidence base.

LETTER FROM AMERICA

The 2014 ASCRS clinical practice guidelines for emergency surgery for acute sigmoid diverticulitis include a strong recommendation based on moderate-quality evidence for urgent sigmoid colectomy in patients with diffuse peritonitis or those in whom non-operative management fails. For patients with Hinchey III or IV diverticulitis, the guidelines committee noted that "operative therapy without resection is generally not an appropriate alternative to colectomy." The committee noted that the "safety of lavage has not been proven or disproven by the published studies to date."

Jon Vogel and Massarat Zutshi

CASE 42

Absolute constipation

Richard Guy

Oxford University Hospitals NHS Foundation Trust, Oxford, UK

A 73-year-old man presented as an emergency with progressive abdominal distension and absolute constipation for 5 days. Past medical history included insulin-dependent diabetes mellitus, hypertension, cerebrovascular accident 6 years previously, and subsequently left carotid endarterectomy. Medications included bendroflumethiazide, simvastatin, doxazosin, aspirin, and insulin. Body Mass Index was $34 \, kg/m^2$.

On admission, he was clinically dehydrated with gross abdominal distension and tenderness in the right iliac fossa but without signs of peritonism. Rectal examination showed an empty rectum. Vital signs were: pulse 98/min regular, BP 148/78 mmHg, temperature 36.2 °C, respiratory rate 18/min. There was left-sided neurological weakness. On digital rectal examination, the lower edge of a rectal tumor was palpable. Blood tests on admission showed: hemoglobin 14.1 g/dL, white cell count 11.5, platelets 258, sodium 138 mmol/L, potassium 3.7 mmol/L, urea 21.5 mmol/L, creatinine 210 µmol/L, C-reactive protein 14, glucose 11.1 mmol/L. A plain abdominal radiograph showed gross colonic dilatation and cecal distension with a diameter of 9 cm (Figure 42.1).

Urgent CT examination revealed a bulky rectal tumor, confirmed a dilated but viable and intact cecum, and showed no evidence of metastatic disease.

DECISION POINT

What would you do now?

The patient clearly needs decompressing, either by stenting or surgery. The obstructing rectal tumor (mid-upper) was considered to be too low to stent. The easiest preliminary surgical option would be to just decompress the colon with a transverse loop colostomy. The alternative would be to resect the tumor with a Hartmann's procedure or perhaps on-table colonic lavage and primary anastomosis with or without a covering ileostomy.

It was decided to just do a loop transverse colostomy. It was felt that rectal resection in the presence of obstruction would be technically difficult, may be oncologically suboptimal and that more detailed imaging would be necessary to decide if preresection radiotherapy was indicated.

Colorectal Surgery: Clinical Care and Management, First Edition.
Edited by Bruce George, Richard Guy, Oliver Jones, and Jon Vogel.
© 2016 John Wiley & Sons, Ltd. Published 2016 by John Wiley & Sons, Ltd.

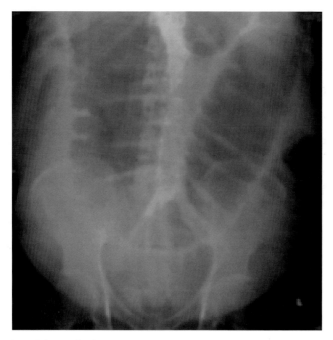

Figure 42.1 Plain abdominal radiograph showing gross colonic dilatation.

Under general anesthesia, a transverse loop colostomy was raised through a transverse muscle-cutting incision in the right upper quadrant. Dilated transverse colon was identified and decompressed proximally and distally by suction through a purse-string colotomy. The stoma was matured over a plastic bridge.

Postoperatively, the patient remained significantly distended and there was little activity via the colostomy. A 30 Fr Foley catheter was inserted into the afferent limb in an attempt to keep the cecum decompressed (Figure 42.2). Insertion of a nasogastric tube into the stomach was required with aspiration of significant gastric volumes. Imaging showed that the colon had been decompressed but there were features of small bowel obstruction.

DECISION POINT

How would you manage this problem?

The patient is functionally obstructed, with dilated loops of small bowel and no stoma output. It is not clear if the problem is due to a paralytic ileus or mechanical obstruction. The CT had shown no evidence of a cause of mechanical obstruction, such as a parastomal hernia.

The options were to continue conservative management or to operate. It was felt that conservative management with correction of electrolytes and possibly TPN would be preferable. A water-soluble contrast follow-through examination was arranged in order to exclude a high-grade mechanical obstruction.

The contrast examination demonstrated that contrast eventually reached the colon. Endoscopic examination of the right colon via the colostomy allowed

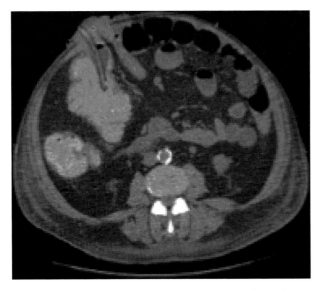

Figure 42.2 CT showing decompressed cecum containing a large Foley catheter.

passage of the scope through the ileocecal valve into the ileum, achieving some decompression. Total parenteral nutrition (TPN) was commenced as well as oral nutritional supplements.

Eventually there was substantial stoma activity, the patient progressed to enteral feeding, and his general condition improved. Flexible sigmoidoscopy was undertaken and an impassable annular tumor was seen, and confirmed on histological examination as an adenocarcinoma. Staging CT showed no evidence of metastatic disease. MRI scanning showed an operable upper mid rectal tumor not threatening the predicted margin of resection. He was discharged home 11 days after this emergency admission.

A month later, after MDT review, the patient underwent laparoscopic-assisted low anterior resection. Some technical difficulties, particularly with port placement, were encountered owing to the position of the transverse colostomy, but the stoma was located sufficiently proximal in the transverse colon that it didn't need to be taken down in order to achieve full mobilization of the splenic flexure. A lower midline incision was made in order to achieve radical rectal excision and low anastomosis, and the transverse colostomy was left in place. Postoperative recovery was uneventful.

Histopathological examination of the resected specimen revealed two cancers, both moderately differentiated adenocarcinomas, one in the sigmoid (T2, Dukes' A) and another in the rectum (T3, Dukes' B). All margins were microscopically clear, all 36 lymph nodes retrieved were free of tumor, and there were no other adverse histological features.

The transverse colostomy was reversed 4 months later, following a satisfactory water-soluble contrast enema examination, without complication.

Could we have done better?

It is generally considered that stenting of obstructing rectal tumors is not feasible due to intractable tenesmus. It is conceivable that if decompression was achieved rapidly by stenting, then early definitive surgery (and putting up with the tenesmus for a week or so) might have been possible.

The small bowel obstruction or ileus following loop colostomy was not really explained and almost necessitated a potentially difficult laparotomy. It may have been precipitated by electrolyte abnormalities, hypoxia or opiates and therefore might have been avoided by better postoperative fluid and analgesic management.

LEARNING POINTS

- Urgent colonic decompression is required when there is "closed loop" large bowel obstruction to avoid cecal ischemia and perforation.
- Malignant large bowel obstruction from rectal cancer may require a staged approach in order to avoid a difficult emergency rectal excision and to optimize oncological outcome.
- CT scanning and water-soluble contrast studies are helpful in the management of patients with ileus/obstruction in the early postoperative period (see page 255–6).

LETTER FROM AMERICA

In cases of an emergency presentation of obstructing rectal cancer, the ASCRS Clinical Practice Guidelines Committee (2013) recommended a proximal loop ostomy for those cases in which endoscopic stenting is impractical and the patient is at risk of closed loop obstruction.

Jon Vogel and Massarat Zutshi

CASE 43

Multiply ischemic parts

Richard Guy

Oxford University Hospitals NHS Foundation Trust, Oxford, UK

A 60-year-old man was transferred from another hospital following the simultaneous sudden onset of acute abdominal pain and a cold blue left hand (Figure 43.1). On examination, he was in atrial fibrillation and was hypotensive. Examination of the left arm revealed it to be cold and pulseless with deteriorating motor function. On examination of the abdomen, he had signs of peritonitis. Following resuscitation with intravenous fluid, oxygen and antibiotics, urgent CT imaging was arranged. This showed free fluid and free intraperitoneal gas from probable perforated and possibly obstructed infarcted small bowel secondary to a cecal carcinoma.

DECISION POINT

How would you manage this patient?

The patient clearly needed vascular embolectomy and laparotomy. The feeling was that if embolectomy and restoration of hand perfusion could be performed swiftly, this would be the preferred choice, particularly as hand ischemia was rapidly worsening. The risk was a lengthy vascular procedure with the potential for worsening of intraabdominal pathology. Conversely, a prolonged laparotomy would potentially result in an unsalvageable limb.

He proceeded to brachial embolectomy which was successful in rapidly restoring hand perfusion. Laparotomy was then undertaken. The findings were of mid-small bowel infarction and necrosis (Figure 43.2), free enteric content, and a partially obstructing cecal cancer.

DECISION POINT

What should be the extent of the resection? What about the cancer – should that be resected now?

There were two pathologies: presumed mesenteric embolus with segmental infarction, necrosis and perforation, and small bowel obstruction from a cecal cancer. The decision taken was to resect the infarcted small bowel and to carry out a right hemicolectomy but not to perform any anastomoses. The cecal cancer could conceivably be left until relook laparotomy, but if a straightforward oncological resection was easily possible, and in view of obstructive features, definitive excision would be better. However, any anastomosis under these conditions would be risky.

Colorectal Surgery: Clinical Care and Management, First Edition.
Edited by Bruce George, Richard Guy, Oliver Jones, and Jon Vogel.
© 2016 John Wiley & Sons, Ltd. Published 2016 by John Wiley & Sons, Ltd.

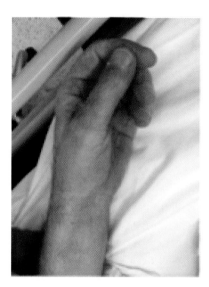

Figure 43.1 Ischemic left hand.

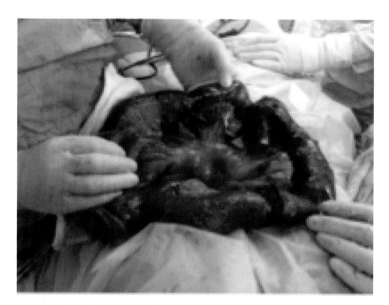

Figure 43.2 Infarcted and necrotic small bowel at initial laparotomy. A linear stapled transection has been carried out prior to resection.

Following bowel mobilization, resection was performed by way of linear staplers, leaving four stapled ends (two jejunal, one ileal, one transverse colon). Foley catheters were inserted into the proximal jejunal end and into the distal ileal end, and brought out separately through the abdominal wall. Temporary abdominal closure was achieved with an ABThera negative-pressure wound dressing. The patient was fully heparinized intravenously in order to reduce the risk of further embolic events.

At relook laparotomy after 48 hours, further small bowel infarction was noted and this was resected. In view of this finding, anastomosis was again considered unwise, Foley catheters were again used, and an ABThera dressing reapplied. After a further 48 hours on ICU, the patient returned to theater once more and all bowel was considered healthy. A jejuno-jejunal anastomosis was performed and an end ileostomy raised, leaving the proximal transverse colon stapled closed. The abdomen was closed definitively. Postoperative recovery was uneventful and the patient was transferred back to the referring hospital.

Could we have done better?

It might have been ideal to carry out simultaneous laparotomy and brachial embolectomy at the time of initial presentation, but the logistical requirements for dual operating of this nature are usually prohibitive.

Superior mesenteric embolectomy was considered at initial laparotomy (see page 250). This is undertaken at emergency laparotomy relatively infrequently, and the results of mesenteric revascularization are generally poor. As the length of bowel resected in this case was relatively short, the length of apparently normally perfused remaining bowel adequate, and in order not to prolong the procedure further, a decision was taken not to explore the superior mesenteric artery (SMA).

The final outcome was satisfactory, although the patient has an ileostomy which itself might be associated with morbidity, such as high output, obstruction, retraction, prolapse, and parastomal hernia. An ileocolic anastomosis could have been undertaken at the third laparotomy, but a second anastomosis was considered too high a risk. Further elective surgery to finally restore bowel continuity would be appropriate.

LEARNING POINTS

- The true extent of small bowel ischemia may not be apparent at initial laparotomy, final demarcation being more obvious at a second examination, and so a relatively conservative resection can be undertaken at first laparotomy, resecting obviously necrotic or infarcted small bowel only.
- DCS techniques with no attempt at anastomosis initially are often necessary in patients with extensive small bowel ischemia.
- Temporary abdominal closure using negative-pressure wound therapy is probably superior to other commonly used techniques.

LETTER FROM AMERICA

No guidelines here. In our limited personal experience, simple stapling of the healthy bowel without external drainage catheters and planned relook laparotomy in 24–72 hours has not been problematic. Waiting 3–6 months for creation of the ileocolostomy seems wise in this case. This reestablishment of bowel continuity is facilitated by implanting the stapled colon stump in the subcutaneous location in the midline wound.

Jon Vogel and Massarat Zutshi

CASE 44

Seriously obscure bleeding

Alistair Myers

Hillingdon Hospital NHS Foundation Trust, London, UK

A 52-year-old postmenopausal woman with no significant past medical history was referred with dark rectal bleeding and diarrhea of a week's duration. Blood tests showed microcytic, iron deficiency anemia (Hb 7.8 g/dL). As the bleeding spontaneously settled, urgent outpatient esophagogastroduodenoscopy (EGD) and colonoscopy were arranged. These examinations were entirely normal, and duodenal, terminal ileal and colonic biopsies were also normal. The patient was prescribed oral iron, but remained anemic on retesting after 2 months. There had been no further overt rectal bleeding.

DECISION POINT

What would you do now? Are any further investigations required?

British Society of Gastroenterology guidelines suggest that a postmenopausal woman presenting with iron deficient anemia with normal EGD and colonoscopy should have the anemia treated and would not need additional investigations unless they become transfusion dependent. However, as this patient had presented with overt blood loss, it was felt necessary to assess the small bowel.

Capsule endoscopy was carried out. This showed a hemi-circumferential ulcerated area at 2 hours and 53 minutes, during a total small bowel transit time of 4 hours and 52 minutes, allowing the location to be estimated as the proximal ileum (Figure 44.1). It was considered atypical for Crohn's disease and not frankly malignant. The patient was keen to avoid surgery.

DECISION POINT

What should be done now? Is this an adequate explanation for the overt blood loss?

It was felt that the ulceration seen may be the cause of blood loss, but that further imaging was required to clarify the cause.

Magnetic resonance enteroclysis (MRE) was normal. Antegrade "push" enteroscopy was performed; this was normal up to the point of insertion, and

---

Colorectal Surgery: Clinical Care and Management, First Edition.
Edited by Bruce George, Richard Guy, Oliver Jones, and Jon Vogel.
© 2016 John Wiley & Sons, Ltd. Published 2016 by John Wiley & Sons, Ltd.

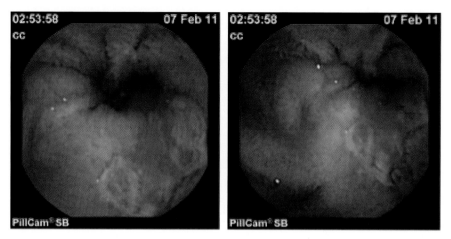

Figure 44.1 Capsule endoscopy images showing discrete ileal ulceration.

an ink tattoo was placed at the limit. Double-balloon enteroscopy was arranged: antegrade examination was normal up to a reported distance of 320 cm beyond the pylorus and a tattoo was placed at this point. A difficult retrograde examination through the ileocecal valve to a distance of 120 cm was also normal, and a further tattoo was placed at the limit. As the tattoo from the antegrade examination was not found, it was assumed that complete visualization of the small bowel had not been achieved.

Over the ensuing 3 months, the patient suffered further episodes of painless, altered rectal bleeding, with symptomatic anemia. Repeat EGD and colonoscopy were, once again, normal.

DECISION POINT

What should be done now in view of persistent symptoms?

It was decided to proceed to surgical assessment. The plan was to undertake a diagnostic laparoscopy and to "run" the small bowel. If no obvious pathology was encountered then intraoperative enteroscopy would be undertaken via a periumbilical incision and enterotomy.

Elective laparoscopy was undertaken through a single port. This showed a 6 cm long Meckel's diverticulum. The three tattoos were seen, all in the ileum proximal to the Meckel's, suggesting that it had been overlooked at retrograde double-balloon enteroscopy.

The ileum was delivered and the segment containing the Meckel's wedge resected. The patient subsequently made an uneventful recovery, with no further reports of rectal bleeding or anemia.

Histological examination of the Meckel's diverticulum showed a large area of ulceration lined by granulation tissue and ectopic gastric pyloric mucosa, assumed to have been the source of bleeding.

Could we have done better?

Earlier intervention would have prevented further bleeding and anemia, but the retrograde double-balloon enteroscopy was falsely reassuring. However, as it was assumed that total small bowel visualization hadn't been achieved, more active management might have been appropriate. Angiographic imaging or nuclear imaging might have been useful, despite their dependency on active bleeding at the time of the examination.

LEARNING POINTS

- Patients with obscure GI bleeding with negative EGD and colonoscopy should undergo capsule endoscopy.
- Patients with pathology or bleeding identified by capsule endoscopy should subsequently undergo push enteroscopy or double-balloon endoscopy.
- If bleeding remains obscure, EGD and colonoscopy should be repeated – lesions commonly overlooked at EGD include Cameron's ulcers (ulcers in a large hiatus hernia), varices, peptic ulcers, and gastric antral vascular ectasia.

LETTER FROM AMERICA

Interesting that the MRE was normal when a Meckel's diverticulum was present. The American Gastroenterological Association (AGA) defines "obscure" GI bleeding as "bleeding from the gastrointestinal tract that persists or recurs without an obvious etiology after upper and lower endoscopy and imaging of the GI tract." Obscure bleeding is subdivided into "occult" and "overt" bleeds with the former defined as a positive fecal occult blood test and no visible evidence of bleeding. The latter is defined as visible bleeding. The patient described in this case would have met the AGA definition for obscure and overt GI bleed. The evaluation of this patient would be similar in the USA. A radionuclide bleeding and/or Meckel's scan are additional tests to consider in cases such as this although the AGA notes that their yield is low (www.gastro.org).

Jon Vogel and Massarat Zutshi

CASE 45

Complicated twist

Richard Guy
Oxford University Hospitals NHS Foundation Trust, Oxford, UK

A 76-year-old woman was admitted with a 5-day history of constipation, abdominal distension, and colicky abdominal pain. She had intermittently passed flatus over this period. The only significant medical history was two spinal operations which had left her with leg weakness, and she had undergone cholecystectomy and hysterectomy for benign disease. On examination, her abdomen was distended, tympanic to percussion but not tender. The rectum was empty on digital examination.

Blood tests showed: hemoglobin 15.3 g/dL, WCC 10.6×10^9/L, potassium 3.1 mmol/L, and CRP 0.6 mg/L. Plain abdominal and chest radiographs were obtained (Figure 45.1).

A diagnosis of large bowel obstruction was made but the cause was uncertain. A CT scan confirmed a closed loop sigmoid volvulus.

Fluid resuscitation and electrolyte correction were instituted. Flexible sigmoidoscopy was carried out in order to decompress the volvulus and exclude other luminal pathology. A good decompression was reported, but within 48 hours the patient was again distended and repeat decompression was performed, leaving a rectal catheter in place. When this became displaced, the volvulus recurred.

DECISION POINT

What would you do now?

Recurrent sigmoid volvulus presents a challenge, especially in medically frail patients. As this lady was reasonably well but had an early recurrent volvulus, it was decided to recommend surgical resection.

The patient underwent a midline laparotomy, at which sigmoid volvulus was confirmed with a hugely dilated sigmoid (Figure 45.2). Sigmoid colectomy was carried out, with colorectal anastomosis using a circular stapler. The anastomosis was formed without twist or tension, was viable, with good anastomotic "doughnuts," and an air leak test was negative.

Three days postoperatively, the patient developed lower abdominal pain and tenderness, a temperature of 37.8°C, and a tachycardia of 110/min. A CT scan

Colorectal Surgery: Clinical Care and Management, First Edition.
Edited by Bruce George, Richard Guy, Oliver Jones, and Jon Vogel.
© 2016 John Wiley & Sons, Ltd. Published 2016 by John Wiley & Sons, Ltd.

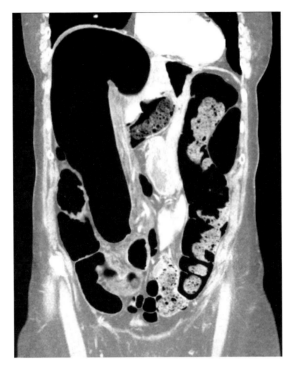

Figure 45.1 CT scan showing sigmoid volvulus.

with rectal contrast was performed. The scan revealed no anastomotic leak, but reported features consistent with an ileus, and rectal fecal loading.

The patient had ongoing pain symptoms for a week postoperatively but eventually settled, with her inflammatory markers normalizing, and she was considered fit for discharge 12 days postoperatively.

Five days later, she was readmitted with abdominal pain and upper abdominal tenderness. Her white cell count was 16 g/dL, and CRP was greater than 156 mg/L. A CT was performed, which showed small bowel dilatation and a transition point adjacent to the previous colonic surgical staple line.

Relaparotomy was performed, at which a leak was found at the colorectal anastomosis, and a loop of small bowel had twisted and become adherent to the defect. A small abscess cavity was noted posteriorly. The anastomosis was taken down, the rectum transsected, and an end colostomy fashioned in the left lower quadrant. Her postoperative recovery was unremarkable, and following stoma training and a period of rehabilitation, she was discharged home a fortnight later.

The patient underwent a successful laparotomy and reversal of Hartmann's a year later, and has been seen and discharged from outpatient care.

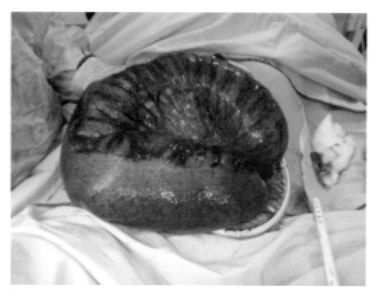

Figure 45.2 Operative image showing grossly distended sigmoid colon.

Could we have done better?

Perhaps a primary anastomosis should not have been performed at the original volvulus operation, or at least a defunctioning stoma brought out. However, with no sepsis and a healthy enough colon, there were no absolute contraindications to primary anastomosis. An earlier laparotomy following re-presentation might have been performed but attempts were made to avoid the morbidity and mortality of repeat laparotomy, and she seemed to settle, although the initial postoperative scan may have been performed too early to identify problems. Perhaps the patient should have been kept in longer and repeat imaging performed.

LEARNING POINTS

- Decompression of sigmoid volvulus should be attempted with a flatus tube at rigid sigmoidoscopy or, preferably, flexible sigmoidoscopy.
- Ischemic mucosa at sigmoidoscopy is an indication for emergency resection.
- Recurrent volvulus during the same inpatient stay may be representative of failed decompression and an indication for laparotomy.
- Attention should be paid to correcting electrolyte imbalances, particularly potassium.
- Persisting pain, cardiac and respiratory complications may be manifestations of a problem with an anastomosis, and whilst leaks classically manifest within the first 2 weeks, "late leaks" may occur following discharge from hospital.

LETTER FROM AMERICA

A report by Swensen *et al.*, published in 2012 in *Diseases of the Colon and Rectum*, included an evaluation of 103 cases of colonic volvulus treated at seven hospitals in Minnesota, USA. There were 50 sigmoid and 53 cecal volvulus cases. The majority of patients were acutely obstructed. Nearly all (98%) cases of cecal volvulus were treated surgically. Of the sigmoid volvulus cases, 79% underwent successful nonoperative reduction and 58% had surgery, of which the majority underwent resection with anastomosis. In cases such as the one described, edema in the colon wall and the great size match between the dilated colon and the decompressed rectum make creation of the colorectal anastomosis a bit more perilous than normal. A side-to-end stapled or sutured anastomosis may be useful in this situation. As with all urgent colorectal operations, the surgeon should have a low threshold for proximal diversion as this often benefits the patient and the surgeon.

Jon Vogel and Massarat Zutshi

CASE 46

Obscure postoperative obstruction

Richard Guy

Oxford University Hospitals NHS Foundation Trust, Oxford, UK

A 56-year-old farm laborer with no significant past medical history was admitted for elective laparoscopic-assisted low anterior resection for a mid-rectal cancer. Preoperative staging had revealed an operable T3 tumor with a clear mesorectal margin and no radiological evidence of mesorectal lymphadenopathy or distant metastases. No preoperative radiotherapy was given.

At surgery, the splenic flexure was completely mobilized from medial to lateral via a submesenteric approach. Early high ligation and division of the inferior mesenteric vein at the lower border of the pancreas was followed by entry into the lesser sac on top of the pancreas through the root of the transverse mesocolon, and then linking up this dissection via detachment of the greater omentum from the transverse colon. The inferior mesenteric artery was approached medially with submesenteric mobilization of the left colon, ligation and division of the artery and then division of lateral colonic attachments. Upper rectal mobilization was performed laparoscopically with a planned lower midline incision to complete a "curative" total mesorectal excision (TME), preparation of the colonic conduit and safe circular stapled coloanal anastomosis. This was tension free and well vascularized; the anastomotic rings were complete and underwater testing with air insufflation revealed no bubbles. In view of this, no loop ileostomy was raised but a size 30 Foley catheter was introduced into the anus and secured to the anal margin, and two low-suction abdominal drains placed in the pelvis.

After 48 hours, the patient reported increasing right iliac fossa (RIF) pain, nausea, and abdominal distension. On examination, the patient was hemodynamically stable but pyrexial (temperature 38 °C) with some tachypnea, poor bibasal air entry, and a distended but soft abdomen. Urinalysis was normal and blood tests showed a CRP of 150 mg/L, white cell count 8×10^9/L, hemoglobin 12 g/dL, and normal lactate and arterial blood gases.

A chest radiograph showed some gas under the diaphragm consistent with recent surgery, and bibasal atelectasis.

The patient was managed with IV antibiotics and additional chest physiotherapy. He remained much the same over the next 24 hours. He complained of RIF pain but examination showed a distended nontender abdomen. A CT scan was reported as showing bibasal lung collapse, a small volume of pelvic fluid but no evidence of anastomotic leak or small bowel injury in the RIF.

By postoperative day 5, chest clinical findings had improved but there was vomiting, the passage of loose stool and increasing abdominal pain and distension. CRP remained above 150 mg/L. Digital rectal examination revealed a palpably intact anastomosis.

DECISION POINT

What would you do now?

He was clearly "not right" although we were reassured by the relatively normal CT scan at day 3. Options considered included immediate relaparotomy or laparoscopy, repeating the CT scan or continuing with expectant management, including adding TPN. We decided to repeat the CT.

Repeat CT showed small bowel dilatation with no obvious transition point. However, rectal contrast was seen to leak through the anastomosis into the pelvis (Figure 46.1).

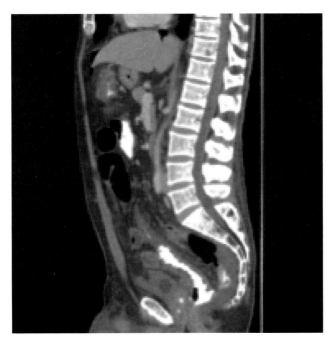

Figure 46.1 Sagittal CT scan image showing anastomotic leak.

DECISION POINT

What would you do now? Should he go straight to surgery? Could this leak be managed conservatively?

It was felt that reoperation was indicated. A nonoperative approach was not appropriate as the patient was significantly unwell and there was still a window of opportunity when relaparotomy was likely to be reasonably safe.

The patient was taken to theater. Under general anesthesia, a rigid sigmoido-scope was inserted. This showed pink mucosa above and below the anastomosis with no obvious major defect. The lower midline wound was reopened. Surprisingly, this revealed herniation of almost the entire small bowel underneath the left colonic mesentery to lie on the left side of the abdomen. The trapped small bowel 10 cm distal to the DJ flexure up to a point 40 cm proximal to the ileocecal valve was profoundly ischemic, with little change after 30 minutes. The colonic mesentery was stretched by the herniated bowel and was under considerable tension. There was a small amount of turbid feculent fluid and fibrin within the pelvis.

Closer examination of the CT images shows a medialized left colon with small bowel to the left of the patient, in keeping with the operative findings (Figure 46.2).

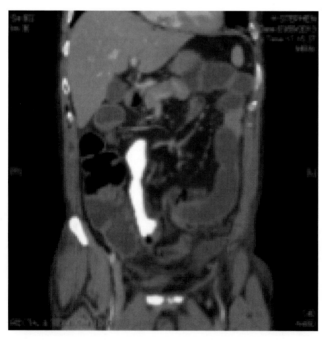

Figure 46.2 Coronal CT image showing the left colonic conduit containing contrast to the right of the midline and most of the small bowel lying in the left of the abdomen, following herniation underneath the colonic mesentery.

The herniated loops were reduced back under the mesentery to the right side of the abdomen and the abdomen filled with warm saline. Rectal air insufflation revealed bubbles in the pelvis. On repalpation of the anastomosis per rectum, a small "divot" was palpable posteriorly which just admitted the tip of an index finger.

DECISION POINT

What would you do now? Should the anastomosis be taken apart? What about the risk of reherniation of small bowel?

The two immediate surgical issues were the very extensive small bowel ischemia and the anastomotic leakage. The small bowel remained dusky despite reduction of the internal hernia. Resection, however, would have left only 50 cm of small bowel. The anastomotic leak was considered to be small and therefore potentially salvageable if simply defunctioned. It was decided to leave the small bowel *in situ* and relook in 24–48 hours.

No resection was performed. The anastomosis was left in place and the pelvis was washed out. An ABThera dressing was inserted. Postoperatively TPN was commenced.

Planned relook laparotomy was performed after a further 48 hours. All of the small bowel had completely recovered and there was no further pelvic contamination. A loop ileostomy was raised, drains were placed in the pelvis and a 30 Fr rectal catheter inserted into the neorectum. Omentum was mobilized and placed between the DJ flexure and along the medial border of the mesenteric defect and the abdomen was closed.

Postoperatively, recovery was complete with gradual introduction of oral diet, satisfactory stoma function, and withdrawal of TPN. Histopathological examination of the resected rectum demonstrated a 45 mm diameter, moderately differentiated adenocarcinoma with invasion beyond the muscularis propria but with no lymphovascular invasion seen and a clear resection margin by 20 mm. Of 28 lymph nodes examined, one was found to contain acellular mucin and was considered positive by TNM criteria (pT3 N1 L0 V0 R0, Dukes' C). The patient went on to receive adjuvant oxaliplatin and capecitabine chemotherapy, and 6 months later the stoma was closed after a satisfactory water-soluble contrast enema examination.

Could we have done better?

The recognition of herniation of small bowel underneath the colonic mesentery was clearly delayed and was not diagnosed prior to surgical intervention, although the CT appearances would fit with the operative findings. Any further delays might have rendered most of the small bowel unsalvageable.

LEARNING POINTS

- Internal hernia through mesenteric defects following laparoscopic surgery is probably underreported, and is likely to be more frequent following full splenic flexure mobilization and submesenteric dissection. Awareness of this type of complication and review of scans with an appropriate radiologist may prevent late diagnosis.
- Slow recovery or unanticipated events after any laparoscopic resection should alert clinicians to potentially serious complications.
- Early imaging should be acquired in patients failing to progress after laparoscopic colonic resection, but complications such as anastomotic leak, intestinal infarction, pelvic abscess or small bowel obstruction or injury may take time to evolve and require repeated evaluation.
- There should be a low threshold for early surgical intervention, with relaparoscopy in the first instance if possible, if there is lack of expected clinical progress following laparoscopic surgery.

LETTER FROM AMERICA

A surgical technique to consider is the retroileal colorectal or coloanal anastomosis. With this, the colon is passed through a window created in the mobilized ileocolic mesentery. This is done to increase length on the colon and also to avoid the problem of small bowel herniation through the defect between the colonic mesentery and the retroperitoneum. This technique was often advocated by Drs Fazio and Remzi at the Cleveland Clinic and described by Hogan and Joyce in *Techniques in Coloproctology*, 2014.

Jon Vogel and Massarat Zutshi

CASE 47

Gynecological disaster

Richard Guy

Oxford University Hospitals NHS Foundation Trust, Oxford, UK

A 60-year-old woman underwent elective laparoscopic bilateral oophorectomy under the gynecologists. In the first five postoperative days, she experienced progressive abdominal distension, pain, and fever. Observations showed a low-grade pyrexia and tachycardia. She was managed by the gynecologists as a "postoperative ileus." Over the next few days, her abdomen became more distended and she was slightly breathless. A colorectal opinion was requested 9 days postoperatively. The patient was found to be unwell with generalized abdominal tenderness. Blood tests showed: Hb 9.5 g/dL, white cell count 19.1, CRP greater than 160 and albumin 27 g/dL. An urgent CT scan demonstrated a large volume of intraabdominal fluid but no sign of free intraperitoneal gas.

Percutaneous radiological drainage under local anesthetic was arranged. This was straightforward and uncomplicated. The drains immediately drained obvious small bowel enteric content and continued to do so over the next 48 hours, with 2–3 liters drained during each 24-hour period. Parenteral nutrition was commenced via a PICC line. Her general condition improved with resolution of breathlessness and slight decrease in white cell count (13.4×10^9/L) and CRP (124 mg/L).

DECISION POINT

What would you do now? Should she go straight to surgery? Could this be treated conservatively?

The patient has clear evidence of an enteric injury. Although her general condition improved slightly following drainage, she remained tachycardic and had low albumin. She was likely to have ongoing intraabdominal sepsis. The options considered were:

- continued nonoperative management with antibiotics, abdominal drainage, and TPN

- early relaparotomy with probably "damage control surgery" and stoma formation.

The decision centered around adequacy of eradication of intraabdominal sepsis with a nonoperative strategy versus the risks of reoperation 11 days postoperatively. Early postoperative fistulae are often associated with fragile, hazardous intraabdominal adhesions, to which the term "obliterative peritonitis" has been applied. It was considered that the priority was to adequately deal with intraabdominal sepsis and so laparotomy was appropriate.

Colorectal Surgery: Clinical Care and Management, First Edition.
Edited by Bruce George, Richard Guy, Oliver Jones, and Jon Vogel.
© 2016 John Wiley & Sons, Ltd. Published 2016 by John Wiley & Sons, Ltd.

Relaparotomy revealed generalized enteric content throughout the abdominal cavity with a hole in an ileal loop, surrounded by matted small bowel loops. The injured segment was resected using linear staplers. The small bowel was edematous with reduced mobility, making exteriorization as an ileostomy difficult. The distal end was left closed in the abdomen, whilst a Foley catheter was inserted into the proximal end and brought out through the abdominal wall. A VAC dressing was applied.

The patient was transferred to the ICU ventilated. She remained stable and returned to theater after 48 hours for planned reexploration. No further injuries were found and the abdomen was washed out. It was decided to exteriorize the two bowel ends with an ileostomy and ileal mucus fistula. Midline fascial closure was impossible in view of retraction and edema, and so fascia and skin were partly closed at the top and bottom of the wound and the VAC reapplied, with the intention of closing the wound serially over the next 2–4 days.

Unfortunately, at reoperation 48 hours later, a perforation in the ileum was found, just proximal to the ileostomy at the level of the abdominal wall, with intraperitoneal contamination. The stoma was taken down and 15 cm of bowel resected to a point just upstream of the perforation. There was an insufficient length of small bowel mesentery to refashion an ileostomy in the right iliac fossa.

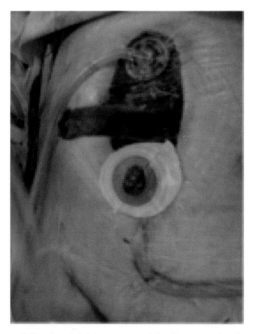

Figure 47.1 Appearance following third laparotomy. The ileostomy has been matured in the lower part of the midline wound and the "mucus fistula" is controlled with a Foley catheter. VAC has been applied to the open wound with a bridge to the previous ileostomy site.

The stoma was matured at the bottom end of the wound and a "mucus fistula" from the distal (efferent) end below this, with a skin bridge fashioned between the two stomas by closing the skin here. Further closure of the fascia and skin was undertaken and a further VAC dressing used, incorporating both wounds and allowing for easier stoma isolation (Figure 47.1).

At a fourth laparotomy 48 hours later, it was clear that complete fascial closure was impossible and vicryl mesh was placed for containment.

The patient subsequently made a steady recovery, enteral feeding being necessary via a PEG tube, and she was discharged from hospital some 36 days after initial laparotomy. Six months later, she underwent elective laparotomy, take-down of stoma and mucus fistula, small bowel anastomosis and abdominal wall repair, with an uneventful recovery. The PEG was subsequently removed.

Could we have done better?

It would clearly have been better to diagnose the original small bowel injury earlier than 9 days post laparoscopic oophorectomy. The relatively late presentation created a challenge in that laparotomy was bound to be difficult. Even in

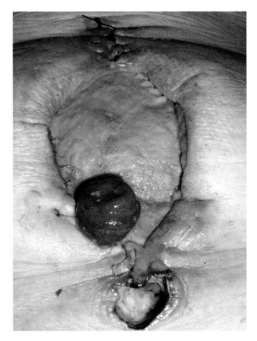

Figure 47.2 At 3 weeks. Fascia and skin have been partly closed and a vicryl mesh used for containment. A skin bridge between ileostomy and mucus fistula facilitated stoma care.

hindsight, it was probably correct to reoperate at this stage rather than risk the consequences of inadequately drained sepsis (Figure 47.2).

It is likely at the time of laparotomy at day 11 that an unrecognized small bowel injury occurred (or was overlooked). Greater care in handling fragile small bowel during this operation may have avoided the additional injury.

LEARNING POINTS

- Failure to recover promptly after apparently straightforward laparoscopic surgery should raise suspicion for iatrogenic bowel injury.
- Reoperation for small bowel injury in the presence of fragile adhesions is hazardous and risks additional injury.
- When reoperating under adverse conditions, a damage control approach should be employed with no anastomoses and temporary/staged abdominal closure if possible.

LETTER FROM AMERICA

No guidelines here. In cases such as this, when surgical therapy is warranted but acute inflammation, vascularized adhesions, and friable bowel make enterolysis and resection risky, operative drainage and proximal bowel diversion, with postoperative TPN as needed, and definitive surgery 6–12 months later is an approach to consider.

Jon Vogel and Massarat Zutshi

CASE 48

Pelvic leak and salvage

Richard Guy

Oxford University Hospitals NHS Foundation Trust, Oxford, UK

A 61-year-old male, who worked as a groundsman, was referred urgently with a 6-week history of altered bowel habit with looser stool, but without rectal bleeding. On examination, he was overweight (weight 112.9 kg, height 1.76 m, BMI 36 kg/m^2) with an old right paramedian scar from appendicectomy. On digital rectal examination, the lower edge of a tumor was just palpable at 9 cm from the anal verge. An MRI scan demonstrated a 5.4 cm long tumor situated 5 cm from the anorectal junction, radiologically staged as T3c N0. A CT scan showed no evidence of metastatic disease. Following MDT discussion, the patient proceeded straight to surgery.

Laparoscopic-assisted anterior resection was undertaken. Following full medial to lateral IMV-first splenic flexure mobilization, high ligation of the IMA and left colonic mobilization, pelvic adhesions and obesity necessitated completion via a lower midline incision. A TME was performed and a tension-free, well-vascularized, side-to-end stapled coloanal anastomosis performed. Doughnuts were complete, the anastomosis was palpably intact, and an underwater leak test was negative. A 30 Fr rectal catheter was inserted, two low suction drains placed in the pelvis, and a loop ileostomy brought out.

On the third postoperative day, the patient had nausea and vomiting with abdominal distension and pain. At day 5, observations were as follows: pulse 130/min, temperature 38.6°C, respiratory rate 18, oxygen saturation 93%. ABG analysis showed PaO$_2$ 8.01 kPa. Venous blood tests showed: hemoglobin 12.3 g/dL, white blood cell count 14.5, and CRP >160. Abdominal and pelvic CT scan revealed a small posterior anastomotic leak with a presacral collection (Figure 48.1).

DECISION POINT

What would you do now?

The priorities were felt to be source control and management of sepsis. As the patient was already defunctioned, it was felt that a trial of nonoperative management was reasonable.

Colorectal Surgery: Clinical Care and Management, First Edition.
Edited by Bruce George, Richard Guy, Oliver Jones, and Jon Vogel.
© 2016 John Wiley & Sons, Ltd. Published 2016 by John Wiley & Sons, Ltd.

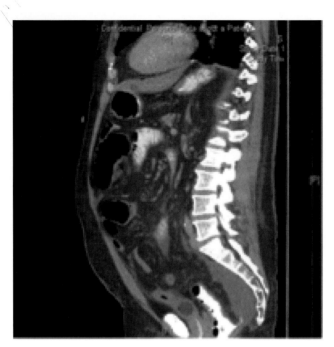

Figure 48.1 Sagittal CT image demonstrating a presacral fluid collection with a wisp of rectally administered contrast leaking from the staple line posteriorly.

Broad-spectrum intravenous antibiotics were commenced. A transgluteal "pigtail" drain was inserted percutaneously into the presacral collection. Some 70 mL of pus was immediately drained and there was clinical improvement over the subsequent 48 hours. Repeat CT after a further 5 days showed stable appearances. TPN was commenced.

Unfortunately, over the next 5 days there was a recurrence of vomiting, abdominal cramps, and high ileostomy output (up to 4 L in 24 hours). A swollen arm necessitated cessation of TPN. The "pigtail" drain was removed. Repeat CT scan showed a 6.7 × 7.3 × 8.6 cm presacral collection containing locules of gas and a separate 7.5 × 2.2 × 3.3 cm RIF collection with an air–fluid level. The patient had "spikes" in temperature and on digital rectal examination, a palpable anastomotic defect was obvious.

An examination under anesthetic (EUA) was carried out. This showed dehiscence of 25% of the circumference of the anastomosis posteriorly with a large pelvic abscess.

DECISION POINT

What would you do now? In view of the enlarging collection and worsening clinical condition, should the patient undergo laparotomy and disconnection of the anastomosis?

This significant dehiscence was of concern and there was clearly ongoing sepsis. Laparotomy and disconnection would have been acceptable treatment but this would have been a major undertaking in a large man who was now just over 2 weeks post-op. It was decided to continue with conservative management but to try to improve sepsis control in the pelvis.

Under anesthetic, a 30 Fr catheter was inserted through the defect into the presacral collection and irrigated, and another similar catheter was inserted into the neorectum in order to reduce contamination. After a further 48 hours, the patient underwent flexible sigmoidoscopy and insertion of two "Endosponge" dressings into the cavity. Subsequently, repeated Endosponge changes were carried out every 2–4 days over the next month, with evidence of good granulation tissue and a reducing cavity size, but an increase in the size of the anastomotic defect to 50% (Figure 48.2). Clinically the patient gradually improved. Serial

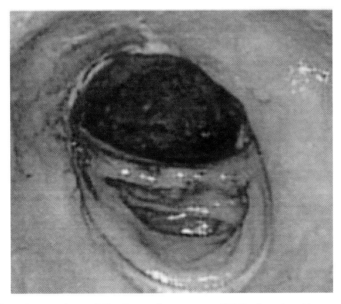

Figure 48.2 Endoscopic image following Endosponge use. Whilst there is evidence of granulation tissue in a clean cavity, the anastomotic defect was 50% of the circumference.

imaging showed resolution of the right iliac fossa collection and reduction of the presacral cavity.

Eventually, after a further 5 months, CT, MRI, and water-soluble contrast enema appearances were satisfactory, and the patient underwent uneventful ileostomy closure exactly 12 months following the original anterior resection. Bowel function at follow-up 4 months later is acceptable. He opens his bowels 4–6 times per day with urgency but no leakage.

Could we have done better?

The anastomotic leak should have been diagnosed earlier, perhaps on the third postoperative day. Active management at this point with radiological percutaneous or peranal drainage may have resulted in a less stormy course.

SECTION F
Surprise cases

Colorectal Surgery: Clinical Care and Management, First Edition.
Edited by Bruce George, Richard Guy, Oliver Jones, and Jon Vogel.
© 2016 John Wiley & Sons, Ltd. Published 2016 by John Wiley & Sons, Ltd.

CASE 49

Radiology 0, Pathology 1

Sara Q. Warraich[1], Marcus Chow[2] & Oliver Jones[1]

[1] *Oxford University Hospitals NHS Foundation Trust, Oxford, UK*

[2] *Tan Tock Seng Hospital, Singapore*

A 37-year-old Caucasian woman was admitted with a 3-month history of left-sided abdominal pain with associated altered bowel habit and weight loss of 15 kg in the same period. She also reported a decreased appetite and night sweats over the last month. Her past medical history included only asthma and she was on no regular medication. Initial investigations in the community included an USS and AXR, which were unremarkable and demonstrated only an IUCD. There was no history of recent foreign travel. Her occupation was as a geologist and she had previously worked in Africa approximately 10 years ago.

On examination, she appeared generally malnourished with conjunctival pallor and there was a palpable mass and tenderness in the LIF. Bloods taken during admission revealed an elevated CRP (133) and WCC (13.05) with microcytic anemia (Hb 7.2). CXR was unremarkable.

An abdominal CT scan (Figure 49.1) showed a 7.5 × 6 cm right adnexal mass and a 5 × 4 cm presacral mass. Several smaller nodules were seen in the pelvis and left iliac fossa. There was bilateral hydronephrosis and small-volume ascites. Multiple small bowel loops were noted to be matted within the pelvis, causing partial obstruction.

This CT scan provided an overwhelming picture of metastatic malignant disease, with unconfirmed primary. A CT chest was normal. Tumor markers (Ca 125, CEA, Ca199, HCG, and AFP) were normal.

The findings were explained to the patient. She was told that the scan was highly suspicious of cancer but that further investigations were needed to confirm this and to determine the site of origin. We decided to proceed to a diagnostic laparoscopy. This revealed multiple adhesions between the omentum and bowel to nodules on the anterior and lateral abdominal wall (Figure 49.2). Several representative biopsies were taken for histology and ascitic fluid sent off for cytology.

Colorectal Surgery: Clinical Care and Management, First Edition.
Edited by Bruce George, Richard Guy, Oliver Jones, and Jon Vogel.
© 2016 John Wiley & Sons, Ltd. Published 2016 by John Wiley & Sons, Ltd.

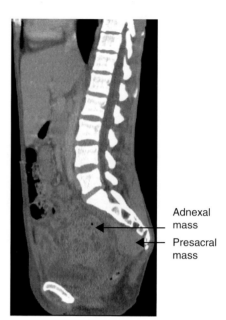

Adnexal
mass

Presacral
mass

Figure 49.1 CT scan showing presacral and pelvic masses. The paucity of body fat makes interpretation difficult.

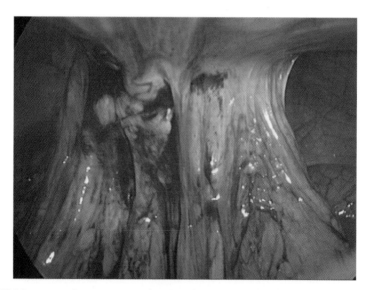

Figure 49.2 Laparoscopic appearances of patient showing tenting of small bowel and omentum to anterior abdominal wall from a peritoneal nodule.

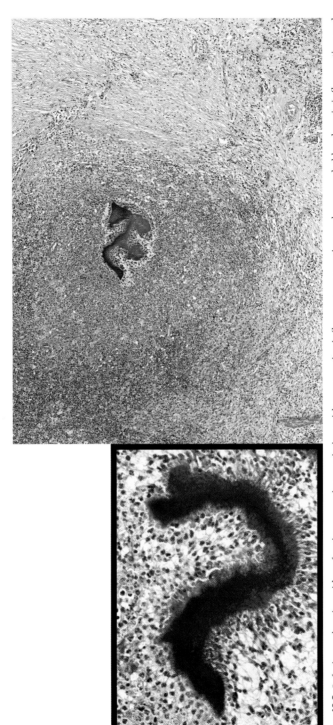

Figure 49.3 Soft tissue showing nidus of actinomyces in association with suppurative inflammatory reaction and surrounded by chronic inflammation and fibrosis. (*Inset*) Periodic acid-Schiff stain highlighting the organized aggregate of delicate bacterial filaments.

DECISION POINT

What would you do now?

The radiological and laparoscopic appearances were suggestive of intraperitoneal malignancy, although the primary site was unclear. The normal tumor markers and operative findings were against an ovarian primary. It was decided to await the final pathology before referring the patient to the appropriate oncologist.

Following laparoscopy, a discussion was held with the patient, explaining that her clinical presentation was most likely due to metastatic malignancy, of either gynecological or colorectal primary. Her main concern, at this point, was her treatment options. These were discussed with her and included the possibility of chemotherapy, radiotherapy, and/or possible further surgery.

However, at this stage, it was emphasized to the patient that the final step before initiation of treatment was awaiting tissue diagnosis, with biopsy results.

The patient and her family were devastated by the diagnosis. She was a young lady with a young family and it later transpired that she had amended her will in preparation for a poor prognosis. Considerable support from colorectal cancer nurse specialists and the psychological medicine department was given at this time.

The histology report was available 5 days after the laparoscopy. Suprisingly, this showed acute fibrosing inflammation, with actinomyces colonies present (Figure 49.3). This suggested that she had severe, disseminated pelvic inflammatory disease with actinomyces infection, associated with her intrauterine device.

There was no dysplasia or malignant cells present.

She was treated immediately wth IV benzylpenicillin. She was subsequently managed at the infectious diseases unit and during her stay there, her symptoms improved with the treatment and her weight increased steadily. Her intrauterine device (IUD) was removed and she was advised not to have another IUD. A PICC line was inserted and she was discharged home, after IV training, with a further course of 4 weeks IV ceftriaxone.

Could we have done better?

The patient was initially given an incorrect diagnosis although at all points we stressed that final test results were awaited. The psychological impact of the diagnosis of probable cancer, which turned out to be wrong, was underestimated.

LEARNING POINTS

- Obtaining a tissue diagnosis is fundamental in the diagnosis and management of every patient presenting with suspected malignancy.

- Benign conditions such as intraabdominal tuberculosis and, very rarely, actinomycosis may mimic intraabdominal malignancy.
- The importance of providing holistic patient management, including psychological support, is highlighted by this case.
- Actinomycosis is an insidiously progressive rare disease resulting from anaerobic, gram-positive Actinomyces bacteria. It usually colonizes the oraphaynx, urogenital tract, and gastrointestinal tract. Colonization of the female genital tract can occur with foreign devices such as IUDs, with other causes including iatrogenic causes (e.g. surgery).

CASE 50

An appendix mass?

Richard Guy

Oxford University Hospitals NHS Foundation Trust, Oxford, UK

A 38-year-old man, who was a smoker with a history of alcohol excess, presented as an emergency at another hospital with a 3-week history of right iliac fossa pain, anorexia, and weight loss. There had been no significant change in bowel habit. There was no past medical or family history. On abdominal examination, there was a tender palpable RIF mass. Blood tests showed a white cell count of 14 and CRP over 156.

The clinical diagnosis was considered to be an appendix mass and CT imaging was arranged (Figure 50.1). Intravenous antibiotics were commenced.

The CT scan showed an inflammatory mass and the radiologists suggested the differential diagnosis was likely between Crohn's disease and appendicitis. Intravenous antibiotics were continued and the patient discharged home after 48 hours on a course of oral antibiotics. A repeat CT scan 5 weeks later showed no significant change.

The patient was treated with continued courses of antibiotics but persisted in having grumbling abdominal pain and lethargy. Four months after initial presentation, he presented acutely to our hospital with severe abdominal pain, fever (38.8°C) and a pointing abscess in the right iliac fossa with cellulitis. An urgent MR scan showed features of terminal ileal inflammation extending over about 25 cm and an abscess presenting subcutaneously.

DECISION POINT

What is the best procedure in the face of sepsis and the catabolic patient: abscess drainage only, laparotomy/resection/stoma or abscess drainage/proximal stoma?

It was decided that the immediate priority was simply to drain the abdominal wall abscess under general anesthesia. Copious pus was drained but no enteric contents. Over the subsequent few days, it was apparent that a fistula was forming, with enteric content draining into a wound bag.

DECISION POINT

What is the next step – immediate further intervention or wait and allow an enterocutaneous fistula to form with a plan for surgery in 3–6 months?

Colorectal Surgery: Clinical Care and Management, First Edition.
Edited by Bruce George, Richard Guy, Oliver Jones, and Jon Vogel.
© 2016 John Wiley & Sons, Ltd. Published 2016 by John Wiley & Sons, Ltd.

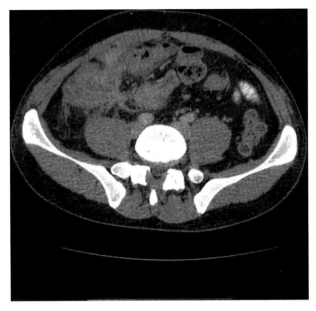

Figure 50.1 CT showing inflammatory mass involving cecum and terminal ileum.

The decision was taken to proceed to urgent/semi-elective resection, as there was concern that the underlying pathology was not known with certainty. Ten days after abscess drainage, he underwent laparotomy through a midline incision. A limited right hemicolectomy with resection of 25 cm of distal ileum was performed. In view of the concurrent sepsis, an end ileostomy was raised and a closed long colonic mucus fistula secured adjacent to the stoma. A drain was inserted into the RIF and the abdomen was closed. Histopathological examination of the resected specimen confirmed severe active Crohn's disease with deep fissuring ulceration and intramural abscess.

Postoperatively, recovery was satisfactory and he was discharged after 10 days. The patient subsequently underwent uncomplicated ileocolic reanastomosis 6 months later, after having undergone colonoscopy demonstrating no downstream abnormalities. Postoperatively, he commenced azathioprine.

Could we have done better?

The major criticism in this case was the failure to appreciate the diagnosis of Crohn's disease at initial presentation and the protracted treatment with antibiotics alone. Although the initial CT report considered the possibility of Crohn's, the clinical management was along the lines of an appendix mass. This resulted in a delay of about 4 months before the diagnosis of Crohn's became obvious with progressive weight loss, sepsis, and general malaise during this period. More detailed review of the radiology, particularly in the first few weeks when there was no clinical improvement, may have prevented this delay.

LEARNING POINTS

- Conservative management of an appendix mass is widely practiced. Classically, there is a delayed presentation and the patient is relatively well, having walled off the inflamed, locally perforated appendix.
- Conservative treatment of an appendix mass fails in about 5–10% of patients. If a patient with a working diagnosis of appendix mass fails to settle quickly or becomes worse, alternative diagnoses including malignancy and Crohn's disease should be considered.
- In Crohn's disease, sepsis, malnutrition, and steroids increase the risk of postoperative complications, most importantly anastomotic leakage. When more than one risk factor is present, anastomosis should be avoided if possible.

CASE 51

A worrying-looking rectal ulcer

Charles Evans

University Hospitals of Coventry and Warwickshire, Coventry, UK

A 52-year-old woman was referred by the gynecologists with a history of sacro-coccygeal pain and a dragging sensation within the pelvis. Her bowel habit was very irregular, often failing to open her bowels for up to 6 days, whilst on some days opening her bowels up to 15 times, with intermittent passage of mucus and blood. She sometimes experienced tenesmus and incomplete evacuation, spending up to 1 hour on the toilet trying to evacuate, including digitating the anus, during which she was able to feel a lump. Past history included irritable bowel syndrome, diagnosed by her GP. Colonoscopy was advised, which showed an ulcerated area in the low rectum anteriorly with the appearances of neoplasia (Figure 51.1).

Histological examination of biopsies taken from this ulcer showed features consistent with solitary rectal ulcer syndrome (SRUS).

Anorectal physiology was normal and endoanal ultrasound showed a slightly thickened internal anal sphincter (3 mm thickness). An evacuation proctogram showed a significant external (Oxford Grade 5) prolapse and enterocele (Figure 51.2).

DECISION POINT

What can you offer this patient? Are there any conservative measures which might help?

Despite the advanced prolapse, it was felt that conservative measures were worth trying in the first instance. Even though surgery was ultimately likely to be required, contact with a specialist nurse with an interest in pelvic floor disorders, and some biofeedback for pelvic retraining and rectal desensitization, would probably be of long-term benefit.

Not surprisingly, biofeedback failed to completely resolve the evacuation difficulties. She was offered a laparoscopic ventral mesh rectopexy and this proceeded uneventfully. At clinic review 6 weeks later, she reported that the prolapsing lump that she had previously thought to be a normal part of defecation had disappeared. There had been significant relief from the dragging sensation and pain, although bleeding and mucus per rectum were still experienced. She was

Colorectal Surgery: Clinical Care and Management, First Edition.
Edited by Bruce George, Richard Guy, Oliver Jones, and Jon Vogel.
© 2016 John Wiley & Sons, Ltd. Published 2016 by John Wiley & Sons, Ltd.

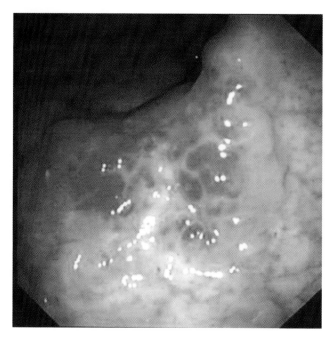

Figure 51.1 Endoscopic appearance of the rectal ulcer.

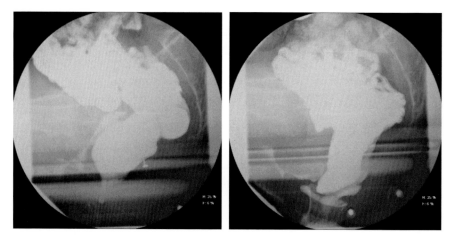

Figure 51.2 Evacuation proctogram. The left-hand image shows the appearances at rest. In the right-hand image, there is invagination of the rectal wall with the lead point outside the anal canal on straining. The small bowel drops down significantly (enterocele), compressing the anterior rectum.

reassured and, at flexible sigmoidoscopy 6 months later, the rectal ulcer was no longer evident.

Could we have done better?

The diagnosis of SRUS was made fairly promptly. Biofeedback preoperatively was probably not necessary and earlier surgery without delay may have been better, potentially supplemented by postoperative biofeedback.

LEARNING POINTS

- Prolapse-related ulceration can look worryingly neoplastic and patients may be mistakenly considered to have rectal cancer until the distinctive histopathological appearances of SRUS are confirmed.
- Rectopexy is the most effective treatment for SRUS.

CASE 52

Think the unthinkable

Bruce George

Oxford University Hospitals NHS Foundation Trust, Oxford, UK

A 29-year-old woman was referred urgently by her GP with a 5-month history of rectal bleeding, frequent loose stools, and abdominal bloating. She also reported weight loss, anorexia, and hip pain. Blood tests arranged by the GP were normal. On examination, she was thin but abdominal examination was otherwise normal. Digital rectal examination was uncomfortable but revealed blood on the finger. Colonoscopy showed severe ulceration with induration in the anterior rectum. The anal canal, perineum, and rest of the colonoscopy were normal, and the initial impression was of Crohn's disease or possible extrarectal pathology. Biopsies, however, showed adenocarcinoma. An MRI scan showed a rectal mass and a metastasis in the L3 vertebra with some cord compression (Figure 52.1). Abdominal CT scan showed liver metastases (Figure 52.2).

DECISION POINT

What would you do now? What are the treatment priorities?

She clearly had rapidly progressive malignant disease. It was felt that the cord compression needed dealing with urgently to prevent neurological disability, and that the help of oncologists and spinal surgeons was required urgently.

The patient was admitted to the emergency surgical unit. On further questioning, she reported significant back pain, difficulty mobilizing, and one episode of urinary incontinence. Neurological examination showed reduced muscle strength in the left leg but no sensory loss. Blood tests showed mild anemia (Hb 11.9 g/dL), raised CRP (105), alkaline phosphatase (444), and CEA (76). She was seen by the acute oncology team and spinal surgeons and received dexamethasone. Spinal surgery was undertaken 5 days after admission and a defunctioning colostomy stoma was created the following week.

Two weeks later, she developed focal seizures and a head CT scan showed cerebral metastases. She received palliative chemotherapy and supportive care but died less than 4 months after her initial outpatient appointment. One of her dying wishes was to increase awareness of cancer, especially bowel cancer, in young people.

Colorectal Surgery: Clinical Care and Management, First Edition.
Edited by Bruce George, Richard Guy, Oliver Jones, and Jon Vogel.
© 2016 John Wiley & Sons, Ltd. Published 2016 by John Wiley & Sons, Ltd.

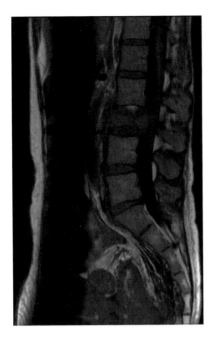

Figure 52.1 Sagittal MRI. The rectal mass is difficult to see but the L3 metastasis is evident.

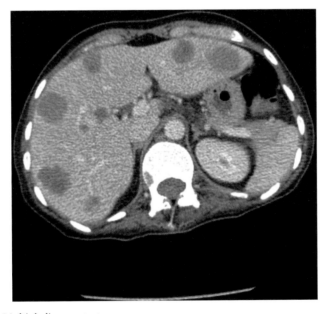

Figure 52.2 Multiple liver metastases.

Could we have done better?

Bowel cancer was not really considered by the GP, in the surgical clinic or even at colonoscopy by an experienced gastroenterologist, leading to inevitable delays in diagnosis and treatment. The severity of her symptoms at initial clinic assessment should probably have prompted hospital admission, although it is unlikely that the final outcome could have been altered. Earlier admission might, however, have allowed clinicians to help the patient and her family to cope more easily with the obvious distress.

> **LEARNING POINTS**
>
> - Colorectal cancer is rare in young people but the incidence is increasing (NAACCR 2013 data, www.cancer.org/research/cancerfactsstatistics).
> - There should always be awareness of potential cancer symptoms even in the young.

SECTION G
New technologies and techniques

Oliver Jones

Oxford University Hospitals NHS Foundation Trust, Oxford, UK

Laparoscopic (multiport) colorectal surgery

The laparoscopic approach to colorectal resection is well established. There have been a number of large randomized trials comparing open and laparoscopic surgery.

The CLASICC trial was a multicenter UK trial which randomized 794 patients on a 2:1 basis between laparoscopic and open approaches to resection for colorectal cancer. The initial short-term results showed a 29% conversion rate in the laparoscopic arm, reflecting the fact that perhaps many surgeons were relatively inexperienced during the period it recruited (1996–2002) and needed to have performed only 20 laparoscopic resections to be able to recruit to the trial [1]. Despite this, mortality did not differ between groups, nor did the proportion of Dukes' C2 tumors. Despite being relatively early in the global experience of laparoscopic colorectal surgery, this trial also recruited patients with rectal cancer and in this group, there was some concern about a higher rate of positive resection margin in the laparoscopic arm. However, a later paper reporting cancer outcomes at a median of 62.9 months after surgery found no differences between study arms in terms of overall survival and disease-free survival [2].

The COST trial was another randomized trial of similar size, with 872 patients. This study included only colon cancer patients and was powered as a noninferiority trial with a primary endpoint of time to recurrence. It confirmed that disease-free and overall 5-year survival was similar in the two groups and that there was no difference in the rate or site of first recurrence [3]. Similar support for the safety of laparoscopic resection for cancer was supplied by the COLOR [4] and Barcelona [5] trials.

More recently, there have been similar trials looking specifically at rectal cancer. The COREAN trial [6] randomized 340 patients on a 1:1 basis, whilst COLOR II [7] randomized 1103 patients on a 2:1 basis. Whilst operating time was longer in both trials for patients undergoing laparoscopic surgery, oncological outcomes, including specimen quality, circumferential margin involvement, lymph node yield, morbidity, and mortality, were similar in both trials. In favor of the laparoscopic approach was less blood loss, a quicker return of bowel function, and a one day shorter hospital stay in both trials.

Longer term oncological outcomes also appear to be sound for the laparoscopic approach. A pooled analysis of the Barcelona, COST, COLOR, and CLASICC trials for patients with colon cancer and at least 3 years of follow-up showed that disease-free survival and overall survival did not differ between open and laparoscopic patients. A similar metaanalysis of six randomized trials for patients with rectal cancer showed similar long-term oncological outcomes [8].

There have been similar studies examining the laparoscopic approach in benign disease, including elective resection for diverticulitis. A randomized trial from a single institution in Geneva showed that despite longer operating times in the laparoscopic group, there was less postoperative pain, quicker return to bowel function, and shorter hospital stay (median 5 versus 7 days) for those receiving the laparoscopic approach [9]. Very similar outcomes were seen in the Sigma trial, which was conducted over five centers and enrolled 104 patients [10]. Similar results have been in seen with the application of laparocopy to inflammatory bowel disease, with benefits in reducing length of stay and morbidity [10, 11].

Single port surgery

Single port surgery reduces the number of operating ports to a single incision, usually around 2 cm long, through which camera and operating ports are introduced. The first reports of its use in colorectal surgery appeared in 2008 [11, 12]. There are a number of commercially available single ports but there have also been descriptions of improvised ports, including the glove port which utilizes a wound retractor and a surgical glove, through the fingers of which reusable laparoscopic ports may be introduced [13].

There are a number of problems with single port surgery. There is crowding of instruments and surgeon/assistant at the operating table itself with camera and instruments in parallel at the site of surgery. Curved instruments have been developed to try to overcome this lack of triangulation whilst flexible laparoscopic cameras have also been employed by some practitioners. Whichever approach is used, it is a challenging approach with its own learning curve separate from that of multiport laparoscopic surgery.

The potential advantages of single port surgery are thought to be improved cosmesis, reduced pain, fewer wound complications, and potentially faster recovery. There are no randomized studies assessing the technique. There have been a number of case comparison studies, case series, and case reports. These have recently been the subject of a systematic review [14]. With the quality of included studies being so heterogenous, it was difficult to draw firm conclusions. The authors concluded, however, that there was no significant reduction in postoperative stay. Lymph node yield was similar but there were no long-term data to assess oncological outcomes for cancer patients. Morbidity and mortality appeared to be improved relative to multiport surgery but such a conclusion should be interpreted with caution due to selection and reporting bias.

Despite the limitations of the published data, there is clear evidence that this is a feasible technique and is possible with a low rate of conversion either to multiport laparoscopic or open surgery and seems relatively safe. Trial data are awaited to see if the single port approach offers a true benefit over conventional laparoscopy.

Three-dimensional (3-D) laparoscopy

There has been increasing interest in the use of 3-D laparoscopy for colorectal surgery. As far back as 1993, Becker *et al.* suggested that 3-D laparoscopy might improve laparoscopic skills [15]. The theory is that the stereoscopic vision gives the surgeon greater depth perception and means that there are fewer errors.

The current systems use a laparoscope with either a dual or single lens system [16]. The image is then projected and synchronized on either a head-mounted or video stack platform.

Papers assessing the value of 3-D laparoscopy have mainly focused on *ex vivo* studies. Many of these studies have looked at laparoscopic novices. One such study looked at 56 novices randomly allocated to 2-D or 3-D practice on a box trainer until they achieved proficiency. Their performance in terms of completion time, number of repetitions, and number of errors was studied for both groups. Completion time showed a trend in favor of the 3-D group (216 versus 247 minutes; p = ns) but there were fewer repetitions (108 versus 121; p = 0.008) and errors (27 versus 105; p = 0.001) in the 3-D group [17]. Other studies have shown that this benefit in the *ex vivo* setting is mirrored amongst experienced surgeons [18].

There have been studies *in vivo* using experienced laparoscopic surgeons. In one such study, the performance of 20 laparoscopic surgeons performing four validated laparoscopic skills tasks, each with 10 repetitions, was compared for 2-D and 3-D. The primary outcome measure was error rate, which was reduced by 62% in the 3-D arm, with the secondary outcome measure of performance time being reduced by 35% [19].

Three-dimensional systems are being used increasingly in colorectal surgery. It is a standard part of the Da Vinci robot (see later), though the stand-alone system is also being used increasingly.

Robotic-assisted surgery

Whilst there has been a progressive adoption of laparoscopic colorectal surgery over the last two decades, there has also been recognition of the limitations of the technique, especially in low rectal cancers (reviewed above). The technical problems of the conventional laparoscopy in the pelvis include working within a confined space with an unstable two-dimensional view, surgeon tremor, retraction difficulties requiring very skilled assistants, fixed straight instruments and poor ergonomics and crowding within the operative field.

Some of these problems can be overcome with the robotic approach. At present, the main system in use is the Da Vinci system. This offers a camera and third arm which can be controlled by the operating surgeon, whilst leaving him or her with two main operating arms, as in conventional surgery. These arms are themselves attached to articulated instruments which have seven degrees of freedom. The surgeon controls these instruments as he or she sits at a console away from the patient and hand movements are translated into the instrument tips, giving better ergonomics and the potential for better training, mentoring, and remote operating. The assistant and scrub nurse assist by facilitating exchange of instruments at the patient's side and may also assist through conventional laparoscopic ports inserted to allow easy use of laparoscopic suction and/or additional laparoscopic retraction.

There are some limitations with the current technology for robotic surgery. One is that the robot needs to be docked to the patient and the ports at the beginning of the procedure. Experienced theater teams may be able to achieve this within a few minutes but for people early in their learning curve, this may take considerably longer. For operations involving more than one part of the abdominal cavity (for example, for colonic mobilization and pelvic dissection in an anterior resection), the robot may need to be redocked. Alternatively, the procedure may be done in a hybrid fashion, being part conventional laparoscopic and part robotic. Furthermore, undocking the robot may be time consuming if urgent conversion is needed in a circumstance such as bleeding.

A further problem is the lack of haptic feedback for the operating surgeon, with the surgeon reliant on visual clues and experience to assess the degree of safe retraction. The surgeon also needs to be careful to avoid inadvertent injury to other structures off screen by the robotic arms.

Finally, there are considerable additional costs associated with robotic surgery. These include the initial capital outlay for the robot, annual servicing costs, and the costs of disposable instruments for the procedure.

There are at present no randomized controlled trials comparing robotic colorectal surgery with conventional laparoscopic surgery or open surgery. The available evidence is limited to case series and comparative studies. The reports on its use have mainly focused on right hemicolectomy [20], rectopexy [21], and low anterior resection. Most of the data relate to its use in low anterior resection [22].

In summary, the available data suggest that the robot is a safe approach to the treatment of rectal cancer. In most series, it seems to be associated with a longer operating time compared to conventional laparoscopic surgery, though interestingly, there are reports that in experienced hands, the robot makes this surgery quicker [23]. Indeed, although the evidence is weak, it may be the case that the learning curve for robotic rectal cancer surgery is attenuated relative to conventional laparoscopy [24].

Reasons for conversion in robotic surgery have been listed as obesity, locally advanced tumors, narrow pelvis and adhesions; indeed, these are all problems encountered with conventional laparoscopic surgery. The rate of conversion in these studies varies from 0% in many of the small series to 7.3% for the study of Baek *et al.* [23]. The two largest series in the literature reported conversion rates of 4.9% of 143 patients [25] and 3.7% of 389 patients [26], which would seem to be representative.

No comparative study to date has shown a significant reduction in anastomotic leak rates between robotic and conventional laparoscopic surgery. The increased dexterity afforded by the robotic platform may, in future, lead to changes in the way in which the anastomosis is formed, with one obvious option, currently employed by some surgeons, being the transabdominal cutting of the low rectum and placement of a purse-string suture in the rectal stump rather than a stapled distal transection. Other potential advantages include an improvement in functional outcomes, including bowel and bladder function as well as sexual function. Most of the reported series on robotic rectal cancer surgery have not reported functional outcomes at all. None has shown a significant difference between approaches, with numbers being small, though there have been reports of a trend to benefit with the robot [27].

In a recent review of comparative studies on robotic surgery for rectal cancer [28], there was no overall difference over 11 comparative studies in terms of circumferential resection margin, distal resection margin, and lymph node harvest. An exception was the study of Baik *et al.* [29] which showed that total mesorectal excision completeness was significantly better in the robotic arm (92.8%) versus the laparoscopic arm (75.4%).

It is hoped that many of the unanswered questions about the role of the robot in rectal cancer surgery will be addressed by the ongoing ROLARR trial which is a multicenter, randomized, unblended, parallel group trial of robotic versus standard laparoscopic surgery for rectal cancer [39]. Preliminary results suggest a reduction in conversion to open surgery in the robotic arm.

NOTES

Natural orifice transluminal endoscopic surgery (NOTES) was heralded as a major advance in minimally invasive surgery. It may be performed through the transvaginal, transgastric, transrectal or transesophageal routes. It is said that the first description of a NOTES procedure was of a transgastric liver biopsy in a pig [31]. It was followed by the first successful human NOTES procedure, a transgastric cholecystectomy, in 2007. There are now several hundred publications on the approach for various surgical operations.

NOTES offers the potential for scarless surgery and the abolition of wound-related complications including infection, pain, and herniation. There are also potential advantages for improved cosmesis.

For all these potential advantages, there has been relatively little progress in the application of the technique in humans. The most commonly performed procedures have been appendicectomy and cholecystectomy. In humans, the transvaginal route has been mainly used, with transgastric approaches (the most favored approach in animal models) placed second. There are risks associated with establishment of the access portal. For transvaginal and transgastric routes, these are most importantly the risk of damage to adjacent structures and vessels. There are similar problems with visceral closure, with various closure techniques being developed.

Modifications of the NOTES approach are becoming established in clinical practice. The first of these is transanal minimally invasive surgery, described in more detail later in this section. A further modification has been the combination of pure NOTES with conventional laparoscopy, known as minilaparoscopy-assisted natural orifice surgery (MA-NOS). This has been used for the transvaginal [32] and transrectal [33] approach to colonic resection. Finally, there have been numerous reports of natural orifice specimen extraction (NOSE). This has been applied particularly in colorectal surgery to the extraction of the specimen transanally prior to anastomosis formation [34].

Transanal minimally invasive surgery (TAMIS)

There has been recent interest in TAMIS, in which an incision is made at or just above the dentate line and a total mesorectal excision is performed from the "bottom up." Intestinal continuity is then restored by performing a coloanal anastomosis [35]. A number of portals have been used to performed the transanal dissection, including the transanal endoscopic microsurgery (TEM) [36] scope and a single port scope. The transanal dissection may be facilitated by multiport or single port [37] assistance from the abdomen and this is also used to perform the more proximal mobilization of, for example, the splenic flexure.

Data supporting the use of this technique is currently limited to case series. The Barcelona group described their first 20 selected patients [38] undergoing the technique, of whom 11 were male and who had a mean body mass index of 25.3 kg/m². All were rectal cancers (seven distal, 10 mid, and three proximal rectum). The coloanal anastomosis was stapled in seven patients and hand sewn in the remainder. The median operative time was 235 ± 56 minutes with a mean lymph node harvest of 16 nodes.

Advocates of the technique suggest that it may have applications in the obese patient with a narrow pelvis. Apart from improving access, it may also allow restorative surgery in an increased number of cases, though this has not yet been proven.

Perfusion studies

Anastomotic leakage remains the most devastating complication in colorectal surgery. It is associated with significant morbidity and mortality and has significant healthcare economic implications [39]. The etiology of leaks is multifactorial but adequate arterial perfusion and tissue oxygenation are repeatedly identified as key [40].

Near-infrared (NIR) laparoscopic technology has been used to confirm variability of colorectal anastomoses using fluorophoric angiography with indocyanine green. This can be used intraoperatively by switching to an NIR laparoscopic system immediately before and after anastomosis to confirm perfusion of the bowel ends. A recent report of 30 cases from Oxford has confirmed that this is a quick procedure (median added procedure time of 5 minutes), and reliable, with fluorescence being demonstrated in 29 of 30 cases [41]. Perfusion was demonstrated to be adequate in every case and indeed, no leaks were seen in this case series.

This technology has also been employed to assess anastomoses endoluminally [42] and via the robotic platform [43].

Lymph node mapping

The sentinel lymph node is considered to be the first draining lymph node within a given lymph drainage area. It is generally identified by the injections of a dye or radiotracer near to the tumor. The sentinel node is then identified by simple visual inspection or by the use of a gamma probe or Geiger counter. Its use is already well established in other cancers, including melanoma and breast cancer. The sentinel node may then be assessed intraoperatively by frozen section. If it is involved with tumor, a more radical lymphadenectomy may be performed immediately.

Near-infrared laparoscopy has also been used for intraoperative lymphatic road mapping. This technique involves initial peritumoral submucosal injection of indocyanine green. This migrates via the lymphatics to the sentinel lymph node and beyond. These can be identified using the NIR laparoscope.

The feasibility of this technique has again been demonstrated in small case series [44]. Our own experience from Oxford has shown that using this technique in a pilot study of 18 patients, a mean of 4.1 nodes was identified in each patient and these nodes were within the standard resection field in 14 patients and outside in a further four patients.

The interest in this area lies in the concept of tailoring surgery to individuals, dependent on tumor stage. This may result in less morbidity and mortality, and better functional outcomes. Detection of lymph nodes outside the standard lymph node basin may also prompt the surgeon to undertake more radical surgery. Saha *et al.* [45] reported on 192 patients undergoing surgery for colon cancer and identified aberrant drainage, outside the standard resection field, in 22% of patients. Nodal positivity was 62% in the patients undergoing the change in operation but only 43% in those having a standard resection.

For all that, the case for sentinel node mapping in colorectal cancer has not yet been made. Retter *et al.*, for example, presented a study of 31 patients with colon cancer, using blue dye. They found the false-negative rate to identify stage III disease was only 67% [46]. They went on to show that in these false-negative tumors, lymphatic and venous invasion by cancer cells was present. This in turn suggests that aberrant lymph node drainage and the presence of skip lesions may be responsible for the inaccuracy of the technique in these settings.

References

1 Guillou PJ, Quirke P, Thorpe H, *et al.* MRC CLASICC Trial Group. Short-term endpoints of conventional versus laparoscopic-assisted surgery in patients with colorectal cancer (MRC CLASICC trial): multicentre, randomised controlled trial. *Lancet* 2005; **365**:1718–26.

2 Green BL, Marshall HC, Collinson F, *et al.* Long-term follow-up of the Medical Research Council CLASICC trial of conventional versus laparoscopically assisted resection in colorectal cancer. *Br J Surg* 2013; **100**:75–82.

3 Fleshman J, Sargent DJ, Green E, *et al.* Clinical Outcomes of Surgical Therapy Study Group. Laparoscopic colectomy for cancer is not inferior to open surgery based on 5-year data from the COST Study Group trial. *Ann Surg* 2007; **246**:655–62.

4 Veldkamp R, Kuhry E, Hop WC, *et al.* Laparoscopic surgery versus open surgery for colon cancer: short-term outcomes of a randomised trial. *Lancet Oncol* 2005; **6**:477–84.

5 Lacy AM, Garcia-Valdecasas JC, Delgado S, *et al.* Laparoscopy-assisted colectomy versus open colectomy for treatment of non-metastatic colon cancer: a randomised trial. *Lancet* 2002; **359**:2224–9.

6 Kang SB, Park JW, Jeong SY, *et al.* Open versus laparoscopic surgery for mid or low rectal cancer after neoadjuvant chemoradiotherapy (COREAN trial): short-term outcomes of an open-label randomised controlled trial. *Lancet Oncol* 2010; **11**:637–45.

7 Van der Pas MH, Haglind E, Cuesta MA, *et al.* Laparoscopic versus open surgery for rectal cancer (COLOR II): short-term outcomes of a randomised, phase 3 trial. *Lancet Oncol* 2013: **14**:210–18.

8 Huang MJ, Liang JL, Wang H, Kang L, Deng YH, Wang JP. Laparoscopic-assisted versus open surgery for rectal cancer: a meta-analysis of randomized controlled trials on oncological adequacy of resection and long-term oncological outcomes. *Int J Colorectal Dis* 2011; **26**:415–21.

9 Gervaz P, Inan I, Perneger T, Schiffer E, Morel P. A prospective, randomized, single-blind comparison of laparoscopic versus open sigmoid colectomy for diverticulitis. *Ann Surg* 2010; **252**:3–8.

10 Klarenbeek BR, Veenhof AA, Bergamaschi R, *et al.* Laparoscopic sigmoid resection for diverticulitis decreases major morbidity rates: a randomized control trial: short term results of the Sigma trial. *Ann Surg* 2009; **249**:39–44.

11 Remzi FH, Kirat HT, Kaouk JH, Geisler DP. Single-port laparoscopy in colorectal surgery. *Colorectal Dis* 2008; **10**:823–6.

12 Bucher P, Pugin F, Morel P. Single port access laparoscopic right hemicolectomy. *Int J Colorectal Dis* 2008; **23**:1010–16.

13 Hompes R, Lindsey I, Jones OM, *et al.* Step-wise integration of single-port laparoscopic surgery into routine colorectal surgical practice by use of a surgical glove port. *Tech Coloproctol* 2011; **15**:165–71.

14 Fung AK-Y, Aly AH. Systematic review of single-incision laparoscopic colonic surgery. *Br J Surg* 2012; **99**:1353–64.

15 Becker H, Melzer A, Schurr MO, *et al.* 3-D video techniques in endoscopic surgery. *Endosc Surg Allied Technol* 1993; **1**:40–6.

16 Mueller-Richter UD, Limberger A, Weber P, *et al.* Possibilities and limitations of current stereo-endoscopy. *Surg Endosc* 2004; **18**:942–7.

17 Alaraimi B, El Bakbak W, Sarker S, *et al.* A randomized prospective study comparing acquisition of laparoscopic skills in three-dimensional (3D) vs. two-dimensional (2D) laparoscopy. *World J Surg* 2014; **38**:2746–52.

18 Storz P, Buess GF, Kunert W, Kirshniak A. 3D HD versus 2D HD: surgical task efficiency in standardized phantom tasks. *Surg Endosc* 2012; **26**:1454–60.

19 Smith R, Schwab K, Day A, *et al.* Effect of passive polarizing three-dimensional displays on surgical performance for experienced laparoscopic surgeons. *Br J Surg* 2014; **101**:1453–9.

20 deSouza AL, Prasad LM, Park JJ, Marecik SJ, Blumetti J, Abcarian H. Robotic assistance in right hemicolectomy: is there a role? *Dis Colon Rectum* 2010; **53**:1000–6.

21 Mantoo S, Podevin J, Regenet N, Rigaud J, Lehur PA, Meurette G. Is robotic-assisted ventral mesh rectopexy superior to laparoscopic ventral mesh rectopexy in the management of obstructed defaecation? *Colorectal Dis* 2013; **15**:e469–75.

22 Aly EH. Robotic colorectal surgery: summary of the current evidence. *Int J Colorectal Dis* 2014; **29**:1–8.

23 Baek JH, Pastor C, Pigazzi A. Robotic and laparoscopic total mesorectal excision for rectal cancer: a case-matched study. *Surg Endosc* 2011; **25**:521–5.

24 Akmal Y, Baek JH, McKenzie S, Garcia-Aquilar J, Pigazzi A. Robot-assisted total mesorectal excision: is there a learning curve? *Surg Endosc* 2012; **26**:2471–6.

25 Pigazzi A, Luca F, Patriti A, *et al.* Multicentric study on robotic tumor-specific mesorectal excision for the treatment of rectal cancer. *Ann Surg Oncol* 2010; **17**:1614–20.

26 Kang J, Min BS, Park YA, *et al.* Risk factor analysis of post-operative complications after robotic-assisted left-sided colon or rectal resection. *World J Surg* 2011; **35**:2555–62.

27 Patriti A, Ceccarelli G, Bartoli A, Spaziani A, Biancafarina A, Casciola L. Short- and medium-term outcome of robot-assisted and traditional laparoscopic rectal resection. *J Soc Laparoendosc Surg* 2009; **13**:176–83.

28 Scarpinata R, Aly EH. Does robotic rectal cancer surgery offer improved early postoperative outcomes? *Dis Colon Rectum* 2013; **56**:253–62.

29 Baik SH, Kwon HY, Kim JS, *et al.* Robotic versus laparoscopic low anterior resection of rectal cancer: short-term outcome of a prospective comparative study. *Ann Surg Oncol* 2009; **16**:1480–7.

30 Collinson FJ, Jayne DG, Pigazzi A, *et al.* An international, multicentre, prospective, randomised, controlled, unblended, parallel-group trial of robotic-assisted versus standard laparoscopic surgery for the curative treatment of rectal cancer. *Int J Colorectal Dis* 2012; **27**:233–41.

31 Kalloo AN, Singh VK, Jagannath SB, *et al.* Flexible transgastric peritoneoscopy: a novel approach to diagnostic and therapeutic interventions in the peritoneal cavity. *Gastrointest Endosc* 2004; **60**:114–17.

32 Lacy AM, Delgado S, Rojas OA, Almenara R, Blasi A, Llach J. MA-NOS radical sigmoidectomy: report of a transvaginal resection in the human. *Surg Endosc* 2008; **22**:1717–23.

33 Lacy AM, Saavedra-Perez D, Bravo R, Adelsdorfer C, Aceituno M, Balust J. Minilaparoscopy-assisted natural orifice total colectomy: technical report of a mini-laparoscopy-assisted transrectal resection. *Surg Endosc* 2012; **26**:2080–5.

34 Wolthuis AM, de Buck van Overstraeten A, Fieuws S, Boon K, D'Hoore A. Standardized laparoscopic NOSE-colectomy is feasible with low morbidity. *Surg Endosc* 2015; **29**:1167–73.

35 Sylla P, Rattner DW, Delgado S, Lacy AM. NOTES transanal rectal cancer resection using transanal endoscopic microsurgery and laparoscopic assistance. *Surg Endosc* 2010; **24**:1205–10.

36 Rouanet P, Mourregot A, Azar CC, *et al.* Transanal endoscopic proctectomy: an innovative procedure for difficult resection of rectal tumours in men with narrow pelvis. *Dis Colon Rectum* 2013; **56**:408–15.

37 Dumont F, Goere D, Honore C, Elias D. Transanal endoscopic total mesorectal excision combined with single-port laparoscopy. *Dis Colon Rectum* 2012; **55**:996–1001.

38 De Lacy AM, Rattner DW, Adelsdorfer C, *et al.* Transanal natural orifice transluminal endoscopic surgery (NOTES) rectal resection: "down-to-up" total mesorectal excision (TME)-short term outcomes in the first 20 cases. *Surg Endosc* 2013; **27**:3165–72.

39 Ashraf SQ, Burns EM, Jani A, *et al.* The economic impact of anastomotic leakage after anterior resections in English NHS hospitals: are we adequately remunerating them? *Colorectal Dis* 2013; **15**:e190–8.

40 Allison AS, Bloor C, Faux W, *et al.* The angiographic anatomy of the small arteries and their collaterals in colorectal resections: some insights into anastomotic perfusion. *Ann Surg* 2010; **251**:1092–7.

41 Ris F, Hompes R, Cunningham C, *et al.* Near-infrared (NIR) perfusion angiography in minimally invasive colorectal surgery. *Surg Endosc* 2014; **28**:2221–6.

42 Sherwinter DA, Gallagher J, Donkar T. Intra-operative transanal near infrared imaging of colorectal anastomotic perfusion: a feasibility study. *Colorectal Dis* 2013; **15**:91–6.

43 Jafari MD, Lee KH, Halabi WJ, *et al.* The use of indocyanine green fluorescence to assess anastomotic perfusion during robotic assisted laparoscopic rectal surgery. *Surg Endosc* 2013; **27**:3003–8.

44 Cahill RA, Anderson M, Wang M, Lindsey I, Cunningham C, Mortensen NJ. Near-infrared (NIR) laparoscopy for intraoperative lymphatic road-mapping and sentinel node identification during definitive surgical resection of early-stage colorectal neoplasia. *Surg Endosc* 2012; **26**:197–204.

45 Saha S, Johnston G, Korant A, *et al.* Aberrant drainage of sentinel lymph nodes in colon cancer and its impact on staging and the extent of operation. *Am J Surg* 2013; **205**:302–5.

46 Retter SM, Herrmann G, Schiedeck TH. Clinical value of sentinel node mapping in carcinoma of the colon. *Colorectal Dis* 2011; **13**:855–9.

Index

Colorectal Surgery: Clinical Care and Management, First Edition.
Edited by Bruce George, Richard Guy, Oliver Jones, and Jon Vogel.
© 2016 John Wiley & Sons, Ltd. Published 2016 by John Wiley & Sons, Ltd.